Sports Biomechanics: Optimizing Human Performance

Sports Biomechanics: Optimizing Human Performance

Editor: Joseph Bowen

FOSTER ACADEMICS
www.fosteracademics.com

www.fosteracademics.com

FOSTER ACADEMICS

Cataloging-in-Publication Data

Sports biomechanics : optimizing human performance / edited by Joseph Bowen.
p. cm.
Includes bibliographical references and index.
ISBN 978-1-64646-620-7
1. Sports--Physiological aspects. 2. Human mechanics. 3. Sports medicine.
4. Performance. I. Bowen, Joseph.
RC1235 .S66 2023
612.044--dc23

Foster Academics,
118-35 Queens Blvd., Suite 400,
Forest Hills, NY 11375, USA

ISBN 978-1-64646-620-7 (Hardback)

Contents

Preface

Biomechanics refers to the study of the motion, structure and function of the mechanical components of biological systems. This can span various levels, from whole organisms to cell organelles, organs and cells by utilizing the methods of mechanics. Sports biomechanics involves quantitative study and analysis of sports activities and professional players. It includes a thorough analysis of sport movements to reduce the risk of injury and enhance athletic performance. The laws of mechanics are used in biomechanics for gaining a better understanding of the athletic performance through computer simulation, mathematical modeling and measurement. Biomechanics facilitates sports players to work on various areas, such as enhancing running technique to improve efficiency or speed, enhancing vehicle aerodynamics and enhancing swimming technique to maximize propulsion. This book contains some path-breaking studies in sports biomechanics. It aims to shed light on the researches focused on optimizing human performance through the application of the principles of sports biomechanics. This book will serve as a reference to a broad spectrum of readers.

The information contained in this book is the result of intensive hard work done by researchers in this field. All due efforts have been made to make this book serve as a complete guiding source for students and researchers. The topics in this book have been comprehensively explained to help readers understand the growing trends in the field.

I would like to thank the entire group of writers who made sincere efforts in this book and my family who supported me in my efforts of working on this book. I take this opportunity to thank all those who have been a guiding force throughout my life.

Editor

A Biomechanical Investigation of Athletic Footwear Traction Performance: Integration of Gait Analysis with Computational Simulation

Kao-Shang Shih [1,2,†], Shu-Yu Jhou [3,†], Wei-Chun Hsu [4], Ching-Chi Hsu [3,*], Jun-Wen Chen [4], Jui-Chia Yeh [5] and Yi-Chun Hung [5]

1 Department of Orthopedic Surgery, Shin Kong Wu Ho-Su Memorial Hospital, Taipei 111, Taiwan; scorelin@gmail.com
2 School of Medicine, College of Medicine, Fu Jen Catholic University, New Taipei City 242, Taiwan
3 Graduate Institute of Applied Science and Technology, National Taiwan University of Science and Technology, Taipei 106, Taiwan; D10622601@mail.ntust.edu.tw
4 Graduate Institute of Biomedical Engineering, National Taiwan University of Science and Technology, Taipei 106, Taiwan; wchsu@mail.ntust.edu.tw (W.-C.H.); M10523102@gapps.ntust.edu.tw (J.-W.C.)
5 Footwear & Recreation Technology Research Institute, Taichung 407, Taiwan; 0811@bestmotion.com (J.-C.Y.); 0852@bestmotion.com (Y.-C.H.)
* Correspondence: hsucc@mail.ntust.edu.tw
† Both authors contributed equally to this work.

Abstract: Evaluations are vital to quantify the functionalities of athletic footwear, such as the performance of slip resistance, shock absorption, and rebound. Computational technology has progressed to become a promising solution for accelerating product development time and providing customized products in order to keep up with the competitive contemporary footwear market. In this research, the effects of various tread pattern designs on traction performance in a normal gait were analyzed by employing an approach that integrated computational simulation and gait analysis. A state-of-the-art finite element (FE) model of a shoe was developed by digital sculpting technology. A dynamic plantar pressure distribution was automatically applied to interpret individualized subject conditions. The traction performance and real contact area between the shoe and the ground during the gait could be characterized and predicted. The results suggest that the real contact area and the structure of the outsole tread design influence the traction performance of the shoe in dry conditions. This computational process is more efficient than mechanical tests in terms of both cost and time, and it could bring a noticeable benefit to the footwear industry in the early design phases of product development.

Keywords: traction; footwear; finite element analysis; plantar pressure; outsole tread pattern

---

1. Introduction

With the significant rise in exercising, the demand for athletic footwear products has grown rapidly. To keep up, the footwear industry has been required to expand product range, accelerate the product development time, and provide customized products. Performing an evaluation is vital in product design, prototyping, biomechanics, and other areas in order to quantify the functions of athletic footwear. These functions include traction, motion control, and the attenuation of impact forces during a motion [1]. Focusing on footwear traction, a proper traction can effectively maximize performance or minimize the risk of injury [2]. The traction is typically measured in terms of the shoe–floor coefficient of friction by various slip testers [3–6]. However, the results of slip testing in predicting the coefficient of friction are inconsistent [7]. On the other hand, experimental tests are time-consuming and expensive, and they cannot keep pace with the growing demand within the footwear market. Developing a numerical simulation could reduce the number of design iterations and improve design quality, and it promises a more efficient and less costly product development process. Previous studies have developed a finite element (FE) model to predict the coefficient of friction between the shoe and floor [8,9]. However, the shoe models had been simplified to a rear part of the outsole. In a previous case study, the outsoles of military boots with five different tread patterns were used to investigate how the tread patterns affect traction-force, which resists slip in a gaiting direction [10]. However, the uniform vertical force of 200 N was applied as the only loading condition. The dynamic simulation was conducted to predict the slip resistant performance by calculating the reaction force [11]. However, the models were simplified to an outsole without complex curves. Oversimplified or unaesthetic models and a lack of subject-specific loading conditions are the primary disadvantages of previous numerical studies of footwear.

In the present study, digital sculpting technology was employed to create the complex curved shapes of a shoe model. Plantar pressure measurement was performed to obtain the personal pressure data. The non-linear FE method was used to simulate the traction performance under subject-specific loading, which was defined by plantar pressure measurement. The mechanical tests were performed to validate the results of the FE analysis. This study aimed to demonstrate an approach that integrated digital sculpting technology and an FE method with gait analysis, and to evaluate the effect of a variety of tread pattern designs on the traction performance during the gait.

2. Materials and Methods

2.1. Development of Shoe Geometry

In this research, we used Geomagic Freeform (3D Systems, Rock Hill, SC, USA), a digital sculpting technology, to create the three-dimensional (3D) shoe model. Geomagic Freeform enables users to easily create a model with complex curves, especially when compared to traditional computer-aided design programs, which struggle to do so [12,13]. The file format conversion was needed before transmitting the file of shoe model to the ANSYS Workbench 18.2 (ANSYS, Inc., Canonsburg, PA, USA). The digital sculpting shoe model was converted by Geomagic Wrap (3D Systems, Rock Hill, SC, USA) then imported in the ANSYS DesignModeler, one of the built-in geometric modelers in Workbench, to accurately create and parametrically control the tread patterns (Figure 1A). The 3D shoe–ground model consisted of elements including ground, outsole, midsole, insole, and upper (Figure 1B). Ten types of outsole tread pattern design were divided into two groups, as shown in Figure 2. Two common outsole tread designs, straight stripe and herringbone, were developed in "group one". The height of the two types of straight stripe design were 3 and 6 mm, respectively; the grooves between each tread were both 3 mm (G1_S_Height-3 and G1_S_Height-6). The tread width of the two types of herringbone design were 10 and 30 mm; the grooves between each tread, the tread height, and the tread angle were 3 mm, 3 mm, and 90° (G1_H_width-10 and G1_H_width-30), respectively. Two commercially available tread pattern designs (G2_A and G2_B) and four original designs (G2_C, G2_D, G2_E, and G2_F) were developed in "group two". The difference between G2_E and G2_F was the height of the straight stripe and the groove in the front part of the outsole.

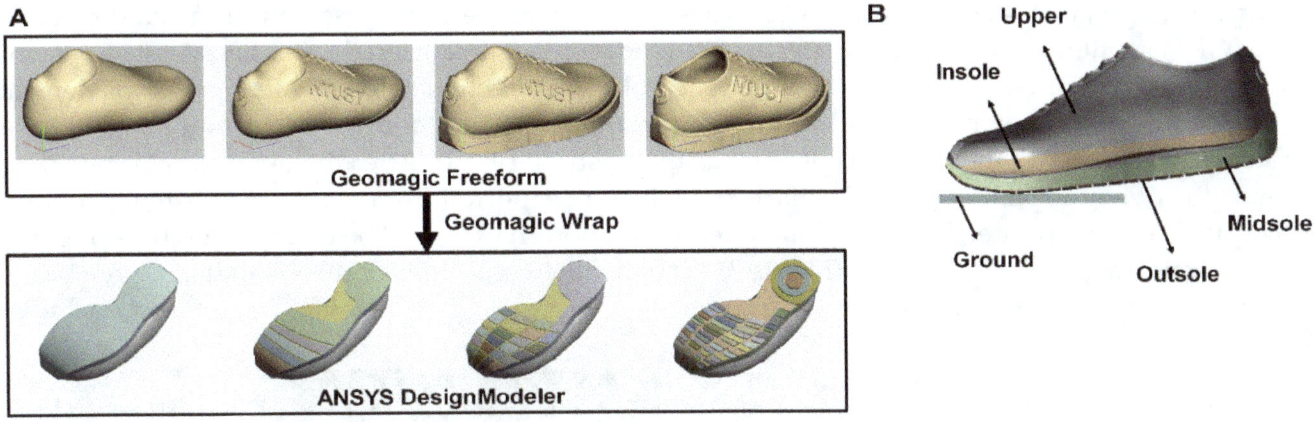

Figure 1. (**A**) The development process of the running shoe model; and (**B**), the anatomy of the 3D shoe and ground model.

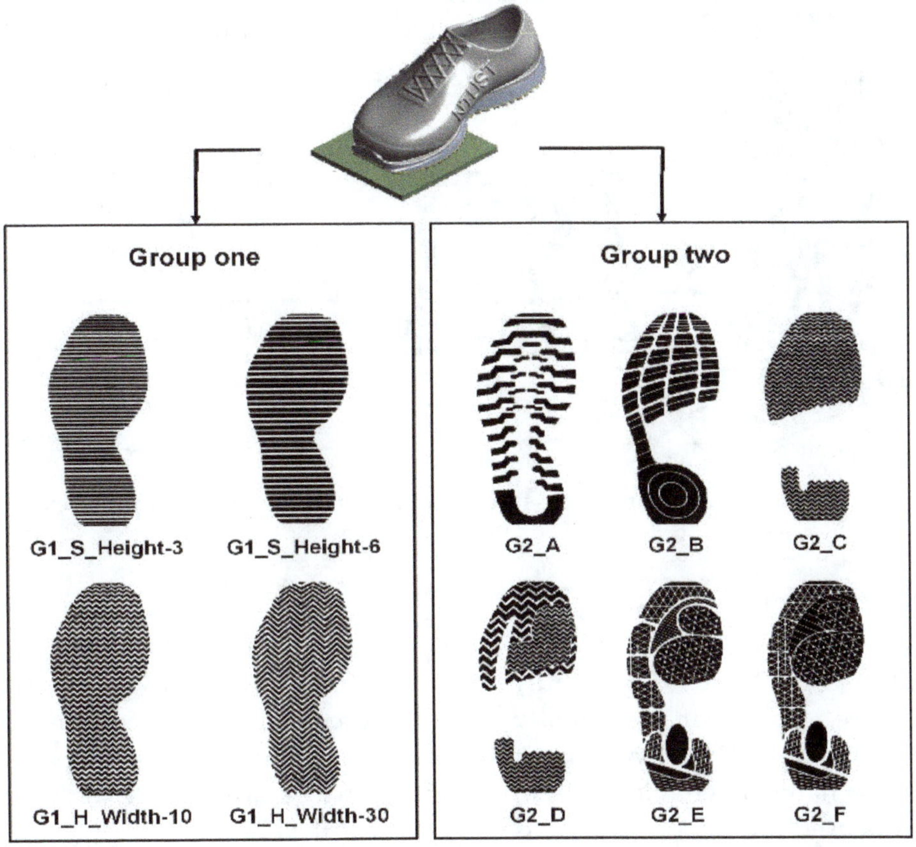

Figure 2. A 3D shoe model, and ten types of tread pattern design.

2.2. *Plantar Pressure Measurements during Gait*

To evaluate the traction performance in a physiological loading condition, plantar pressure was measured during a gait. Data of dynamic plantar pressure were recorded using an in-shoe pressure measurement system called the F-Scan Wireless System (Tekscan, Inc., South Boston, MA, USA), and synchronized with force plates (Kistler, Inc., Winterthur, Switzerland). The F-Scan Wireless System consists of an in-shoe sensor and software for data analysis. In this study, the sensing region of a 3000 Esport in-shoe sensor was 2.5 mm × 2.5 mm × 0.406 mm, and the pressure-sensitive area of the sensor was 305 mm × 107 mm. The total number of sensels was 954 (resolution: 3.9 sensel/cm^2), with a 75–125 psi pressure range. The F-Scan Wireless System was attached to one subject (male, aged 24, 58 kg weight and 166 cm height), who performed level walking at a naturally self-selected pace across the force plates (Figure 3). Three major phases of a right foot gait cycle were identified and selected:

loading response, mid-stance, and push-off. These phases were selected based on the ground reaction force (GRF) profiles from the force plates and the foot contact area from the F-Scan Wireless System. The maximum GRF in the anteroposterior and mediolateral direction before the first peak was defined as the loading response phase; the maximum foot contact area was defined as the mid-stance phase; and the second peak of the GRF was defined as the push-off phase. After the definition of the major phases, the dynamic plantar pressure charts of each were exported from the F-Scan System program. According to the literature, the plantar pressure distribution charts could be divided into three regions: forefoot, mid-foot, and rearfoot [14] (Figure 3). The loading conditions of the FE analysis were based on the pressure distribution charts.

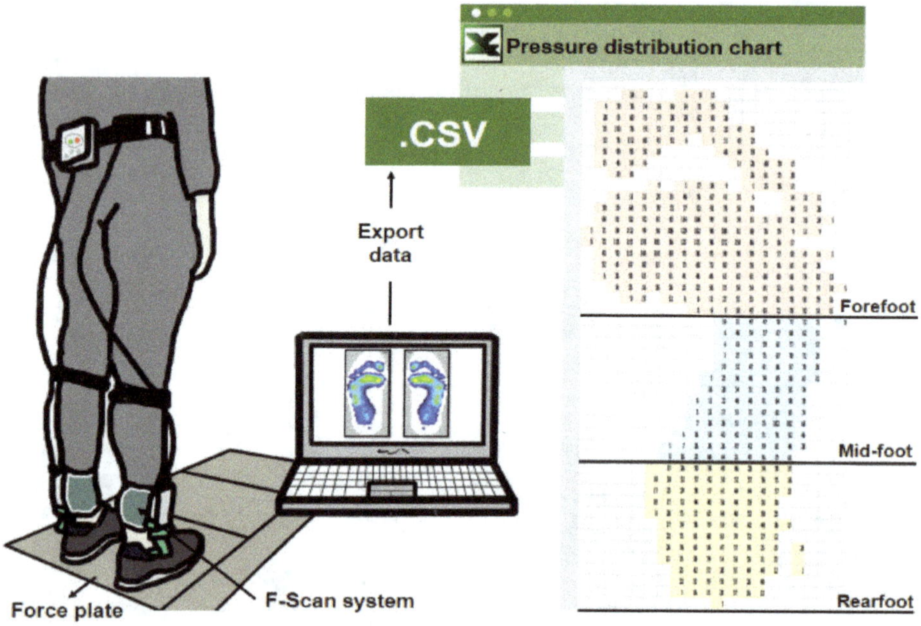

Figure 3. Experimental setup for plantar pressure measurements during gait, and the exporting plantar pressure distribution chart.

2.3. *Finite Element Model*

After model preparation in the ANSYS DesignModeler, the ANSYS Workbench 18.2 static structural module (ANSYS, Inc., Canonsburg, PA, USA) was employed to simulate the footwear traction performance. Footwear is normally manufactured using very compressible rubber-like materials that can be modelled by a hyperelastic material model, and a strain-energy function is needed to describe their mechanical behavior [15–20]. In the current study, an Ogden foam second-order material model was used for the footwear, and the values of the elastomeric Ogden foam parameters are shown in Table 1 [21]. The Young's modulus of the ground was 17,000 MPa, while the Poisson's ratio was 0.1 [21]. In terms of element types, the ground and the outsole were modelled with hex dominant elements, whereas the upper, insole, and midsole sections were modelled with tetrahedron elements. The convergence analysis was conducted by manually refining the mesh size of the outsole and the ground until the difference between the results of the reaction force and real contact area were less than the convergence criterion, with an allowance of error of 0.5%. Through this convergence process, the optimal mesh density was determined. The element size of upper, insole, and midsole were 4 mm, while the outsole and ground were 1.7 mm. Each FE model contained approximately 858,074 to 1,014,773 nodes, and 377,489 to 465,000 elements. The frictional contact between the relevant surfaces of the outsole and the ground was applied by using CONTA 174 and TARGE 170 elements. The contact elements with the default settings were used. The coefficient of friction was 0.6, as a static coefficient of friction of 0.5 was recommended by James Miller as the minimum slip-resistant standard [22], and others have proposed an optimal coefficient of friction for various sports between 0.5

and 0.7 [23]. The foot angles in three different positions were defined to mimic level walking (Figure 4). The foot angle was set to 6°, as the average foot angle is between 5° and 7° [24]. The contact angle between the bottom of the heel and the ground was 7° during the loading response phase. The contact angle between the bottom of the shoe and the ground was 7° during the push-off phase. The footwear was parallel with the ground during the mid-stance phase (Figure 4).

Table 1. The parameters of the Ogden foam material model used for footwear materials.

Material	μ_1	μ_2	α_1	α_2	β_1	β_2
Upper	0.213	−0.06209	10.3	−3.349	0.32	0.32
Insole	0.213	−0.06209	10.3	−3.349	0.32	0.32
Midsole	1.037	−0.3044	7.181	−2.348	0.32	0.32
Outsole	8.874	−7.827	2.028	1.345	0.32	0.32

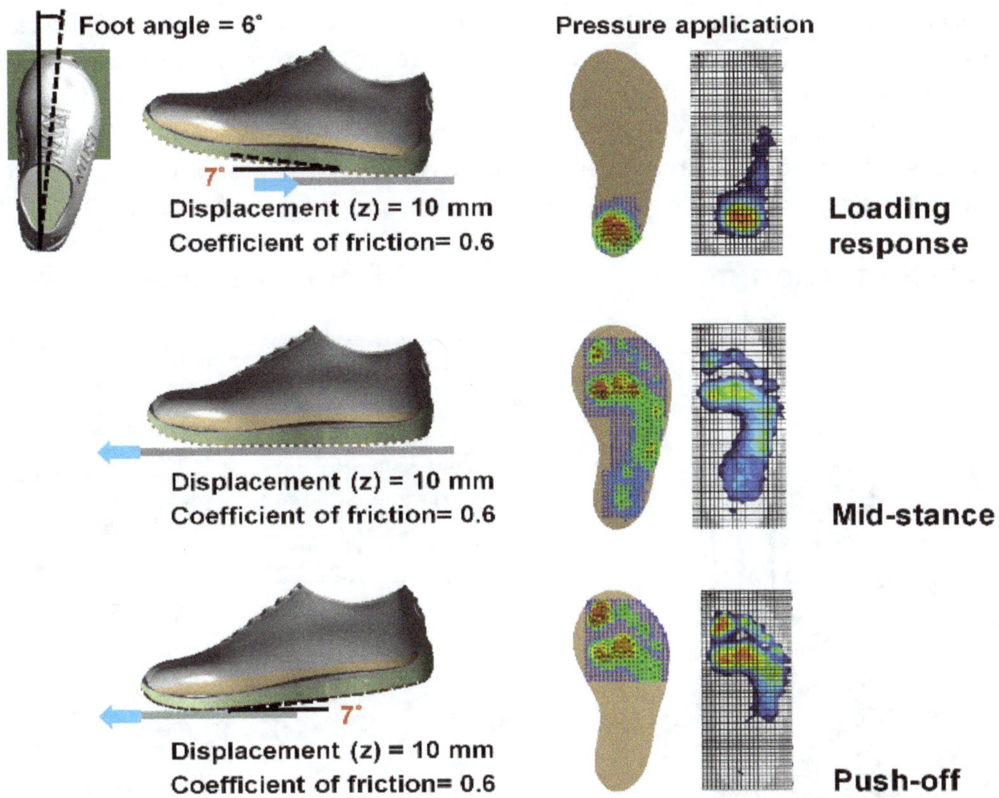

Figure 4. The position, boundary, and loading conditions of the finite element (FE) analysis three major phases of a gait cycle.

2.4. Simulation Condition and Data Output

In this research, a total of thirty FE analyses were conducted using ten types of tread pattern design with three positions: loading response, mid-stance, and push-off. The traction analysis was performed by fully constraining both ends of the shoe throughout the simulation. The horizontal displacement was applied to the bottom surface of the ground to mimic the sliding behavior. The moving directions of the ground were defined based on the international standard ISO 13287 [25]. All of the data from the dynamic plantar pressure were applied as the loading conditions. We used the time-effective ANSYS Application Customization Toolkit (ANSYS ACT), an add-on module to the Workbench Environment based on Python and XML, to create the automatic pressure generator on the insole (Figure 4). In this FE analysis process, two steps were considered: loading application and ground movement. The dynamic plantar pressure was applied at the first step, and the displacement of the ground was applied at the second step. In post-processing, the horizontal reaction force of the bottom surface of the ground was calculated and considered as the friction force to evaluate the traction performance [26]. A higher value reaction force indicated better traction performance. Additionally, the real contact area of the outsole was calculated to understand the contact area of the shoe after the loading application and ground movement.

2.5. Experiment for FE Model Validation

An experimental test was conducted to validate the feasibility and applicability of the numerical simulation. Four types of tread design (straight stripe with 3 mm height, straight stripe with 6 mm height, herringbone with 3 mm height, and herringbone with 6 mm height) predicted by the FE method in group one were selected for the slip-resistance test. Before performing any tests, a horizontal surface was needed on which to place the testing machine. The specimen was placed parallel to both the floor with the dry condition and the test holder. Initially, the test was performed by leaving the rotating support in the vertical position and the weight was released using the trigger. It was noted visually whether the specimen slipped when it contacted the floor surface. Without moving the tester, the steps described above were repeated, increasing the angle of rotating support until the slip just occurred. The corresponding value of the coefficient of friction was obtained and recorded. The operational procedure was followed using a previous slip-resistance standard test (ASTM F 1677 for Mark II) [27] (Figure 5). Each test was repeated three times, and the average coefficient of friction was reported. The experimental measurements of the coefficient of friction were compared to their FE results.

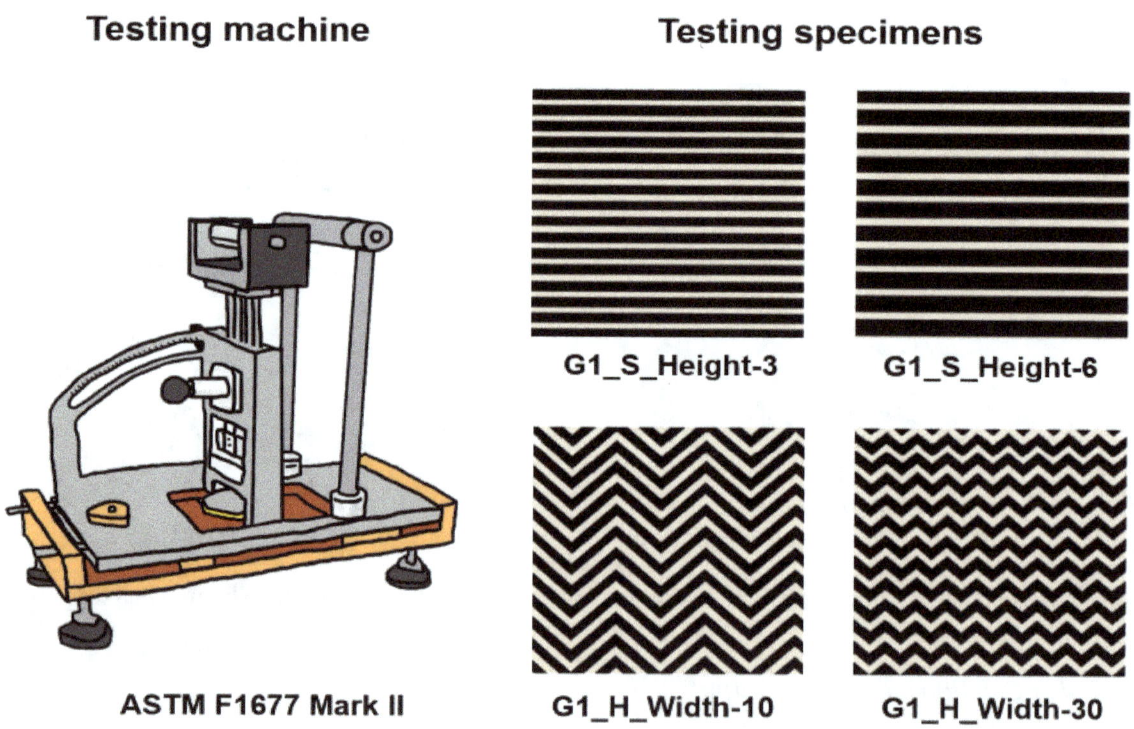

Figure 5. The configuration of the experiment and the specimens.

2.6. Experimental–Computational Correlation

The flowchart of the experimental–computational process is illustrated in Figure 6. The four types of tread design (straight stripe with 3 mm height, straight stripe with 6 mm height, herringbone with 3 mm height, and herringbone with 6 mm height) were first selected to compare their FE predicted results to the experimental data. As strong positive correlations between the FE prediction and the mechanical testing measurement were found, the traction simulations of new designs, group two, were then conducted.

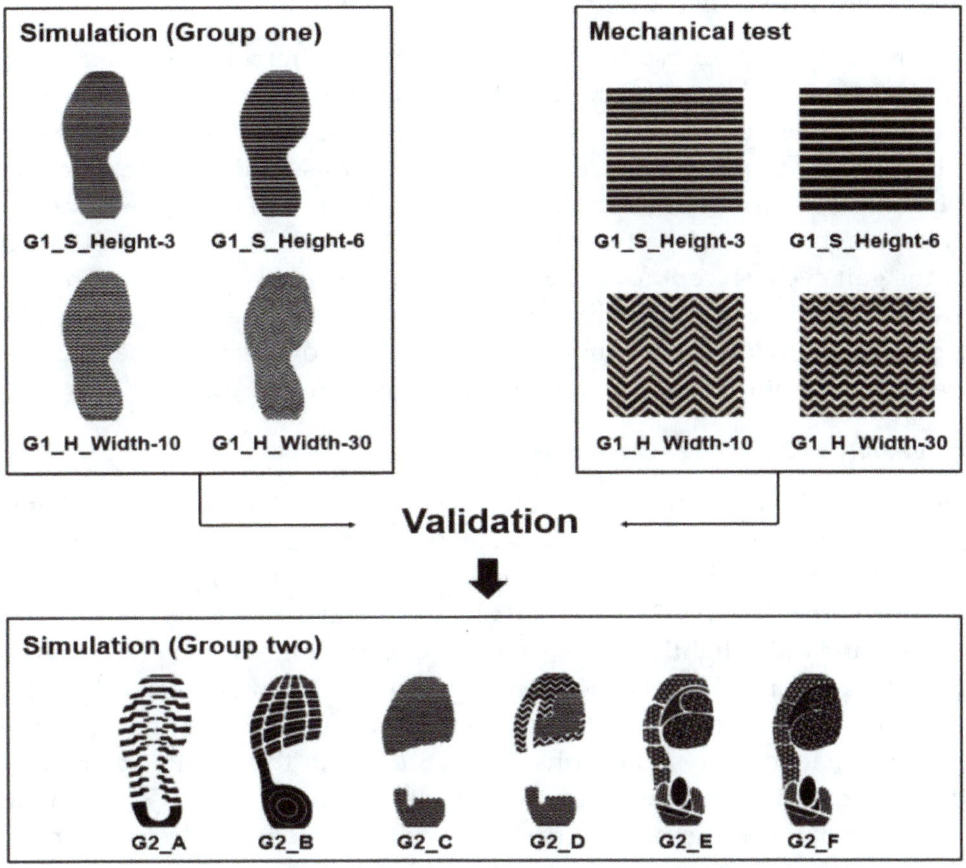

Figure 6. Flowchart of the experimental–computational process.

3. Results

3.1. FE Model Validation

The FE analyses in this research were conducted for the loading response, mid-stance, and push-off phases, which represent the entire stance phase of a gait cycle. The experimental measurements of the coefficient of friction for the four testing specimens were compared to their FE predicted reaction force, group one. The predicted FE reaction forces in group one were found to reasonably comply with the experimental measurement of the coefficient of friction. Strong positive correlations existed between the reaction force during the entire stance phase of the gait cycle in the FE analysis and the coefficient of friction in mechanical testing: $R^2 = 0.936$ at loading response, $R^2 = 0.920$ at mid-stance, and $R^2 = 0.935$ at push-off (Figure 7).

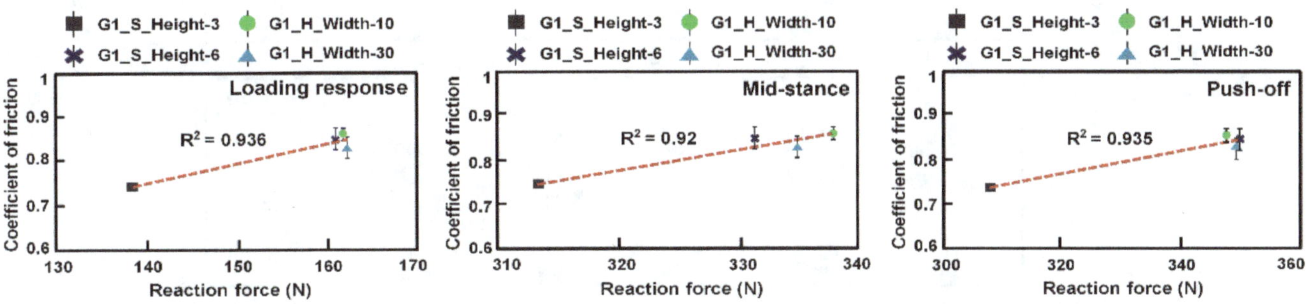

Figure 7. The relationship between the FE predicted ground reaction force of group one and the experimentally measured coefficient of friction.

3.2. Traction Performance Evaluation of Group One

The reaction force of the four types of straight stripe and herringbone tread pattern design in group one is shown in Figure 7. It is observed that G1_S_Height-3 had the lowest value reaction force during the entire stance phase of the gait cycle. The results of the reaction force in the moving direction revealed slightly different trends between the loading response, mid-stance, and push-off phases. The straight stripe tread pattern (G1_S_Height-3 and G1_S_Height-6) had a lower value reaction force than that of the herringbone tread pattern (G1_S_Width-10 and G1_S_Width-30) during the entire stance phase of the gait cycle, except for G1_S_Height-6 at the push-off phase. The higher height of straight stripe (G1_S_Height-6) had a higher reaction force during the entire stance phase of the gait cycle. In terms of the tread width of herringbone, the results show that a higher value of tread width had a higher reaction force at the loading response and push-off phases.

3.3. Traction Performance Evaluation of Group Two

Figure 8 represents the reaction force of the two commercially available designs and the four original designs in group two. The results of the reaction force in the moving direction revealed the different trends between the loading response, mid-stance, and push-off phases. The reaction force of the commercially available design G2_A was smaller than that of the others in the loading response and push-off phases, and only slightly higher than G2_C in the mid-stance phase. As compared with the two commercially available designs, the reaction force of G2_B was greater than that of the G2_A during the entire stance phase of the gait cycle. The four original designs showed similar results for the reaction force at the loading response phase. Distinct from the results at the loading response phase, the wide straight stripe and thin groove tread design in the front (G2_F) had a higher value reaction force than that of the thin straight stripe and wide groove tread design in the front (G2_E) at the push-off and mid-stance phases. As the tread width was increased, the reaction force could be increased, and this trend can be found both in the mechanical test and the FE analysis.

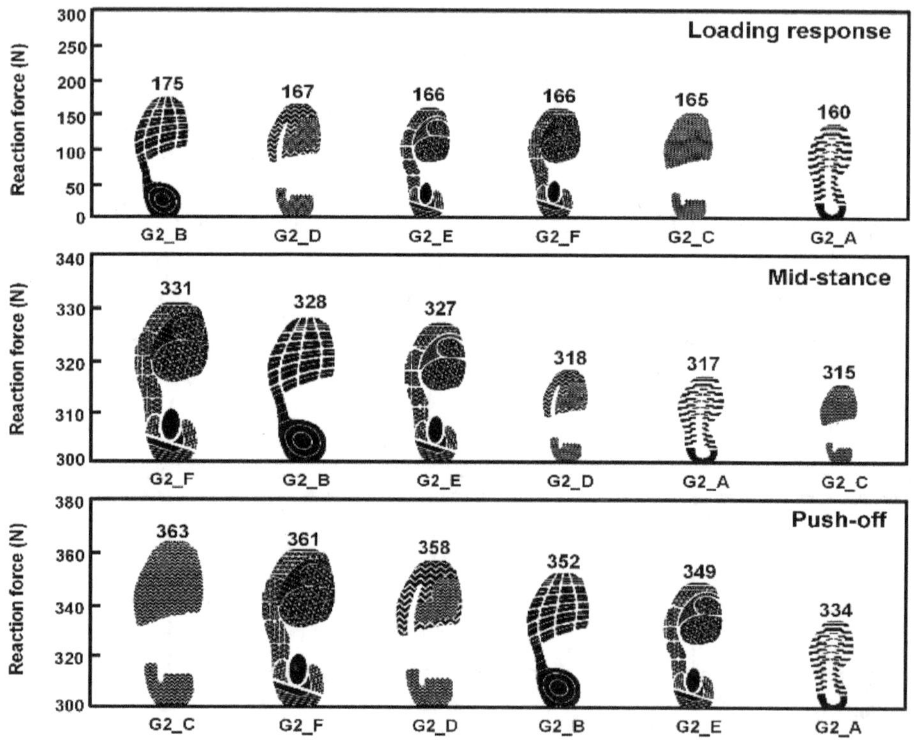

Figure 8. The reaction force chart for group two.

3.4. The Correlation between Contact Area and Traction Performance

The predictions for the real contact area where the outsole made contact with the ground surface at push-off are presented in Figure 9. The results show the significant effect of tread pattern design on the real contact area. Linear regression was used to establish the relationship between two variables, real contact area and reaction force. As shown in the linear regressions graphs (Figure 10), strong positive correlations were observed between the reaction force of the ground and the shoe–ground real contact area during the entire stance phase of the gait cycle in the FE analysis: R = 0.84 at loading response, R = 0.76 at mid-stance, and R = 0.80 at push-off. Overall, a higher value of shoe–ground real contact area could have a greater reaction force.

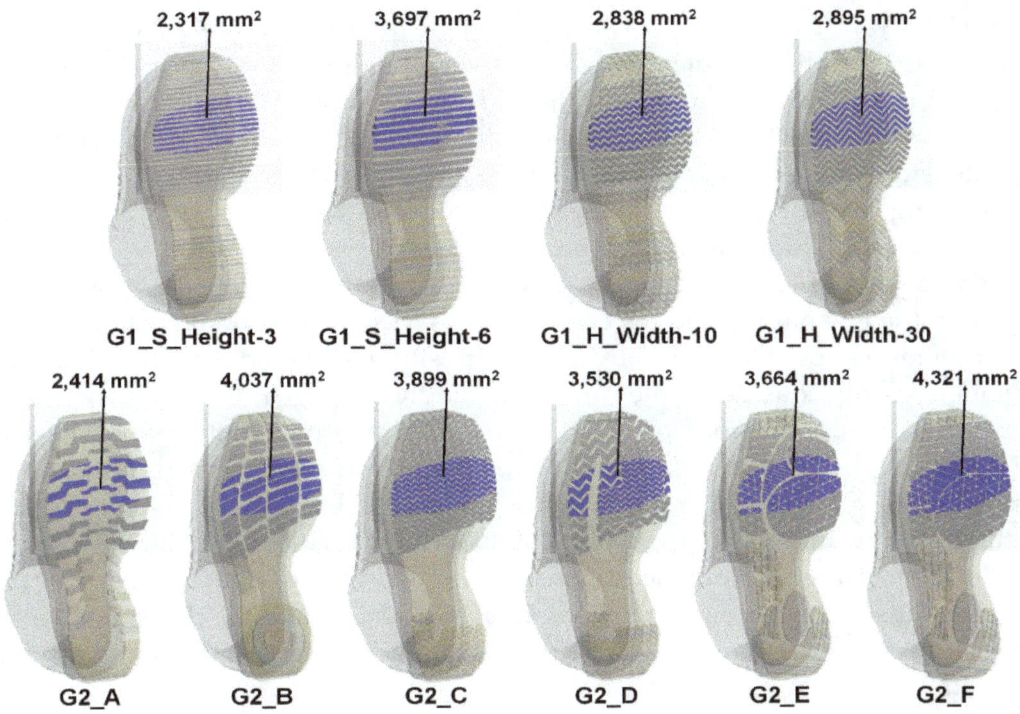

Figure 9. The predicted real contact area at push-off.

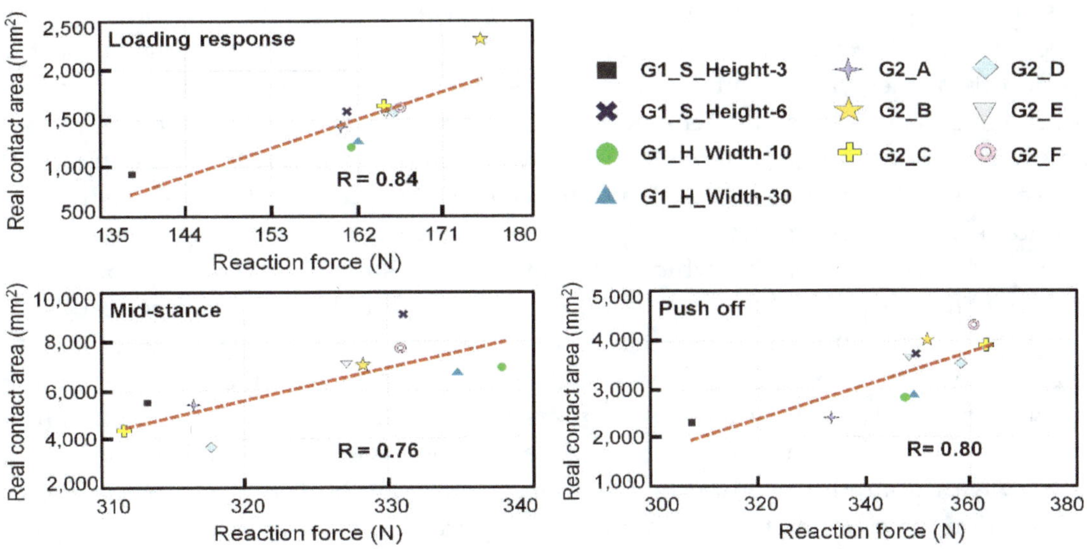

Figure 10. The relationship between ground reaction force and real contact area.

4. Discussion

The influence of oversimplified models and the lack of actual circumstances have been underestimated in recent experimental research and simulation analysis of footwear traction [10,28–32]. For example, a simplified outsole pad model could lead to an overly constrained boundary condition. The lack of actual loading conditions and shoe position lead to the inability to mimic human weight, pressure distribution, and foot angle in normal gait. To the best of our knowledge, the model development and FE analysis setting process in this research could improve the feasibility and applicability of traction performance simulation.

One of the most prominent features of this research was the automatic pressure application, which could provide new insights for computational simulation. Instead of the built-in manual pressure generator, the ANSYS ACT extension was used to create an automatic plantar pressure generator. The manual pressure time settings were 4 h at the mid-stance phase, 2.5 h at the push-off phase, and 1 h at the loading response phase. The automatic pressure application time was significantly reduced to 8 min at the mid-stance phase, 3 min at the push-off phase, and 50 s at the loading response phase. The ANSYS ACT extension for the automatic plantar pressure generator is an efficient tool for mimicking physiological loading conditions during the gait motion, and it is particularly advantageous to the footwear industry, especially for customized products.

Trend differences have been found between the reaction force calculation during the entire stance phase of the gait in the FE analysis and the coefficients of friction measurements in the experimental test. The trend differences could be caused by the shoe position, sliding direction, or loading condition. The experimental test only considered the condition that the specimen was parallel with the ground and slid in one direction under a load of 4.5 kg. To mimic the human gait motion, the contact angle between the bottom of the shoe and the ground was 7° at the loading response phase and 7° at the push-off phase. The footwear was parallel with the ground at the mid-stance phase. The foot angle was 6° at all three phases. In terms of the ground sliding direction, the horizontal displacement of the ground was from toe to heel at the loading response phase, and was from heel to toe at the push-off and mid-stance phases. Instead of a uniform loading of 4.5 kg, the data of the dynamic plantar pressure were used in the FE analysis. Therefore, the FE results of reaction force had different trends from the experimental test.

According to the classical Amontons–Coulomb friction law, the friction force is independent of the apparent contact area [33]. However, this theory could only be correct at the macroscopic scale. Previous research has proven that the real contact area between sliding surfaces plays a role in friction at a microscopic scale, especially for an elastic material during sliding [34–36]. Some important aspects may be gained from the graph of linear regressions shown in Figure 10. The higher value of the shoe–ground real contact area could achieve a higher traction performance. Some of the results that did not follow this observation perfectly could be caused by the geometry of the tread. When the surfaces of ground and outsole tread push against one another, a shear force is needed to break the adhesive bond of the contacting surfaces [37–39]. The geometry of the tread may have contributed to the formation and strength of bonds, which could affect the results of the reaction force.

The potential limitations of this research should be noted. Firstly, for the surface condition, neither contamination conditions nor the roughness of the surface of the ground were tested. A dry and flat concrete ground was applied in the FE model. Secondly, the loading condition in the FE model was based on a single-subject dynamic plantar pressure measurement, and was applied to the insole. Thirdly, the coefficient of friction between the outsole and the ground was fixed at 0.6, and the traction performance was evaluated by comparing the horizontal reaction forces of the ground. Fourthly, the ground reaction forces in the medial–lateral and superior–inferior directions were ignored, as we considered the magnitudes of the friction force and ground reaction force in the anterior–posterior direction to be equal. The friction types of the current analysis only focus on static friction. Finally, the simplified testing specimens based on ASTM F 1677 were manufactured and used in the present study. Further tests using the whole shoe specimens are needed to validate the numerical outcomes in a future study.

5. Conclusions

Evaluation is essential to quantifying the function of traction performance. The findings of this research suggest that the real contact area and the structure of the outsole tread design influence the traction performance of the shoe in dry conditions. This computational process provides a lower cost and more time-efficient method evaluating traction performance in an actual-person situation during a gait motion. This research can be applied to product development in the early design phases in the footwear industry to improve product performance or achieve the goals of customized products.

Author Contributions: Conceptualization, K.-S.S., W.-C.H. and C.-C.H.; Formal analysis, S.-Y.J., J.-W.C., J.-C.Y. and Y.-C.H.; Funding acquisition, K.-S.S. and C.-C.H.; Investigation, K.-S.S., S.-Y.J., C.-C.H., J.-W.C., J.-C.Y. and Y.-C.H.; Methodology, W.-C.H. and C.-C.H.; Validation, K.-S.S., W.-C.H. and C.-C.H.; Writing–original draft, S.-Y.J. and C.-C.H.; Writing–review & editing, K.-S.S., W.-C.H. and C.-C.H. All authors have read and agreed to the published version of the manuscript.

Acknowledgments: The authors would like to express their appreciation for the supports from the Footwear & Recreation Technology Research Institute (FRT, Taiwan, R.O.C.).

References

1. McPoil, T.G. Athletic Footwear: Design, Performance and Selection Issues. *J. Sci. Med. Sport* **2000**, *3*, 260–267. [CrossRef]
2. Gronqvist, R.; Chang, W.-R.; Courtney, T.K.; Leamon, T.B.; Redfern, M.S.; Strandberg, L. Measurement of Slipperiness: Fundamental Concepts and Definitions. *Ergonomics* **2001**, *44*, 1102–1117. [CrossRef] [PubMed]
3. ASTM. *Standard Test Method for Measuring the Coefficient of Friction for Evaluation of Slip Performance of Footwear and Test Surfaces/Flooring Using a Whole Shoe Tester*; ASTM International: West Conshohocken, PA, USA, 2011.
4. Hanson, J.P.; Redfern, M.S.; Mazumdar, M. Predicting Slips and Falls Considering Required and Available Friction. *Ergonomics* **1999**, *42*, 1619–1633. [CrossRef] [PubMed]
5. Chang, W.-R.; Grönqvist, R.; Leclercq, S.; Brungraber, R.J.; Mattke, U.; Strandberg, L.; Thorpe, S.C.; Myung, R.; Makkonen, L.; Courtney, T.K. The Role of Friction in the Measurement of Slipperiness, Part 2: Survey of Friction Measurement Devices. *Ergonomics* **2001**, *44*, 1233–1261. [CrossRef] [PubMed]
6. Burnfield, J.M.; Powers, C.M. Prediction of Slips: An Evaluation of Utilized Coefficient of Friction and Available Slip Resistance. *Ergonomics* **2006**, *49*, 982–995. [CrossRef]
7. Powers, C.M.; Brault, J.R.; Stefanou, M.A.; Tsai, Y.-J.; Flynn, J.; Siegmund, G.P. Assessment of Walkway Tribometer Readings in Evaluating Slip Resistance: A Gait-Based Approach. *J. Forensic Sci.* **2007**, *52*, 400–405. [CrossRef]
8. Moghaddam, S.R.M.; Acharya, A.; Redfern, M.S.; Beschorner, K.E. Predictive Multiscale Computational Model of Shoe-Floor Coefficient of Friction. *J. Biomech.* **2018**, *66*, 145–152. [CrossRef]
9. Beschorner, K.E. Development of a Computational Model for Shoe-Floor Contaminant Friction. Mechanical Engineering. Ph.D. Thesis, University of Illinois Urbana-Champaign, Champaign, IL, USA, 2004.
10. Sun, Z.; Howard, D.; Moatamedi, M. Finite Element Analysis of Footwear and Ground Interaction. *Strain* **2005**, 113–117. [CrossRef]
11. Huang, Q.; Hu, M.; Xu, B.; Wu, J.; Zhou, J. Feasibility of Application of Finite Element Method in Shoe Slip Resistance Test. *Leather Footwear J.* **2018**, *18*, 139–148. [CrossRef]
12. Kim, S.H.; Cho, J.R.; Choi, J.H.; Ryu, S.H.; Jeong, W.B. Coupled Foot-Shoe-Ground Interaction Model to Assess Landing Impact Transfer Characteristics to Ground Condition. *Interact. Multiscale Mech.* **2012**, *5*, 75–90. [CrossRef]
13. Qiu, T.-X.; Teo, E.-C.; Yan, Y.-B.; Lei, W. Finite Element Modeling of a 3d Coupled Foot-Boot Model. *Med. Eng. Phys.* **2011**, *33*, 1228–1233. [CrossRef] [PubMed]

14. Cavanagh, P.R.; Rodgers, M.M.; Liboshi, A. Pressure Distribution under Symptom-Free Feet During Barefoot Standing. *Foot Ankle* **2016**, *7*, 262–278. [CrossRef] [PubMed]
15. Miehe, C.; Goktepe, S.; Lulei, F. A Micro-Macro Approach to Rubber-Like Materials? Part I: The Non-Affine Micro-Sphere Model of Rubber Elasticity. *J. Mech. Phys. Solids* **2004**, *52*, 2617–2660. [CrossRef]
16. Verdejo, R.; Mills, N.J. Heel–Shoe Interactions and the Durability of Eva Foam Running-Shoe Midsoles. *J. Biomech.* **2004**, *37*, 1379–1386. [CrossRef] [PubMed]
17. Goske, S.; Erdemir, A.; Petre, M.; Budhabhatti, S.; Cavanagh, P.R. Reduction of Plantar Heel Pressures: Insole Design Using Finite Element Analysis. *J. Biomech.* **2006**, *39*, 2363–2370. [CrossRef] [PubMed]
18. Sissler, L.; Jacques, A.; Rao, G.; Berton, E.; Gueguen, N. A 3-D Finite Element Model of the Foot-Shoe Structure During a Walking Cycle for Shoe Sole Design. *Footwear Sci.* **2013**, *5*, S36–S37. [CrossRef]
19. Benkahla, J.; Baranger, T.N.; Issartel, J. Experimental and Numerical Simulation of Elastomeric Outsole Bending. *Exp. Mech.* **2012**, *52*, 1461–1473. [CrossRef]
20. Chen, W.M.; Lee, S.J.; Lee, V.S. Plantar Pressure Relief under the Metatarsal Heads—Therapeutic Insole Design Using Three-Dimensional Finite Element Model of the Foot. *J. Biomech.* **2015**, *48*, 659–665. [CrossRef]
21. Cheung, T.M.; Zhang, M. Finite Element Modeling of the Human Foot and Footwear. In Proceedings of the ABAQUS Users' Conference, Boston, MA, USA, 23–25 May 2006.
22. Miller, J.M. "Slippery" Work Surface: Towards a Performance Definition and Quantitative Coefficient of Friction Criteria. *J. Saf. Res.* **1983**, *14*, 145–158. [CrossRef]
23. Nigg, B.M.; Segesser, B. The Influence of Playing Surfaces on the Load on the Locomotor System and on Football and Tennis Injuries. *Sports Med.* **1988**, *5*, 375–385. [CrossRef]
24. Menz, H.B.; Latt, M.D.; Tiedemann, A.; Mun San Kwan, M.; Lord, S.R. Reliability of the Gaitrite® Walkway System for the Quantification of Temporo-Spatial Parameters of Gait in Young and Older People. *Gait Posture* **2004**, *20*, 20–25. [CrossRef]
25. ISO. *Personal Protective Equipment-Footwear-Test Method for Slip Resistance*; International Organization for Standardization: Geneva, Switzerland, 2012.
26. Ali, A.S.; Badran, A.H.; Ali, W.Y. Friction Behavior of Epoxy Floor Tiles Filled by Carbon Nanoparticles. *J. Egypt. Soc. Tribol.* **2018**, *15*, 1–10.
27. ASTM. *Standard Test Method for Using a Portable Inclineable Articulated Strut Slip Tester (Plast)*; ASTM International: West Conshohocken, PA, USA, 2005.
28. Li, K.W. Friction between Footwear and Floor Covered with Solid Particles under Dry and Wet Conditions. *Int. J. Occup. Saf. Ergon.* **2014**, *20*, 43–53. [CrossRef] [PubMed]
29. Mohamed, M.K.; Samy, A.M.; Ali, W.Y. Friction Coefficient of Rubber Shoes Sliding against Ceramic Flooring. *KGK-Rubberpoint* **2012**, *65*, 52–57.
30. Moghaddam, M.; Reza, S. Finite Element Analysis of Contribution of Adhesion and Hysteresis to Shoe-Floor. Science in Engineering. Master Thesis, University of Wisconsin-Milwaukee, Milwaukee, WI, USA, 2013.
31. Shibataa, K.; Abe, S.; Yamaguchi, T.; Hokkirigwa, K. Evaluation for Slip Resistance of Floor Sheets and Shoe Sole with Newly Developed Mobile Friction Measurement System. In Proceedings of the 19th Triennial Congress of the IEA, Melbourne, Australia, 9–14 August 2015.
32. Li, K.W.; Chen, C.J. The Effect of Shoe Soling Tread Groove Width on the Coefficient of Friction with Different Sole Materials, Floors, and Contaminants. *Appl. Ergon.* **2004**, *35*, 499–507. [CrossRef]
33. Popova, E.; Popov, V.L. The Research Works of Coulomb and Amontons and Generalized Laws of Friction. *Friction* **2015**, *3*, 183–190. [CrossRef]
34. Etsion, I.; Kogut, L. A Static Friction Model for Elastic-Plastic Contacting Rough Surfaces. *J. Tribol.* **2004**, *126*, 34–40.
35. Krim, J. Resource Letter_Fmmls-1_Friction at Macroscopic and Microscopic Length Scales. *Am. Assoc. Phys. Teach.* **2002**, *70*, 890–897.
36. Kanaga Karuppiah, K.S.; Bruck, A.L.; Sundararajan, S. Evaluation of Friction Behavior and Tts Contact-Area Dependence at the Micro- and Nano-Scales. *Tribol. Lett.* **2009**, *36*, 259–267. [CrossRef]
37. Johnson, K.L.; Kendall, K.; Roberts, A.D. Surface Energy and the Contact of Elastic Solids. *Proc. R. Soc. A. Math. Phys. Eng. Sci.* **1971**, *324*, 301–313.
38. Strandberg, L. The Effect of Conditions Underfoot on Falling and Overexertion Accidents. *Ergonomics* **1985**, *28*, 131–147. [CrossRef] [PubMed]

2

Evolution of the Hurdle-Unit Kinematic Parameters in the 60 m Indoor Hurdle Race

Pablo González-Frutos [1,*], Santiago Veiga [2], Javier Mallo [2] and Enrique Navarro [2]

1 Faculty of Health Sciences, Universidad Francisco de Vitoria, 28223 Madrid, Spain
2 Health and Human Performance Department, Technical University of Madrid, 28040 Madrid, Spain; santiago.veiga@upm.es (S.V.); javier.mallo@upm.es (J.M.); enrique.navarro@upm.es (E.N.)
* Correspondence: p.gfrutos.prof@ufv.es;

Featured Application: Coaches and athletes should implement their training programs to have an impact on some of these variables according to the specific demands of each hurdle-unit phase and gender.

Abstract: The aims of this study were to compare the five hurdle-unit split times from the deterministic model with the hurdle-to-hurdle model and with the official time, to compare the step kinematics of each hurdle-unit intervals, and to relate these variables to their respective hurdle-unit split times. The temporal and spatial parameters of the 60 m hurdles race were calculated during the 44th Spanish and 12th IAAF World Indoor Championships (men: n = 59; women: n = 51). The hurdle-unit split times from the deterministic model showed a high correlation (r = 0.99; $p < 0.001$) with the split times of the hurdle-to-hurdle model and faster split times were related to shorter step and flight times in hurdle steps for both genders. At the first hurdle, male athletes tended to increase their flight and contact times while the tendency of female athletes was to decrease their contact and flight times. In addition, at the first hurdle, both genders presented shorter take-off distance, shorter landing distance, and greater step width than in the remaining hurdles of the race. Therefore, coaches should implement training programs that have an impact on these key variables according to the specific demands of each hurdle-unit phase and gender.

Keywords: track and field; kinematics; performance analysis; competition; DLT algorithms

---

1. Introduction

The hurdles events have been analyzed through different approaches such as biomechanics, conditional, teaching and learning, talent identification, psychological, or medical [1,2]. Within biomechanical analyses, two types of studies stand out: temporal and spatial. The ubication of the hurdles serves as a useful reference for the division of the event into the following phases [3]: approach run phase (from the starting line to the first hurdle), hurdle unit phase (race and clearance of the hurdles), and run-in phase (from the last hurdle to the finishing line).

Temporal analyses are commonly focused on the split times between each hurdle clearance (foot landing) [4–7]. The times from the athlete's foot landing after one hurdle to the following hurdle are employed for practical reasons, as it allows an easy visual identification of the splits. Tsionakos et al. [6] showed that the correlation between intermediate times and final performance was decisive from the fifth obstacle onwards in the 110 m obstacle event (r = 0.77 to 0.98), while Panoutsakopoulos et al. [7] found a correlation between split times with the official time in the 60 m indoor event in most of the intervals, both for elite men (r = 0.65 to 0.84) and women (r = 0.55 to 0.87). Similarly, González Frutos et al. [8] found an almost perfect correlation (r = 0.99) between the mean of the hurdle-unit split time and the official time in the 60 m hurdle race. In addition to the split time analysis, it is frequent to refer to the flight time over the hurdle (from take-off to landing) in temporal studies. Panoutsakopoulos et al. [7] found a correlation in not all of the hurdles between the flight time and the official time, while González Frutos et al. [8] found a very large correlation (r = 0.82) between the mean flight time of the five hurdle steps and the official time.

Among the spatial analyses, three-dimensional (3D) studies stand out, even though they are habitually carried out in a single hurdle-unit interval (between the second and fifth hurdle), in a training situation or employing a small sample of subjects due to the costly analysis of the data [9–16]. The organization of the steps that make up the hurdle-unit phase within the studies depends on the selection of the phase of interest: following a deterministic model which comprises the preparatory, hurdle, landing and recovery steps [9,17], only the hurdle and landing steps [10,11,13–15], or from hurdle to hurdle [12]. There is a single precedent of the analysis of all ten hurdles during the 110 m hurdle event [18], who performed a two-dimensional analysis and calculated take-off (2.04 ± 0.07 m) and landing (1.47 ± 0.03 m) distances. Complementarily, González-Frutos et al. [8] analyzed the average of every step of the hurdle-unit phase, in addition to the approach run and run-in phases, finding differences between international and national hurdlers in various parameters during 60 m hurdles event, for both men and women.

Most of these kinematical studies indicate that an efficient hurdle clearance technique is associated with the take-off contact time, take-off and landing distances, take-off angle, and to the hurdle flight time. However, the differences found between some studies may be due to the analysis of different single hurdle intervals, since the kinematic parameters in hurdles and sprint events change as the running speed varies [18,19]. Also, differences could rely on the different criteria when defining the split times of each hurdle-unit [11,13–15] as not many studies consider both the preparatory and recovery steps on it.

Therefore, the aims of the present research were: (1) to compare the five hurdle-unit split times from a deterministic model with the hurdle to hurdle model and with the official time, (2) to compare the step kinematics of each hurdle-unit intervals, and (3) to relate these variables to their respective hurdle-unit split times. Our hypothesis is that both models correlate with each other and with the final result in the race, while there should be differences in the registered values of each hurdle-unit interval. Additionally, we hypothesize that these differences between hurdle-unit phases, and the correlations between variables and their hurdle-unit split times, will be diverse for men and women.

2. Materials and Methods

2.1. Subjects

All the races were filmed during the 60 m hurdle event of the 44th Spanish Indoor Championship and 12th IAAF World Indoor Championship (2008) with the license of both organizing committees. The best performance of each athlete (men, n = 59; women, n = 51) from the heat, semifinal, and final rounds was included in the study. All experimental procedures were carried out in accordance with the Declaration of Helsinki and were approved by the Ethics Committee of the Technical University of Madrid.

2.2. Procedures

The races were filmed with six fixed JVC GY-DV300 video cameras (Japan Victor Company, Yokohama, Japan) located at the main stands and operating at 50 fps (frames per second; shutter speed: 1/1000), similar to that previously used in other studies [5,9,11,12,15]. Four cameras had a predominantly side view: camera one recorded the first 13 m; camera two from 13 to 30 m; camera three from 30 to 47 m; camera four the last 13 m (47 to 60 m) of the race. To avoid visual occlusion of the athletes, cameras five and six were placed to capture the frontal view: camera five recorded the first 30 m (including the referees' starting shot) and camera six the last 30 m. A common event (foot landing or take-off) in the field of view of two different cameras were employed for the camera synchronization.

An experienced observer manually digitized the hurdlers' foot landing and take-off points from the race footage using Photo 23D software (Technical University of Madrid, Spain) [20]. The official lane marks were employed as control points (six in each camera) for calibration purposes and direct lineal transformation algorithms [21] were used to reconstruct the real coordinates (in meters) from the screen coordinates (in pixels). Thirty points of known spatial coordinates (different from those used for calibration purposes) represented by the official lane marks and uniformly distributed in the field of view were used for error estimation. The root mean square error [22] was less than 0.04 m for the step length (x-axis) and less than 0.02 m for the step width (y-axis) on the six cameras, providing a validity of the measurements similar to those of other previous research on race analysis [23]. The step length and step width were calculated by the difference on the x (longitudinal) or y (transverse) axes, respectively, of the most forward point of the foot on the ground during successive contacts on it.

The definition (Figure 1) proposed by McDonald and Dapena [9] was used for the organization of the temporal and spatial parameters of the five hurdle-unit phases of the 60 m hurdles, which integrated the preparatory step, hurdle step (divided into take-off distance and landing distance), landing step, and recovery step. The calculation of the split times used the same sequence, including the time elapsed from the beginning of the preparatory step to the beginning of the next preparatory step. Alternatively, the split times were also calculated from the landing step to the next landing step as done by the temporal studies [4–7], for comparative purposes.

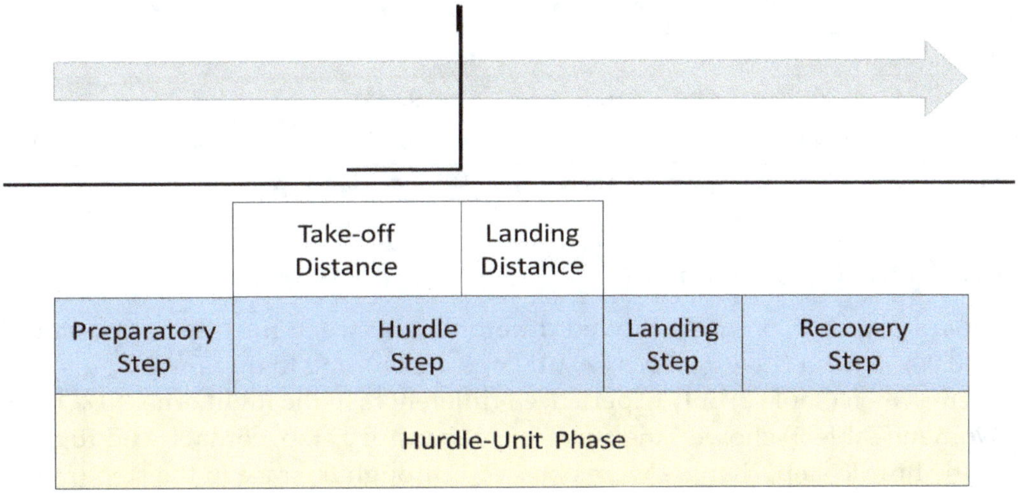

Figure 1. Definitions employed for the hurdle-unit phase analysis according to McDonald and Dapena [9].

2.3. Statistical Analysis

All results are expressed as the mean ± standard deviation (SD). Split times, step times, contact times, flight times, step lengths, and step width of the athletes were compared with a repeated measures analysis of variance according to the hurdle-unit phase (first, second, third, fourth, and fifth hurdle, and mean of the five hurdles) for both genders of athletes (male or female). Planned repeated contrast tests between successive laps were carried out. Post hoc tests were used to determine statistical effects ($p < 0.05$) between factors using Bonferroni corrections and were interpreted using effect sizes ($\eta p2$) with 0.2, 0.5, and 0.8 threshold values for small, medium, and large effects [24]. Cohen d effect sizes between the hurdle-unit phases and mean hurdle-unit phase were calculated to display practical significance. Effect sizes of 0.00 to 0.19, 0.20 to 0.59, 0.60 to 1.19, 1.20 to 1.99, 2.00 to 3.99, and ≥4.00 were interpreted as trivial, small, moderate, large, very large, and nearly perfect, respectively [25]. Pearson correlation coefficients were used to relate all the kinematic race parameters to the hurdle-unit split time or race result, being 0.1, 0.3, 0.5, 0.7, and 0.9, the threshold values that represented small, moderate, large, very large, and nearly perfect correlations [25]. Statistical analyses were performed using the IBM Statistical Package for Social Sciences Statistics, version 22.0 (IBM Inc., Armonk, NY, USA).

3. Results

3.1. Split Times

The mean split times on the hurdle-unit phase (men: 1.10 ± 0.06 s; women: 1.09 ± 0.07 s) measured from preparatory to the next preparatory step showed nearly perfect relationships with the split times measured from landing to the next landing step (r = 0.99; $p < 0.001$), and also with the race results (r = 0.99; $p < 0.001$) both for men and women.

Hurdle-unit split times changed along the 60 m hurdles race (men: $F_{3.718} = 3.28$, $p = 0.014$, ηp2 = 0.05, and women: $F_{3.299} = 6.60$, $p = 0.001$, ηp2 = 0.12) with the greatest differences observed in hurdle one for both gender and hurdle five for men (Table 1). Split times in all the hurdles showed very large to nearly perfect correlations with the race results, with correlation coefficients increasing from the first to the fourth hurdle (Table 1).

Table 1. Evolution of the hurdle-unit split times (s) and relationships (r) with the 60 m hurdle race results during the 44th Spanish Indoor and 12th IAAF World Indoor Championships.

	Hurdle 1	Hurdle 2	Hurdle 3	Hurdle 4	Hurdle 5
Split Time					
Men	1.11 ± 0.06 ^{*4}	1.10 ± 0.06	1.10 ± 0.08	1.09 ± 0.07	1.11 ± 0.07 ^{*4}
Women	1.10 ± 0.06 $^{*34\#5}$	1.09 ± 0.07	1.09 ± 0.08	1.08 ± 0.09	1.08 ± 0.07
Correlation					
Men	0.906 $^{\#}$	0.914 $^{\#}$	0.927 $^{\#}$	0.955 $^{\#}$	0.874 $^{\#}$
Women	0.942 $^{\#}$	0.970 $^{\#}$	0.975 $^{\#}$	0.980 $^{\#}$	0.944 $^{\#}$

Inter-hurdle-unit phase differences and correlations: * $p < 0.05$, # $p < 0.001$. Superscripts numbers indicate the hurdle-unit (1–5) where differences exist.

3.2. Kinematic Differences between Hurdles

In the preparatory step, women showed differences between hurdles in the step ($F_{3.50} = 4.15$, $p = 0.005$, ηp2 = 0.08), contact ($F_{3.77} = 3.23$, $p = 0.015$, ηp2 = 0.06), and flight times ($F_{3.74} = 10.84$, $p = 0.001$, ηp2 = 0.18), whereas men (Table 2) only experienced differences in the flight time ($F_{3.95} = 2.92$, $p = 0.023$, ηp2 = 0.05). Women (Table 3) showed the shortest preparatory step, contact, and flight times on the first hurdle. In the hurdle step, changes were observed through the race in the step (men: $F_{3.53} = 6.35$, $p = 0.001$, ηp2 = 0.10; women: $F_{3.37} = 5.26$, $p = 0.001$, ηp2 = 0.10) and flight (men: $F_{3.33} = 5.92$, $p = 0.001$, ηp2 = 0.09; women: $F_{3.69} = 3.19$, $p = 0.017$, ηp2 = 0.06) times, with the greatest values observed in the first hurdle both for men (Table 2) and women (Table 3). In the landing step, men (Table 2) showed differences along the race in the step ($F_{4.00} = 4.35$, $p = 0.002$, η2 = 0.07) and contact times ($F_{3.96} = 3.04$, $p = 0.018$, ηp2 = 0.05), while, in the recovery step, changes were observed for women (Table 3) in step time ($F_{3.69} = 6.20$, $p = 0.001$, ηp2 = 0.11), with maximum step times accounting in the first hurdle.

When compared to the mean race values, the greatest differences for women were observed in the first hurdle for contact (moderate effect, Figure 2D) and flight times (large effect, Figure 2F) of the preparatory step, and in the third hurdle for preparatory flight time (moderate effect, Figure 2F). However, the differences regarding the mean race values for men hurdlers did not show a moderate effect size for the step, contact, and flight times (Figure 2A–C,E).

Step length also changed through the 60 m hurdle race in every step of the hurdle-unit phase, except for the landing step in the women's race. The greatest changes were observed in the landing distance during the men's race ($F_{3.82} = 27.91$, $p = 0.001$, ηp2 = 0.33) and in the take-off distance of the women's race ($F_{3.74} = 62.29$, $p = 0.001$, ηp2 = 0.56). Step width also displayed meaningful differences according to the hurdle order, specifically in the hurdle step for men ($F_{2.99} = 11.97$, $p = 0.001$, ηp2 = 0.17) and women ($F_{3.04} = 11.64$, $p = 0.001$, ηp2 = 0.19).

Table 2. Evolution of the spatial-temporal variables of men hurdlers participating in the 44th Spanish Indoor and 12th IAAF World Indoor Championships.

		Hurdle 1	Hurdle 2	Hurdle 3	Hurdle 4	Hurdle 5
Step Time	Preparatory step	0.20 ± 0.00	0.20 ± 0.00	0.20 ± 0.00	0.20 ± 0.00	0.20 ± 0.00
	Hurdle Step	0.51 ± 0.01	0.50 ± 0.01	0.50 ± 0.01	0.49 ± 0.01 $^{\#125}$	0.50 ± 0.01
	Landing Step	0.16 ± 0.00	0.15 ± 0.00	0.15 ± 0.00	0.16 ± 0.00 $^{¥2\#3}$	0.16 ± 0.00
	Recovery Step	0.25 ± 0.00	0.25 ± 0.00	0.24 ± 0.00	0.24 ± 0.00	0.25 ± 0.00
Contact Time	Preparatory step	0.11 ± 0.00	0.11 ± 0.00	0.11 ± 0.00	0.11 ± 0.00	0.11 ± 0.00
	Hurdle Step	0.12 ± 0.00	0.12 ± 0.00	0.12 ± 0.00	0.12 ± 0.00	0.12 ± 0.00
	Landing Step	0.09 ± 0.00 $^{¥3}$	0.08 ± 0.00	0.08 ± 0.00	0.09 ± 0.00	0.09 ± 0.00
	Recovery Step	0.12 ± 0.00	0.12 ± 0.00	0.12 ± 0.00	0.12 ± 0.00	0.12 ± 0.00
Flight Time	Preparatory step	0.09 ± 0.00	0.09 ± 0.00	0.09 ± 0.00	0.09 ± 0.00	0.09 ± 0.00
	Hurdle Step	0.39 ± 0.01 $^{\#4}$	0.38 ± 0.00	0.38 ± 0.01	0.37 ± 0.01	0.38 ± 0.01 $^{¥3}$
	Landing Step	0.07 ± 0.00	0.07 ± 0.00	0.07 ± 0.00	0.08 ± 0.00	0.07 ± 0.00
	Recovery Step	0.12 ± 0.00	0.13 ± 0.00	0.12 ± 0.00	0.12 ± 0.00	0.12 ± 0.00
Step Length	Preparatory step	1.82 ± 0.01 $^{*24\#3}$	1.88 ± 0.02	1.91 ± 0.02	1.87 ± 0.02	1.86 ± 0.01 $^{¥3}$
	Hurdle Step	3.76 ± 0.03	3.73 ± 0.02	3.89 ± 0.03 $^{\#1245}$	3.71 ± 0.02	3.72 ± 0.02
	Take-off distance	2.01 ± 0.02 $^{*4\#235}$	2.11 ± 0.02	2.14 ± 0.02	2.08 ± 0.02 $^{¥35}$	2.12 ± 0.02
	Landing distance	1.74 ± 0.03 $^{\#245}$	1.62 ± 0.03	1.75 ± 0.03 $^{\#245}$	1.63 ± 0.03	1.60 ± 0.02
	Landing Step	1.42 ± 0.02 $^{¥5\#4}$	1.46 ± 0.02	1.45 ± 0.02 ^{*4}	1.50 ± 0.02	1.48 ± 0.02
	Recovery Step	1.98 ± 0.01 ^{*4}	2.01 ± 0.02	1.98 ± 0.01 ^{*4}	2.03 ± 0.01	2.02 ± 0.02
Step Width	Preparatory step	0.13 ± 0.01	0.14 ± 0.01	0.15 ± 0.01 ^{*4}	0.12 ± 0.01	0.13 ± 0.01
	Hurdle Step	0.16 ± 0.01 $^{¥23\#45}$	0.09 ± 0.01	0.10 ± 0.01	0.08 ± 0.01	0.08 ± 0.01
	Landing Step	0.13 ± 0.01	0.12 ± 0.01	0.12 ± 0.01	0.12 ± 0.01	0.16 ± 0.01 $^{*1¥2\#34}$
	Recovery Step	0.21 ± 0.01	0.24 ± 0.01	0.23 ± 0.01	0.24 ± 0.01	0.29 ± 0.01 $^{*2¥34\#1}$

Inter-hurdle difference: * $p < 0.05$; $^{¥}$ $p < 0.01$; $^{\#}$ $p < 0.001$. Superscripts numbers indicate the hurdle-unit (1–5) where differences exist.

Table 3. Evolution of the spatial-temporal variables of women hurdlers participating in the 44th Spanish Indoor and 12th IAAF World Indoor Championships.

		Hurdle 1	Hurdle 2	Hurdle 3	Hurdle 4	Hurdle 5
Step Time	Preparatory step	0.20 ± 0.00 $^{¥3}$	0.21 ± 0.00	0.21 ± 0.00	0.21 ± 0.00	0.21 ± 0.00
	Hurdle Step	0.46 ± 0.01	0.46 ± 0.01	0.45 ± 0.01 ^{*12}	0.45 ± 0.01	0.45 ± 0.01
	Landing Step	0.18 ± 0.00	0.17 ± 0.00	0.17 ± 0.00	0.17 ± 0.00	0.17 ± 0.00
	Recovery Step	0.26 ± 0.00 $^{*2\#5}$	0.25 ± 0.00	0.25 ± 0.00	0.25 ± 0.00	0.25 ± 0.00
Contact Time	Preparatory step	0.11 ± 0.00 $^{*4¥5}$	0.11 ± 0.00	0.11 ± 0.00	0.11 ± 0.00	0.11 ± 0.00
	Hurdle Step	0.11 ± 0.00	0.11 ± 0.00	0.11 ± 0.00	0.11 ± 0.00	0.11 ± 0.00
	Landing Step	0.09 ± 0.00	0.09 ± 0.00	0.09 ± 0.00	0.09 ± 0.00	0.09 ± 0.00
	Recovery Step	0.12 ± 0.00	0.11 ± 0.00	0.11 ± 0.00	0.12 ± 0.00	0.11 ± 0.00
Flight Time	Preparatory step	0.09 ± 0.00 $^{\#2345}$	0.10 ± 0.00	0.10 ± 0.00	0.10 ± 0.00	0.10 ± 0.00
	Hurdle Step	0.35 ± 0.01	0.34 ± 0.01	0.34 ± 0.01	0.34 ± 0.01	0.34 ± 0.01
	Landing Step	0.09 ± 0.00	0.09 ± 0.00	0.09 ± 0.00	0.09 ± 0.00	0.09 ± 0.00
	Recovery Step	0.14 ± 0.00	0.14 ± 0.00	0.14 ± 0.00	0.14 ± 0.00	0.13 ± 0.00

Table 3. *Cont.*

		Hurdle 1	Hurdle 2	Hurdle 3	Hurdle 4	Hurdle 5
Step Length	Preparatory step	1.63 ± 0.01 [#2345]	1.76 ± 0.02	1.78 ± 0.01	1.79 ± 0.01	1.79 ± 0.01
	Hurdle Step	3.18 ± 0.03	3.21 ± 0.02	3.33 ± 0.02 [#1245]	3.20 ± 0.02	3.22 ± 0.02
	Take-off distance	1.79 ± 0.02 [#2345]	1.93 ± 0.02	2.01 ± 0.02 [#24]	1.93 ± 0.02	1.97 ± 0.02
	Landing distance	1.40 ± 0.03 [¥3#245]	1.28 ± 0.03	1.32 ± 0.03 [#5]	1.27 ± 0.03	1.25 ± 0.03
	Landing Step	1.48 ± 0.02	1.45 ± 0.02	1.50 ± 0.01	1.49 ± 0.01	1.50 ± 0.02
	Recovery Step	1.93 ± 0.01 [¥4]	1.98 ± 0.01	1.95 ± 0.01	1.98 ± 0.01	1.91 ± 0.01 [*2¥4]
Step Width	Preparatory step	0.10 ± 0.01	0.10 ± 0.01	0.09 ± 0.01	0.10 ± 0.01	0.09 ± 0.01
	Hurdle Step	0.13 ± 0.01 [¥5#234]	0.07 ± 0.01	0.06 ± 0.01	0.06 ± 0.01	0.07 ± 0.01
	Landing Step	0.12 ± 0.01	0.10 ± 0.01	0.11 ± 0.01	0.11 ± 0.01	0.13 ± 0.01
	Recovery Step	0.20 ± 0.01	0.19 ± 0.01	0.20 ± 0.01	0.20 ± 0.01	0.23 ± 0.01 [*2]

Inter-hurdle difference: * $p < 0.05$; ¥ $p < 0.01$; # $p < 0.001$. Superscripts numbers indicate the hurdle-unit (1–5) where differences exist.

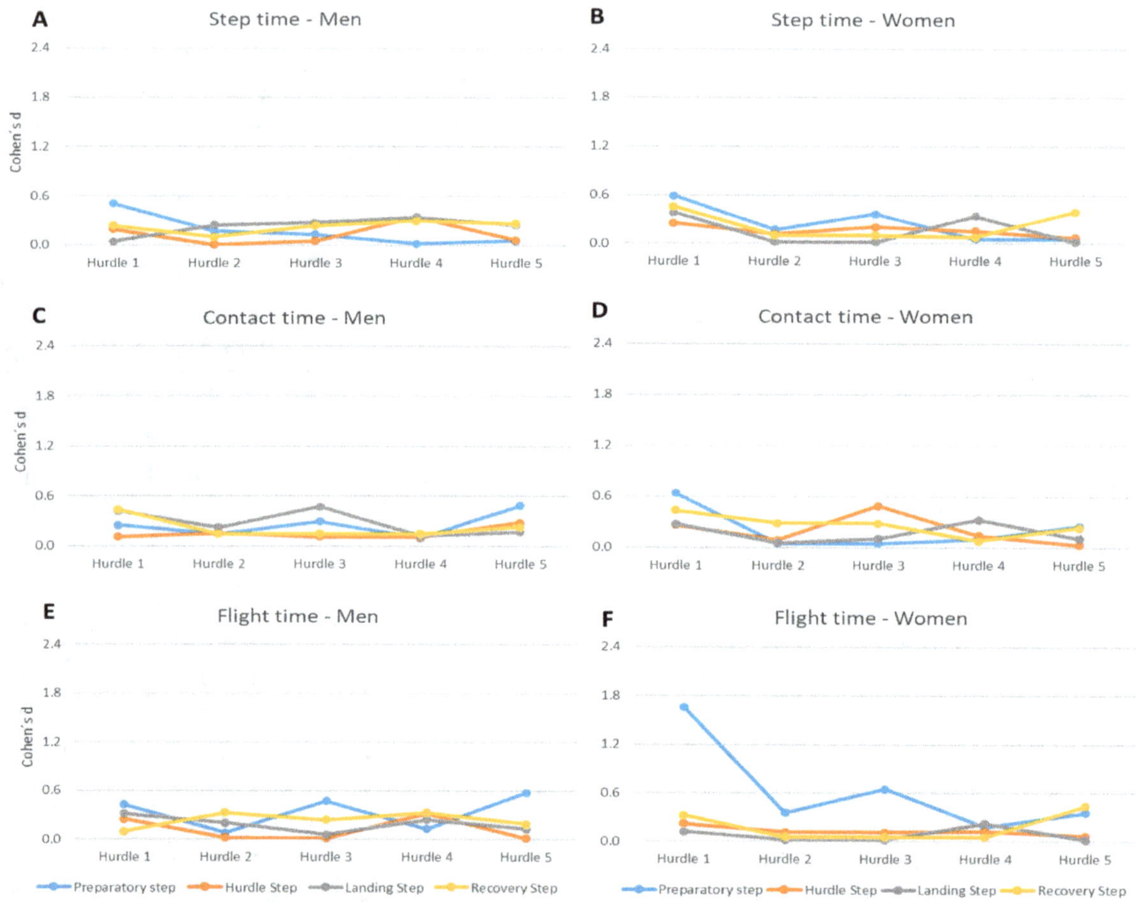

Figure 2. Magnitude of differences (Cohen's d) for the temporal parameters ((**A**,**B**) step time; (**C**,**D**) contact time; and (**E**,**F**) flight time) in relation to mean race values for men and women. An effect size greater than 0.6 or 1.2 was considered as moderate or large, respectively, by Hopkins et al. [25].

The differences in the spatial parameters with respect to the mean race values showing moderate, large, or very large effect sizes on step length in every step, except for the landing step, both for men and women. Moreover, the greatest values were achieved in the first and third hurdle (Figure 3A,B). The step width also showed moderate (men's recovery step), large (men's hurdle step), or very large (women's hurdle step) differences at the first hurdle (Figure 3C,D).

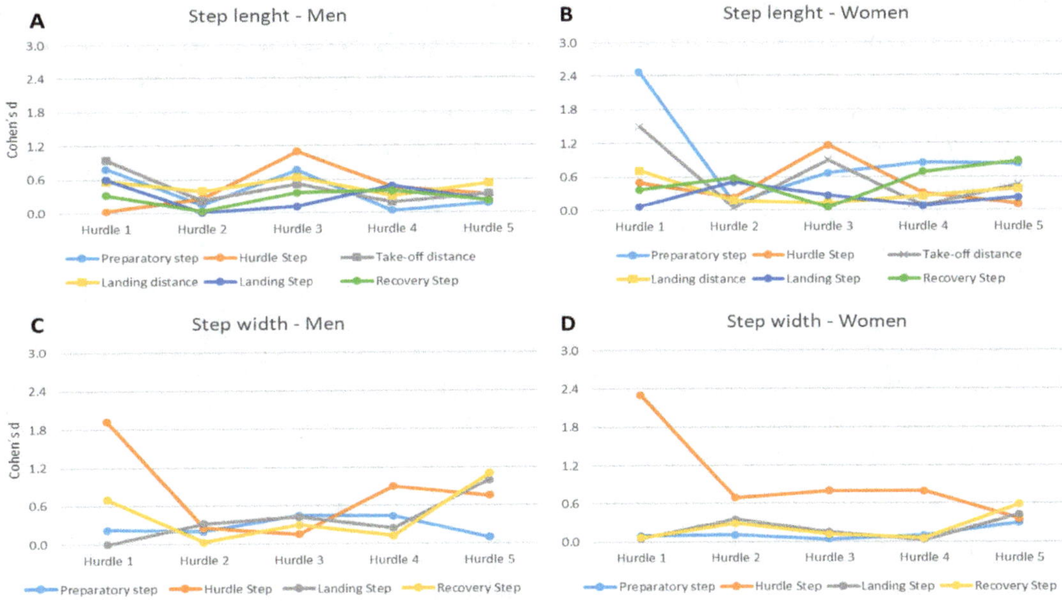

Figure 3. Magnitude of differences (Cohen's d) for the spatial parameters ((**A**,**B**) step length; (**C**,**D**) step width) in relation to mean race values for men and women. An effect size greater than 0.6 or 1.2 was considered as moderate or large, respectively, by Hopkins et al. [25].

3.3. Correlations of Kinematic Parameters with Hurdle-Unit Times

Step and flight times during the hurdle step showed very large relationships with the split times both for men (Figure 4A–E) and women (Figure 4B,F). Additionally, the step time during the recovery step showed a very large correlation with the split times for women (Figure 4B).

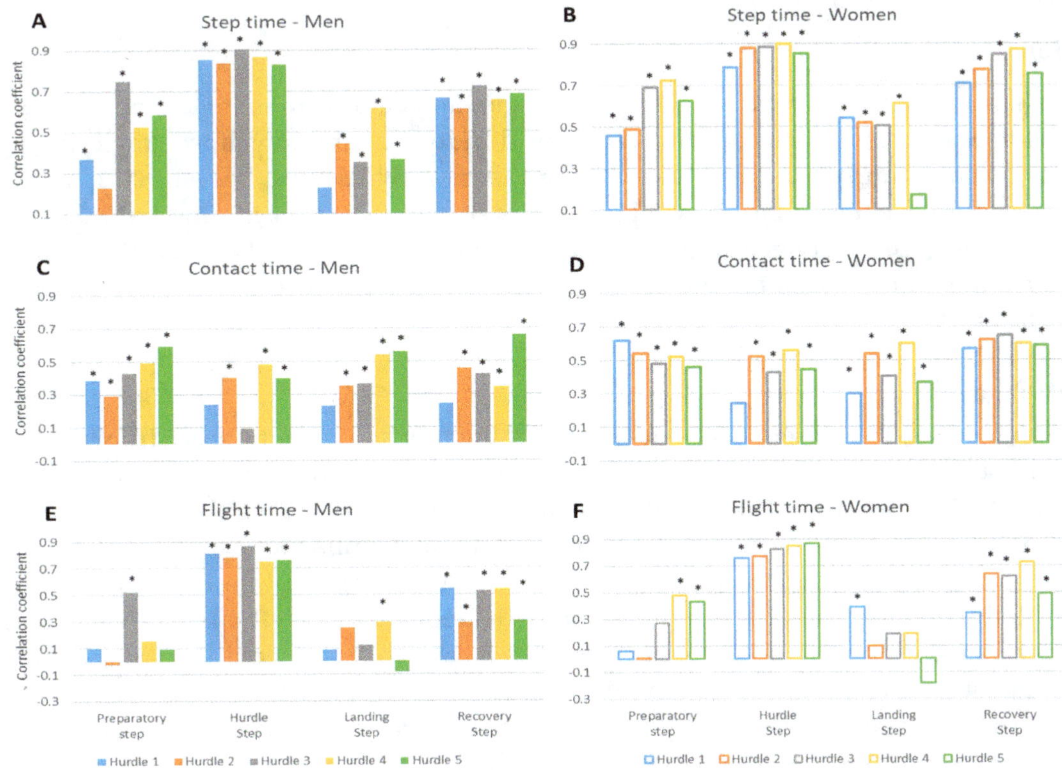

Figure 4. Pearson's correlation coefficient (r) between temporal parameters ((**A**,**B**) step time; (**C**,**D**) contact time; and (**E**,**F**) flight time) and the hurdle-unit splits times during the 44th Spanish Indoor and 12th IAAF World Indoor Championships. Correlations: * $p < 0.05$.

Every landing distance showed moderate to large (first and third hurdle) relationships with their respective split times in the men's race, while take-off distance showed moderate to large (fourth hurdle) correlations from the third to the fifth hurdle (Figure 5A). In the case of women athletes, the highest correlations were observed in the landing and recovery step of the last hurdle (moderate). The hurdle step width of men (Figure 5C) and women (Figure 5D) hurdlers showed moderate relationships with their respective split times in the first hurdle.

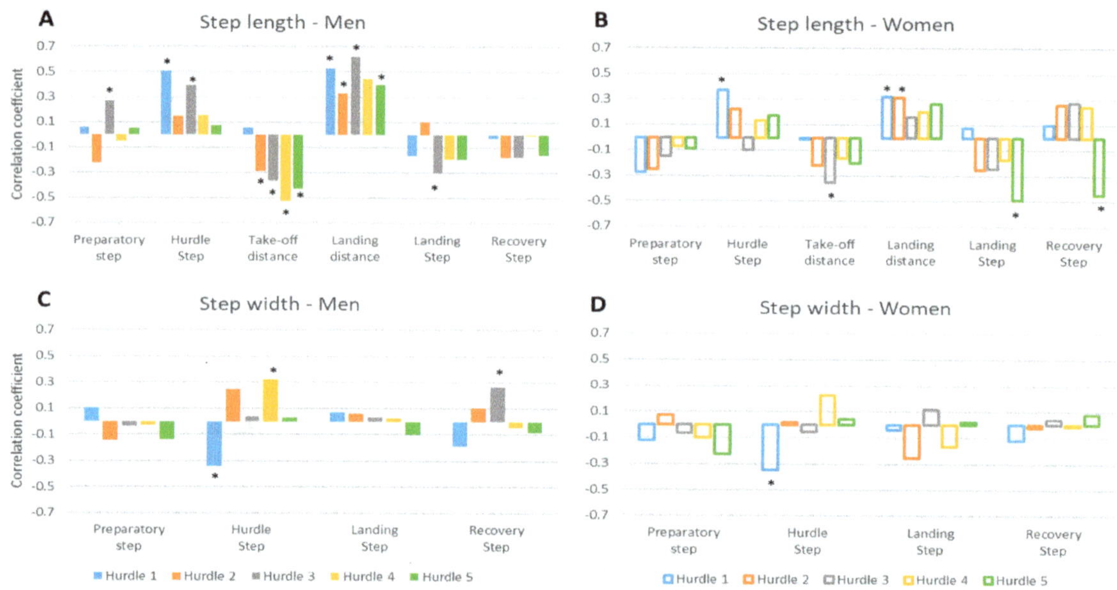

Figure 5. Pearson's correlation coefficient (r) between spatial parameters ((**A**,**B**) step length; and (**C**,**D**) step width) and the hurdle-unit split times during the 44th Spanish Indoor and 12th IAAF World Indoor Championships. Correlations: * $p < 0.05$.

4. Discussion

The present research examined the evolution of the kinematic parameters during the 60 m hurdle races of the 44th Spanish Indoor and 12th IAAF World Indoor Championships. Previous studies have focused on an isolated hurdle-unit analysis during the race, which could presumably have left a big knowledge-gap for coaches and athletes. The results of the present study indicate that each of the hurdle-units of the race presents a high correlation with the race result. Nevertheless, there were differences on some of the temporal and spatial parameters of the hurdle-unit subphases (especially the first and last ones).

4.1. Split Times

For the split times, the present research organized the hurdle-unit subphases from the preparatory to the recovery steps [9]. This hurdle-unit division allowed the inclusion of all performance criteria of the hurdle event in a more rational way following a deterministic model [17]. Split times calculated in the current investigation showed greater correlations with race results than values reported in previous studies [7,26], although, in all the cases, correlations were very large. Interestingly, correlation values increased from the first to the fourth hurdle in line with Tsionakos [6] in the 100/110 m event, whereas the values decreased in the fifth interval of the men's races. This may be due to the shorter distance between the last hurdle and the finish line, which could cause technical modifications (i.e., advance the trunk) in the last hurdle-unit phase to prepare for the run-in phase [27] or by the fatigue created by the greater relative height of the hurdles in men races [8,9,28].

Mean split times were slightly greater than the values of the finalists of international competitions [4–7,29–32], probably because of a greater sample size in the present research as it included both international and national standard level athletes. For both genders, there was a tendency in the first hurdle-unit to be the slowest of the race in line with previous studies [6]. However, in the case of men, the fifth (last) hurdle-unit was slower than the previous ones. This gender-dependent evolution in the split times coincides with that observed by Panoutsakopoulos et al. [7] and Kuitunen and Poon [26] and could be explained by the highest hurdle height of men. According to McDonald and Dapena [9], Salo et al. [11], and González-Frutos et al. [8], this height difference would represent a greater effort for men and would cause a loss of speed from the fourth hurdle on, whereas women can fasten up to the last hurdle.

4.2. Kinematic Differences between Hurdles

The first hurdle presented most of the kinematic differences throughout the race, even though the pattern was different from men to women. Male athletes presented a greater flight time in the hurdle step and a greater contact time on the landing step of the first hurdle, whereas female athletes presented a shorter step, contact, and flight times on the preparatory step. These differences could be explained by the relative differences in height and distance between hurdles in men and women hurdlers [9,28]. Indeed, the greater height of the hurdle in the male event could hinder the adjustments to the first hurdle with a possible greater take-off angle to avoid falling and its subsequent landing from a greater height [8,9,11]. For both genders, the take-off distance was the shortest and the step width was the greatest in the first hurdle step, which could be related to the need to avoid contact with the lead leg [29,30] by means of a lateral displacement. This could represent an important finding of the present research, as previous studies [9–12,15] have only focused on the study from the second to the fifth hurdle without providing information about the step width.

For the remaining hurdles, the longest take-off distance was observed in the third hurdle, which seems to be one of the most important performance indicators [8,9,11,15]. In the last (fifth) hurdle, male athletes increased their landing and recovery step length while female athletes presented a shorter recovery step length. These spatial differences in the last hurdle are in line with the temporal modifications mentioned above and suggest that gender differences, due to different distance and number of steps to the finish line, should be acknowledged by coaches when addressing this hurdle unit. Since previous studies have analyzed the second [10], third [11], fourth [9,12,15], or fifth hurdle [9,12] in isolation, our data clearly show that kinematics differences exist between hurdle units in a single race.

4.3. Correlations of Kinematic Parameters with Hurdle-Unit Times

The very large correlations of the step and flight times during the hurdle step with the hurdle-unit performance were in line with the very large correlations of these parameters with the race result [8]. These data reinforce the idea that shorter hurdle clearance times favor the maintenance of the horizontal velocity of the athletes [11]. Previous studies have not reported such large correlations [6] or have only observed high correlations in the men's race [26] or in some specific hurdle-units [7]. The differences with the current study might be due to a wider sample of athletes who were examined during the present research. For the female hurdlers, and as a difference to their male counterparts, very large correlations were observed between the recovery step and the split times. It is probable that the lower parabola observed for women [9] in the hurdle step, required the lengthening of the three inter-hurdle steps and highlighted the role of the recovery step. These gender differences somehow support the idea proposed by Mann [28] of increasing the distance between hurdles in the men's races and the hurdle height in the women's races. In the case of women, this would increase the importance of the technical ability [33], contributing to an upgrading of this event [34].

Regarding spatial variables, the correlations found between the take-off and landing distances with the split times of male hurdlers support the influence of the hurdle height on kinematics [8,9,11,34]. The fastest male hurdlers showed a clear ability to produce a longer take-off but shorter landing distances throughout the race. Furthermore, landing distances obtained greater correlations with the split times on the first half of the race, while take-off distances showed greater correlations with the split times in the second half of the race. Therefore, it could be understood that the lack of technical control in the landing distance during the first part of the race leads to fatigue in the second part, which might have a technical impact translating into a shorter take-off distance. Women hurdlers, on the other hand, presented the largest correlations between the split times in the landing and recovery step of the last hurdle. That is, a longer length of the landing and recovery after the last hurdle was related to a better split indicating the importance of the sprint ability [35]. Interestingly, for both genders, a greater step width over the first hurdle was related to a better split time. This had not been previously measured in competition, even though other studies focused on the approach run phase [36–38] and provides clear information on how the best hurdlers perform at the beginning of the race and negotiate the short take-off distance to the first hurdle.

4.4. Practical Applications and Research Limitations

According to the present results, coaches and practitioners should consider the key role of the first hurdle-unit and its technical demands with a greater step width and changes on the flight-contact times depending on gender. Also, the technical evolution throughout the race should be considered by maximizing the take-off distances at the beginning and minimizing the landing distances as the race progresses. Split times both in a training and competition setup should be recorded comprising the entire hurdle-unit structure (from preparatory to recovery steps).

Future research on the 60 m hurdle events could also consider the effect of contacting the hurdle during the flight phase on the kinematic parameters [39] or the differences in the race evolution according to the athletes' competitive level. Also, studies employing data recordings with a greater temporal resolution would be advisable to increase the uncertainty related to contact and flight times.

5. Conclusions

The results of this study provide solid evidence on the kinematic differences that competitive hurdlers present through the race. Split times improve from the first hurdle onwards and present gender-specific differences on the last (fifth) hurdle. In the first hurdle, men tend to increase their flight and contact times and women tend to decrease their contact and flight times. Also, both genders present shorter take-off distance, shorter landing distance, and greater step width than in the remainder of the race.

Faster split times were related to shorter step and flight times of the five hurdle steps for both genders. However, greater take-off distances for men in the first half of the race and shorter landing distances in the second half were related to faster performers. For women, longer recovery steps on the last hurdle were related to faster performers. The hurdle-unit split times from the preparatory to the recovery step present a more rational race division (according to a deterministic model) and can be compared with the split times of temporal studies.

From all of the above, coaches and athletes should implement their training programs considering the differences between men and women, to have an impact on the key variables according to the specific demands of each hurdle-unit phase.

Author Contributions: Conceptualization, P.G.-F., S.V., J.M., and E.N.; Data curation, P.G.-F.; Formal analysis, P.G.-F. and S.V.; Investigation, P.G.-F., S.V., and E.N.; Methodology, P.G.-F., S.V., J.M., and E.N.; Project administration, P.G.-F. and S.V.; Resources, E.N.; Software, E.N.; Supervision, E.N.; Validation, P.G.-F., J.M., and E.N.; Visualization, P.G.-F.; Writing—original draft, P.G.-F. and S.V.; Writing—review & editing, P.G.-F., S.V., J.M., and E.N. All authors have read and agreed to the published version of the manuscript.

Acknowledgments: The author would like to acknowledge José Campos as the coordinator of the biomechanical studies developed during the 44th Spanish Indoor Championship and 12th IAAF World Indoor Championship, as well as the Royal Spanish Athletics Federation (RFEA) and the International Association of Athletics Federations (IAAF) for promoting, facilitating access and location for data collection, and managing the stay during the championships.

References

1. Schiffer, J. Hurdles (Part I). *New Stud. Athl.* **2006**, *21*, 71–104.
2. Schiffer, J. Hurdles (Part II). *New Stud. Athl.* **2006**, *21*, 97–122.
3. Brüggemann, G.-P.; Glad, B. Time Analysis of the 110 Metres and 100 Metres Hurdles. Scientific Research Project at the Games of the XXIVth Olympiad—Seoul 1988. *New Stud. Athlet.* **1990**, *5*, 91–131.
4. Muller, H.; Hommel, H. Biomechanical research project at the VIth world championships in athletics, Athens 1997. *New Stud. Athl.* **1997**, *12*, 43–73.
5. Graubner, R.; Nixdorf, E. Biomechanical analysis of the sprint and hurdles events at the 2009 IAAF world championships in athletics. *New Stud. Athlet.* **2011**, *26*, 19–53.
6. Tsiokanos, A.; Tsaopoulos, D.; Giavroglou, A.; Tsarouchas, E. Race pattern of women's 100-m hurdles: Time analysis of olympic hurdle performance. *Int. J. Kinesiol. Sports Sci.* **2017**, *5*, 56–64. [CrossRef]
7. Panoutsakopoulos, V.; Theodorou, A.S.; Kotzamanidou, M.C.; Fragkoulis, E.; Smirniotou, A.; Kollias, I.A. Gender and event specificity differences in kinematical parameters of a 60 m hurdles race. *Int. J. Kinesiol. Sports Sci.* **2020**, *20*, 668–682. [CrossRef]
8. González-Frutos, P.; Veiga, S.; Mallo, J.; Navarro, E. Spatiotemporal comparisons between elite and high-level 60 m hurdlers. *Front. Psychol.* **2019**, *10*, 2525. [CrossRef]
9. McDonald, C.; Dapena, J. Linear kinematics of the men's 110-m and women's 100-m hurdles races. *Med. Sci. Sports Exerc.* **1991**, *23*, 1382–1391.
10. McLean, B. The biomechanics of hurdling: Force plate analysis to assess hurdling technique. *New Stud. Athl.* **1994**, *9*, 55–58.
11. Salo, A.; Grimshaw, P.N.; Marar, L. 3-D biomechanical analysis of sprint hurdles at different competitive levels. *Med. Sci. Sports Exerc.* **1997**, *29*, 231–237. [CrossRef]
12. Coh, M. Biomechanical analysis of Colin Jackson's hurdle clearance technique. *New Stud. Athl.* **2003**, *18*, 37–45.
13. Park, Y.J.; Ryu, J.K.; Ryu, J.S.; Kim, T.S.; Hwang, W.S.; Park, S.K.; Yoon, S. Kinematic analysis of hurdle clearance technique for 110-m men's hurdlers at IAAF world championships, Daegue 2011. *Korean J. Sport Biomech.* **2011**, *21*, 529–540. [CrossRef]
14. Ryu, J.K.; Chang, J.K. Kinematic analysis of the hurdle clearance technique used by world top class women's hurdler. *Korean J. Sport Biomech.* **2011**, *21*, 131–140. [CrossRef]
15. Coh, M.; Iskra, J. Biomechanical studies of 110 m hurdle clearance technique. *Sport Sci.* **2012**, *5*, 10–14.
16. Čoh, M.; Bončina, N.; Štuhec, S.; Mackala, K. Comparative biomechanical analysis of the hurdle clearance technique of Colin Jackson and Dayron Robles: Key Studies. *Appl. Sci.* **2020**, *10*, 3302. [CrossRef]
17. Chow, J.W.; Knudson, D.V. Use of deterministic models in sports and exercise biomechanics research. *Sport Biomech.* **2011**, *10*, 219–233. [CrossRef]
18. Ho, C.S.; Chang, C.Y.; Lin, K.C. The wearable devices application for evaluation of 110 meter high hurdle race. *J. Hum. Sport Exerc.* **2020**, *15*, 34–42. [CrossRef]
19. Ito, A.; Ishikawa, M.; Isolehto, J.; Komi, P.V. Changes in the step width, step length, and step frequency of the world's top sprinters during 100 metres. *New Stud. Athl.* **2006**, *21*, 35–39.
20. Cala, A.; Veiga, S.; García, A.; Navarro, E. Previous cycling does not affect running efficiency during a triathlon world cup competition. *J. Sport Med. Phys. Fitness* **2009**, *49*, 152–158.
21. Abdel-Aziz, Y.I.; Karara, H.M. Direct linear transformation from comparator coordinates into space coordinates in close range photogrammetry. In *Proceedings of the Symposium on Close Range Photogrammetry*; The American Society of Photogrammetry: Falls Church, VA, USA, 1971; pp. 1–18.
22. Allard, P.; Blanchi, J.P.; Aíssaqui, R. Bases of three-dimensional reconstruction. In *Three Dimensional Analysis of Human Movement*; Allard, P., Stokes, I.A.F., Bianchi, J.P., Eds.; Human Kinetics: Champaign, IL, USA, 1995; pp. 19–40.
23. Veiga, S.; Cala, A.; Mallo, J.; Navarro, E. A new procedure for race analysis in swimming based on individual distance measurements. *J. Sports Sci.* **2013**, *31*, 159–165. [CrossRef]
24. Cohen, J.A. Power primer. *Psychol. Bull.* **1992**, *112*, 155–159. [CrossRef] [PubMed]
25. Hopkins, W.; Marshall, S.; Batterham, A.; Hanin, Y. Progressive statistics for studies in sports medicine and exercise science. *Med. Sci. Sports Exerc.* **2009**, *41*, 3–13. [CrossRef]

26. Kuitunen, S.; Poon, S. Race pattern of 60-m hurdles in world-class sprint hurdles: A biomechanical analysis of World Indoor Championships 2010. In Proceedings of the International Conference on Biomechanics in Sports, Marquette, MI, USA, 19–23 July 2010.
27. Kugler, F.; Janshen, L. Body position determines propulsive forces in accelerated running. *J. Biomech.* **2009**, *43*, 343–348. [CrossRef] [PubMed]
28. Mann, R. Rules-related limiting factors in hurdling. *Track Coach* **1996**, *136*, 4335–4337.
29. Pollitt, L.; Walker, J.; Bissas, A.; Merlino, S. Biomechanical report for the IAAF world championships 2017: 110 m hurdles men's in 2017. In *IAAF World Championships Biomechanics Research Project*; International Association of Athletics Federations: London, UK, 2018.
30. Pollitt, L.; Walker, J.; Bissas, A.; Merlino, S. Biomechanical report for the IAAF world championships 2017: 100 m hurdles women's in 2017. In *IAAF World Championships Biomechanics Research Project*; International Association of Athletics Federations: London, UK, 2018.
31. Walker, J.; Pollitt, L.; Paradisis, G.P.; Bezodis, I.; Bissas, A.; Merlino, S. *Biomechanical Report for the IAAF World Indoor Championships 2018: 60 Metres Hurdles Men*; International Association of Athletics Federations: Birmingham, UK, 2019.
32. Walker, J.; Pollitt, L.; Paradisis, G.P.; Bezodis, I.; Bissas, A.; Merlino, S. *Biomechanical Report for the IAAF World Indoor Championships 2018: 60 Metres Hurdles Women*; International Association of Athletics Federations: Birmingham, UK, 2019.
33. Bedini, R. Technical ability in the women's 100m hurdles. *New Stud. Athl.* **2016**, *31*, 117–132.
34. Stein, N. Reflections on a change in the height of the hurdles in the women's sprint hurdles event. *New Stud. Athl.* **2000**, *15*, 15–20.
35. Mackala, K. Optimisation of perfomance through kinematic analysis of the different phases of the 100 meters. *New Stud. Athl.* **2007**, *22*, 7–16.
36. López del Amo, J.L.; Rodríguez, M.C.; Hill, D.W.; González, J.E. Analysis of the start to the first hurdle in 110 m hurdles at the IAAF world athletics championships Beijing 2015. *J. Hum. Sport Exerc.* **2018**, *13*, 504–517. [CrossRef]
37. Hücklekemkes, J. Model technique analysis sheets for the hurdles. Part IV: The women's 100 m hurdles. *New Stud. Athl.* **1990**, *5*, 33–58.
38. Bezodis, I.N.; Brazil, A.; von Lieres und Wilkau, H.C.; Wood, M.A.; Paradisis, G.P.; Hanley, B.; Tucker, C.B.; Pollitt, L.; Merlino, S.; Vazel, P.-J.; et al. World-Class male sprinters and high hurdlers have similar start and initial acceleration techniques. *Front. Sports Act. Living* **2019**, *1*, 23. [CrossRef]
39. Iwasaki, R.; Shinkai, H.; Ito, N. How hitting the hurdle affects performance in the 110 m hurdles. *ISBS Proc. Arch.* **2020**, *38*, 268–271.

3

Effects of Differential Jump Training on Balance Performance in Female Volleyball Players

Philip X. Fuchs [1,2,*], Andrea Fusco [1,2,*], Cristina Cortis [2] and Herbert Wagner [1]

1 Department of Sport and Exercise Science, University of Salzburg, Schlossallee 49, Hallein-Rif, 5400 Salzburg, Austria; spowi@sbg.ac.at
2 Department of Human Sciences, Society and Health, University of Cassino e Lazio Meridionale, Viale dell'Università, 03043 Cassino FR, Lazio, Italy; c.cortis@unicas.it
* Correspondence: philip.fuchs@sbg.ac.at (P.X.F.); andrea.fusco@unicas.it (A.F.)

Featured Application: The presented training concept can be applied to combine two seemingly contradictory desired effects that are associated with increased jump performance and injury prevention in an effective and efficient way without adding excess physiological stress.

Abstract: The purpose of this study was to determine whether coordinative jump training that induces neuromuscular stimuli can affect balance performance, associated with injury risk, in elite-level female volleyball players. During the competitive season, the balance performance of 12 elite female players (highest Austrian division) was obtained via a wobble board (WB; 200 Hz) placed on an AMTI force plate (1000 Hz). Three identically repeated measurements defined two intervals (control and intervention phases), both comparable in duration and regular training. The intervention included 6 weeks of differential training (8 sessions of 15–20 min) that delivered variations in dynamics around the ankle joints. Multilevel mixed models were used to assess the effect on postural control. WB performance decreased from 27.0 ± 13.2% to 19.6 ± 11.3% during the control phase and increased to 54.5 ± 16.2% during the intervention ($\beta = 49.1 \pm 3.5$; $p < 0.001$). Decreased sway area [cm^2] ($\beta = -7.5 \pm 1.6$; $p < 0.001$), anterior–posterior ($\beta = -4.1 \pm 0.4$; $p < 0.001$) and mediolateral sway [mm] ($\beta = -2.7 \pm 0.6$; $p = 0.12$), and mean velocity [$mm \cdot s^{-1}$] ($\beta = -9.0 \pm 3.6$; $p < 0.05$) were observed during the intervention compared with the control phase. Inter-limb asymmetry was reduced ($\beta = -41.8 \pm 14.4$; $p < 0.05$). The applied training concept enhanced balance performance and postural control in elite female volleyball players. Due to the low additional physiological loads of the program and increased injury risk during the competitive season, we recommend this intervention for supporting injury prevention during this period.

Keywords: postural control; center of pressure; in-season intervention; injury risk; ankle sprain prevention

1. Introduction

Sport-specific performance training is required in all sports to achieve a high international level. In volleyball, an important performance criterion correlating with competition level and a main objective in volleyball conditioning programs is to increase jump height [1]. This is commonly achieved through various types of strength and power training [2,3]. On the other hand, volleyball is known for its severe risk of ankle injuries during jumping [4] that cannot be prevented by strength training alone [5]. Therefore, traditional performance training should be accompanied by additional injury prevention programs [4]. The most frequent injury is ankle sprains [4], which are associated with chronic ankle instability and an increased chance of recurrence [5]. Neuromuscular impairment due to traumatized mechanoreceptors of the ligaments and muscles in the ankle is expected to cause the recurrence of sprains [5]. Unsurprisingly, neuromuscular and proprioceptive training has shown positive effects and is recommended to prevent ankle injuries [5,6]. Such training consists of balance exercises on stable and unstable platforms or the combination of, e.g., balance, plyometric, and sport-specific exercises [6]. The objective is to improve proprioception and neuromuscular responses. Thus, mechanoreceptors and stabilizing muscles around the ankle sense and process the risk of balance loss early and can react in time to prevent falls and injuries.

Recent technical-coordinative jump training [7] may have targeted both performance and prevention aspects during volleyball spike jumping. The concept was based on differential training [8,9], which applies movement variability and allows for adaptations in neuromuscular activation patterns [10]. Differential training has been shown to provide good transferability of training effects on sport-specific jump performance when compared with traditional concepts [11]. The program focused on spike jump performance determinants [12], centering around approach velocity, feet position, and velocity conversion strategy through the dominant leg (i.e., side of the striking arm). The conversion strategy is associated with neuromuscular activation patterns in the lower limbs [13]. Therefore, the emphasis and implementation of numerous variations in these movement characteristics is expected to constantly create proprioceptive and neuromuscular stimuli for ankle stabilization. The effect of such differential jump training on prevention can be operationalized via balance assessment, since reduced balance performance can be associated with an increased risk of injury [14]. Both injury prevention and balance performance are affected by the proprioceptive and neuromuscular systems that stabilize and maintain balance [5,6,15,16]. Therefore, a transfer of effects on balance performance during such differential jump training can be presumed.

For balance assessment, quantitative posturography via force platforms is considered the gold standard and superior to functional balance tests with respect to sensitivity and objectivity [17]. The most frequently analyzed characteristic is the excursion of the center of pressure (CoP) [18]. However, there are many variables that can be calculated from the CoP. A systematic review of 32 published articles involving CoP analyses recommended including both distance (e.g., sway area) and time–distance (e.g., mean velocity) based variables [19]. Its authors advised against the usage of minimal, maximal, and peak-to-peak values as they represent severe data reduction, great variance, and low reliability [19]. It seems unclear whether to alternatively prioritize analyses on fractal dimensions or on resultant horizontal data [19]. The drawbacks of posturography via CoP are the numerous variables and uncertainty about the best choice among variables to reflect balance performance [19]. Moreover, the high costs, complex handling, and space required for the equipment often complicate its usage in clinical settings [17].

A handy and validated alternative with fair to excellent reliability is found in computerized wobble boards (WBs) [20]. WBs are unstable platforms frequently used in clinical and therapeutic settings. They can be equipped with, e.g., accelerometers to collect the WB tilt angle that can then be processed by software and displayed on a screen in real time. Besides their practical handling, the strength of WBs is the single output variable of balance performance (i.e., time spent at ~0° tilt). Moreover, classical assessment of the CoP when standing on a force platform can also be applied to standing on a WB [21]. Poor correlation between WB performance and the outcome of one of the most frequently used validated balance tests, the Y Balance Test [20], can be explained by the complexity of the underlying mechanisms of postural control [14] and different test-specific skills of postural control [20]. Since WBs are a common tool in sprain prevention programs [5] and are suitable for balance assessment in individuals with chronic ankle instability [16], their usage is reasonable for the context of the current study (i.e., injury prevention in high-risk individuals).

The objective of this study was to determine the effect of a differential-training-based jump intervention on postural control in high-level female volleyball players. It was hypothesized that a 6-week differential jump training regimen that induces proprioceptive and neuromuscular stimuli for ankle stabilization would improve WB balance performance and CoP characteristics.

2. Materials and Methods

2.1. Participants

A female volleyball team (n_{team} = 12) from the highest league in Austria participated in this study (age: 22.8 ± 3.7 years; training experience: 11.8 ± 3.8 years; body height: 1.78 ± 0.09 m; mass: 69.9 ± 9.4 kg; body mass index: 22.0 ± 1.9 kg·m^{-2}; spike jump height: 0.44 ± 0.09 m). Depending on player positions and associated jumping skills, players were categorized as spikers (n_1 = 6), blockers (n_2 = 2), or setters and libera (n_3 = 4). The individual's preferred striking arm during the volleyball spike defined the dominant side. In accordance with the Declaration of Helsinki, the study was approved by the local institutional research ethics committee (approval code: 29/2014). All players were informed about the risks, benefits, and procedure of the study. They signed a consent form and reported being free of injuries at the beginning of the investigation. The sample size was determined by the size of the team and the accessibility of such high-level athletes.

2.2. Study Design and Training Intervention

Three identical testing sessions were conducted during the competitive season (i.e., 1. Control, 2. Post-Control = Pre-Intervention, 3. Post-Intervention). Post-Control and Post-Intervention testing took place 5.5 ± 0.5 and 4.5 ± 0.5 days after the most recent match, respectively. The first interval (6.5 weeks) defined the control phase. The second interval (6 weeks) included an intervention with no systematic differences in the regular training scheme, training loads (8.8 ± 0.3 vs. 7.7 ± 0.2 h per week), and competition loads (both phases: 1 international, 7 national matches). This approach to assess training effects by comparing control and intervention phases has been used before [7,22]. A control group was not feasible for ethical reasons and due to the limited numbers of accessible elite female volleyball players [22].

The intervention consisted of eight sessions of differential training [8,9], 15–20 min per session, and focused on the volleyball-specific spike jump movement. Differential training implements movement variations to allow for individual adaptations towards an individual optimum. The concept was described by its founder [8]; the methodology and positive effects across sports, ages, and levels have been reported [23–25]. The objective of the applied training was to induce coordinative adaptations in previously identified performance determinants [12]. Variations in approach speed (thus, dynamics), feet positioning (thus, joint angles), and the distribution of weight and time-related power development through both legs (thus, neuronal activation patterns) create neuromuscular stimuli for stabilizing muscles around the ankles. In contrast to traditional balance training, these variations exploit system fluctuations [26] at the kinematic and kinetic levels. For instance, the athletes were instructed to vary the length of the penultimate step, the ankle joint angle at planting, and the pressure perceived at the left and right feet during planting. The exercises followed two concepts: (1) the athletes alternatingly performed two opposing, detrimental extremes, reducing the discrepancy between both variations after each pair of trials; and (2) starting from one detrimental extreme, the players approached an individual optimum. A detailed description of the program and a full list of variations are available [7].

2.3. Data Collection and Processing

Three identical repeated measurements were made, following a validated protocol and instructions [20].

The participants performed test trials for familiarization with a validated mediolateral and anterior–posterior tilting WB equipped with tri-axis accelerometers (GSJ Service, Rome, Italy) [20]. Subsequently, three trials per leg (30 s per trial) of a single-leg stance on the WB, hands at the hips, were measured at 200 Hz. The sequence was blocked for legs and randomized for participants. In real time, validated software (GSJ Service, Rome, Italy) [20] displayed a motion marker based on the WB tilt angle and circles around a central area (~0° WB tilt) on a screen in front of the participants. Participants aimed to keep the motion marker within the central area for as long as possible over the full span of each trial. To prevent fatigue, there was approximately one minute of break time between trials.

Simultaneously, a force platform (120 × 60 cm; AMTI, Watertown, MA, USA) recorded ground reaction forces at 1000 Hz. The CoP was calculated in Visual3D (C-Motion, Inc., Rockville, MD, USA). Based on residual analyses [27] of the current data and a recommendation for CoP filtering [19], a fourth-order zero-lag Butterworth low-pass filter at 10 Hz was applied (Supplementary Materials).

2.4. Criterion Variables and Definitions

WB performance was defined as the time for which the WB was kept at ~0° tilt, divided by the trial duration [%]. In agreement with a CoP review [19], ground reaction forces were used to compute the sway area (i.e., 95% confidence ellipse; see Figure 1), mediolateral and anterior–posterior sway (i.e., fractal standard deviation), and mean velocity of sway (i.e., total CoP path distance, divided by trial duration). As a characteristic associated with injury risk, the inter-limb asymmetry [%] was also calculated [28]. Development during the phases was defined as the difference between two measurements. Development in WB performance and asymmetry is displayed as percentage points (e.g., a rise from 20% to 40% equals a development of +20% points). For all variables, outliers [mean ± 2 times the standard deviation (SD)] within participants were removed.

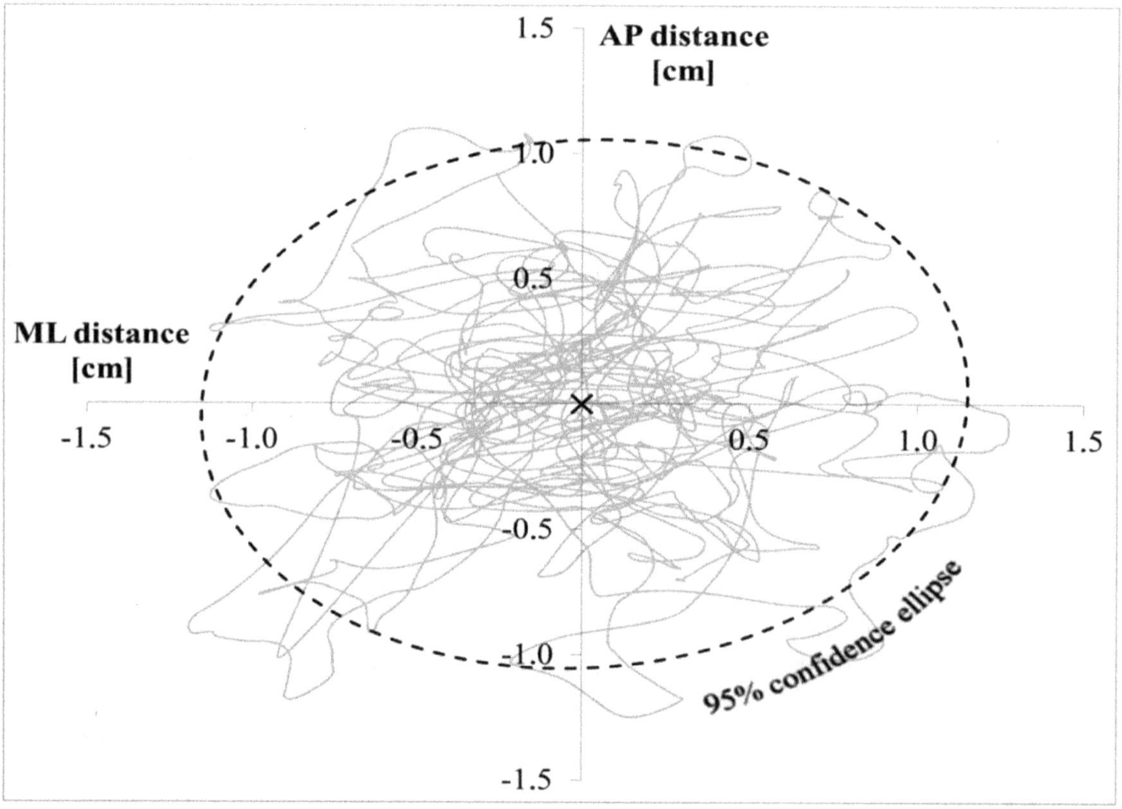

Figure 1. Exemplary path of the center of pressure of one participant during one trial and the sway area defined as a 95% confidence ellipse. Note: AP, anterior–posterior; ML, mediolateral.

2.5. Statistical Analyses

PASW Statistics (version 18.0; SPSS Inc, Chicago, IL, USA) was used for statistical analyses and Office Excel 2019 (Microsoft Corporation, Redmond, WA, USA) was used for visualization. For WB performance, as the primary interest of this investigation, linear multilevel mixed model analyses accounting for the repeated effect of trials were applied. The superiority of such an approach over traditional analysis of variance has been explained by reviews, technical reports, and empirical assessments with real data [29–31], and the reasons include the way of handling missing data and interindividual variance. Since both were observed in the current data, this approach was suitable for the specific set of data and purpose. Such a model predicts a dependent variable (i.e., WB performance) in consideration of fixed and random effects of intercepts and independent variables (i.e., measurement session, phase, leg used during the trial, player position). A random intercept was considered for participants and fixed and random effects for independent variables. A fixed intercept was defined as a pre-intervention measurement to allow for comparison with control and post-intervention measurements. Effects were included one after another, and the fit of the derived models was assessed for effects and specifications of covariances via chi-square (X^2) statistics based on -2 log-likelihood and degrees of freedom (*df*) [30,31]. The covariance structures for independent variables were defined after assessment of the correlation matrix and confirmed by the fit of the model when compared to alternative models. The covariance structure of the random intercept was specified as the variance component for all models. Depending on the data type, collinearity was checked via Pearson or Spearman correlation analyses, and none was found. Among models of comparable fit, the one with the smallest number of parameters was accepted as the final model. All analyses were performed using maximum-likelihood estimation [31]. The same statistical approach was applied for comparison of the developments between the control and intervention phases, with development during the control phase as a fixed intercept. Following the same procedure as for WB performance, the most successful single-predictor models with variable-specific specification of the covariance structure were calculated for each other dependent variable (i.e., inter-limb asymmetry, sway area, mediolateral sway, anterior–posterior sway, and CoP velocity). The performances at all measurement sessions are presented as mean ± SD and 95% confidence intervals (CIs). The results are presented as *F*-value, degree of freedom (*df*), estimate (β), and standard error (SE). *p*-values below 0.05 were considered significant.

3. Results

One ankle sprain occurred during the control phase, with no effect on data collection and presentation. One participant missed the first measurement; removal from analyses was not required thanks to the statistical approach.

The performances at the three measurement sessions, covariance specifications of the final models, and the effects of measurements are presented in Table 1.

Table 1. Means ± standard deviations (SDs), 95% confidence intervals (CIs), *F*-statistics for the main effect of measurements, estimates (β), and standard error (SE) for effects between single measurements.

Variable	Control Phase		Intervention Phase					
	Control	Post-Control = Pre-Intervention			Post-Intervention			
	Mean ± SD / 95% CI	β / SE	Mean ± SD / 95% CI	β / SE	Mean ± SD / 95% CI	*F*	*df*	*p*
WB performance [%] †	27.02 ± 13.18	(−5.20)	19.60 ± 11.31	42.87	59.49 ± 16.16	88.03	2, 14.17	<0.001
	18.17 – 35.87	(2.71)	12.00 – 27.19	3.05	48.64 – 70.35			
Sway area [cm^2] §	8.03 ± 3.28	6.35	10.91 ± 3.42	−6.63	8.02 ± 2.89	23.41	2, 2.90	<0.05
	5.82 – 10.23	1.01	8.61 – 13.21	1.31	6.01 – 9.96			
AP sway [mm] †	7.04 ± 1.61	(1.03)	9.18 ± 1.93	(−0.79)	7.09 ± 1.47	1.53	2, 3.33	0.34
	5.96 – 8.12	(0.66)	7.88 – 10.47	(0.81)	6.10 – 8.08			
ML sway [mm] ‡	6.02 ± 1.23	0.98	6.34 ± 0.98	−1.24	5.82 ± 1.12	8.41	2, 9.58	<0.01
	5.19 – 6.85	0.29	5.69 – 7.00	0.30	5.06 – 6.58			
CoP velocity [$mm \cdot s^{-1}$] †	68.54 ± 6.86	(3.51)	67.88 ± 8.12	−5.85	64.08 ± 7.88	4.77	2, 14.47	<0.05
	63.93 – 73.15	(2.18)	62.42 – 73.34	2.11	58.78 – 69.37			
Asymmetry [%] ¥	23.64 ± 17.33	(6.38)	32.69 ± 23.30	−25.89	10.15 ± 8.26	9.62	2, 52.33	<0.001
	11.24 – 36.03	(6.76)	16.02 – 49.36	6.23	4.24 – 16.07			

Note: Control, Post-Control, Pre-Intervention, and Post-Intervention denote measurement timings; WB, wobble board; AP, anterior–posterior; ML, mediolateral; CoP, center of pressure; *df*, degrees of freedom for the numerator and denominator, separated by a comma; β is converted so that negative values indicate decreased values from the previous to the subsequent measurement; β and SE relate to two adjacent measurements and are in parentheses if the effect was not significant ($p > 0.05$); Covariance structure specification: †, antedependence first order; §, unstructured; ‡, factor analytic first order; ¥, heterogeneous autoregressive first order.

The best model with measurement as the only predictor for WB performance included a fixed and a random intercept, a fixed slope for measurement, and an error. It detected a main effect for measurements ($F(2,58.24) = 173.83$, $p < 0.001$), decrease from control to pre-intervention ($\beta = -8.86$, SE = 2.36, $p < 0.001$), and increase from pre- to post-intervention ($\beta = 40.69$, SE = 2.29, $p < 0.001$). The random intercept for participants yielded 65.95% of this model's overall variance ($p < 0.05$).

The final model with the best fit consisted of 18 parameters ($X^2 = 29.29$, $\Delta df = 13$, $p < 0.01$, compared with the initial model). It was expressed by the following equation, where Y_{is} (WB performance), X_{is} (measurement), Z_{is} (leg), and ε_{is} (error) vary as functions of individual observations (i; level 1 variable) and participants (s; level 2 variable). b_0 and u_{0s} represent a fixed and a random intercept, respectively; b_1, b_2, and b_3 define the gradients.

$$Y_{is} = (b_0 + u_{0s}) + b_1 X_{is} + b_2 Z_{is} + b_3 X_{is} Z_{is} + \varepsilon_{is}$$

Besides the effects of measurements (Table 1), no effect was found for leg ($F(1,26.10) = 0.33$, $p = 0.57$), but an effect was found for the interaction of measurement by leg ($F(2,20.19) = 6.98$, $p < 0.01$). The random intercept for participants yielded 0.41% of this model's overall variance ($p < 0.05$).

Additional fixed and random effects did not produce significantly improved models (best alternative model including player position as a random effect, compared with the final model: $X^2 = 1.14$, $\Delta df = 1$, $p = 0.28$).

Model-based effects between the control and intervention phases are displayed in Figure 2.

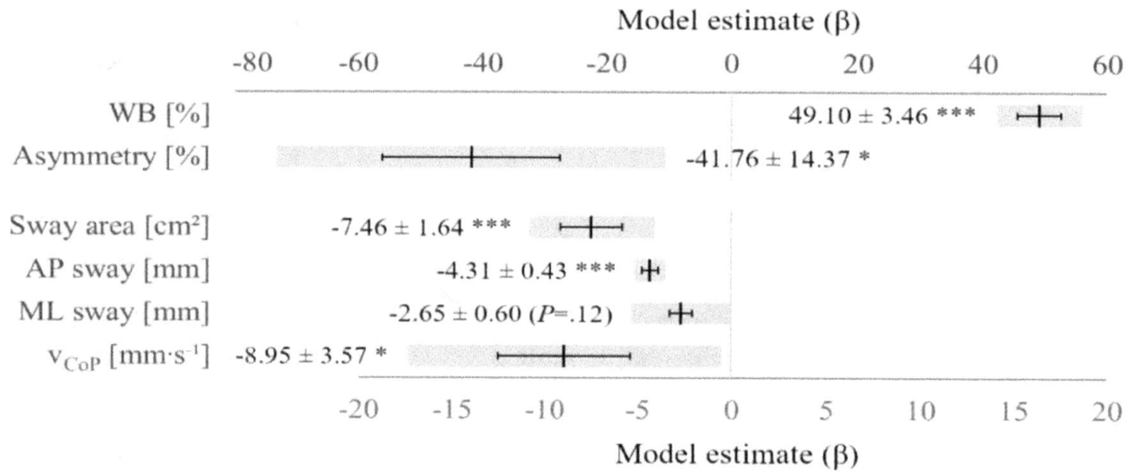

Figure 2. Discrepancies between development during the control and intervention phases, displayed as the model estimate (β) ± standard error and 95% confidence interval (i.e., grey bars). Note: WB, wobble board performance; Asymmetry, inter-limb asymmetry; AP, anterior–posterior; ML, mediolateral; v_{CoP}, mean velocity of the center of pressure; * $p < 0.05$; *** $p < 0.001$.

The final model for WB performance over the phases consisted of three parameters and was expressed by the following equation, where Y_i (WB performance), X_i (phase), and ε_i (error) vary as functions of individual observations (i). b_0 represents a fixed intercept and b_1 represents the gradient.

$$Y_i = b_0 + b_1 X_i + \varepsilon_i$$

The inclusion of random intercept, phase, leg, player position, and interactions as fixed and/or random effects did not deliver improved models (best models for each additional effect in comparison with the final model: $0 \leq X^2 \leq 8.06$, $1 \leq \Delta df \leq 20$, $0.09 \leq p \leq 1$). In these alternative models, no effects were found for leg ($F(1,46) = 2.87$, $p = 0.10$), leg by phase ($F(2,46) = 1.53$, $p = 0.23$), position ($F(1,46) = 2.24$, $p = 0.14$), or position by phase ($F(2,46) = 1.48$, $p = 0.24$).

For all other criterion variables, the final models included significant random intercepts for participants.

4. Discussion

The objective of this study was to investigate the effects of sport-specific differential jump training on balance performance and associated injury risk in elite female volleyball players. A mixed model analysis was deemed suitable because it is superior to traditional statistical approaches in the current scenario [29–31]. The first reason for this was increased power, as mixed models are capable of handling missing data instead of removing a participant from analyses. This applied in the current data since one participant missed the first measurement session. Second, mixed models differentiate between interindividual variance and random error variance. Ignoring occurrent interindividual variability leads to over- or underestimation of statistical significance in repeated measures analysis of variance; in fact, this generates inaccurate results and can affect the overall interpretation [31]. The significant effects of the random intercept for participants indicated interindividual variance [29,31] in the current study and supported the usage of mixed models. In the simple model for WB performance, the random intercept explained two-thirds of the overall variance. This is a great but not exceptional amount (e.g., values of >50% are systematically reported in sleep deprivation) and underlines the relevance of accounting for interindividual variance [31]. The reduced (yet significant) variance in the more complex model is probably due to the added effects explaining variance that was previously absorbed by the random intercept.

The results showed decreased balance performance during the control phase. This was not surprising as decreased performance during the competitive season is known in volleyball and is explained by increased physiological loads [7,22]. Sway area and ML sway increased significantly, which is considered detrimental for postural control. Also, WB performance, AP sway, mean CoP velocity, and inter-limb asymmetry tended ($0.08 \leq p \leq 0.36$) to develop unfavorably. During the intervention, all variables improved significantly (except for AP sway, only indicating ($p = 0.35$) a beneficial development).

WB performance is a valid single outcome reflecting postural control [20], and it was found to be decreased in subjects with chronic ankle instability, which is associated with increased risk of ankle sprains [16]. Previous data showed that healthy limbs scored 19.6–21.8 s (i.e., 65.33–72.66%) in WB performance [16]. In the current study, WB performance was comparably low during the control (27.02 ± 13.18%) and pre-intervention (19.60 ± 11.31%) measurements. This indicates and corroborates the assertion that volleyball players are at high risk for ankle sprains [4], since reduced balance performance is associated with increased ankle instability [16] and injury incidence [6]. After the 6-week intervention, WB performance (59.49 ± 16.16%) almost reached the level of the previously reported healthy limbs [16]. Interestingly, there is some evidence that it takes 8–10 weeks of neuromuscular training to reduce injury risk to a baseline level [5]. Therefore, it can be presumed that a prolonged intervention of the current type may have closed the gap between the currently achieved WB performance and the baseline level of healthy limbs.

CoP variables were considered insightful in addition to WB performance and were selected in agreement with a review on CoP analyses [19]. This review recommends the consideration of multiple variables because reports are controversial, no single gold standard is apparent, and various variables may reflect different aspects of postural control [19]. In the case of conflicting findings, individual assessment of the CoP variables allowed for specific interpretation of single characteristics. However, the developments of all CoP variables were in line with the change in WB performance, showing detrimental trends during the control phase and beneficial changes during the intervention phase. Based on this, we cannot conclude that specific CoP variables were more suitable for WB performance than others. Moreover, the data do not indicate that specific CoP variables reflect different aspects of postural control on WB. Despite mean velocity being the most reliable CoP variable [19], its values should be interpreted with caution. Mean velocity easily gives the misleading impression of reflecting adaptability (i.e., quick adjustment of CoP to keep the center of mass within the base of stability). However, the mean velocity is calculated as the total path of the CoP normalized by time [19]. Therefore, it reflects total sway and does not provide additional information about adaptability. No recommendation was found in the literature to properly quantify adaptability in balance performance.

Decreased inter-limb asymmetry is considered desirable. Therefore, a detrimental trend during the control phase and a beneficial change during the intervention phase were observed. The recommended equation to calculate asymmetry includes the smaller of the two values from both legs as the denominator [28]. Thus, asymmetry values rapidly approach 100% if the smaller value is close to 0, even when only a small absolute discrepancy between both values exists. Such values usually do not occur in the analyses of net peak vertical ground reaction forces where this equation was applied previously [28]. However, this problem was identified in one case during the current study and should be considered in future investigations. This data point was excluded from further analyses. Removal of this data point did not change the statistical outcome.

The results of the comparison of developments during both phases (Figure 2) are in line with the analyses across the three measurement sessions (Table 1). Throughout all variables, beneficial trends were observed during the intervention when compared with the control phase. ML sway was the only variable where this trend did not reach statistical significance ($p = 0.12$). However, the full range of the 95% CI was found to be on the negative (i.e., beneficial) side of the scale. Therefore, it can be stated with 95% confidence for this study that the intervention induced a beneficial effect on ML sway compared with the control phase. Considering the large sizes of the model estimates in comparison with the baseline values during the control and pre-intervention measurements, the intervention produced a great, beneficial effect on postural control and inter-limb asymmetry.

The lack of a main effect of leg on performance implies that any leg-specific factors contributing to balance performance (e.g., previous injuries, chronic instability) were distributed equally to both legs. This result indicates that, in general, both legs performed comparably. However, the training program specifically stressed the usage of the dominant leg for approach velocity conversion, and an interaction effect of measurement by leg was observed. Probably, the focus of the jump training on the dominant leg induced different stimuli and resulted in different adaptations in the two legs.

For player position, no main or interaction effects were found. This suggests that, first, position was not a crucial factor in balance performance for volleyball players and, second, training stimuli do not need to be position-specific to achieve improvements.

Neuromuscular prevention training may only be effective in individuals with previous injuries [5]. Volleyball players are known to be a high-risk group with frequent ankle injuries [4]. The current data suggest that the participants' balance performance prior to intervention was poor, even in comparison with individuals with chronic ankle instability [16]. Therefore, the same effects of training may not be expected in individuals with no history of injuries. However, transferability of the current findings to other high-risk sports and previously injured individuals seems reasonable.

The primary focus of the training program was to improve sports-specific jump performance via coordinative adaptations [7]. Jump height increased by 11.9%, and promising effects on biomechanical determinants were reported in detail [7]. Improvements in balance performance and ankle stabilization were expected side-effects thanks to neuromuscular stimuli that accompanied the implemented movement variations in the program. The positive effects of the differential jump training program on both jump and balance performance support its potential for combining two effects that are usually targeted separately. A repeated effect for balance performance may be expected, as a review on ankle sprains [5] suggested increased risk and training effects after reoccurring injuries. After every ankle sprain, the injury risk can be reduced to baseline risk via neuromuscular training within 8–10 weeks [5]. However, the repeated effect of the same program was not tested in the current study.

The longitudinal design of this study could be discussed as a limitation. This is a common difficulty; previously published investigations [7,22] applied the same study design and, thus, these data serve as a suitable reference. The control and intervention phases were comparable in terms of factors that were deemed potentially influential (except for the intervention program itself). All factors were reported and accounted for during the statistical analyses and interpretations. We are not aware of other factors that contributed to the training effects in a phase-specific fashion. A cross-sectional approach was not feasible for ethical reasons and due to the accessibility of such high-level female athletes.

To achieve the observed improvement in spike jump height, biomechanical understanding of specific performance determinants is required, which could be a challenge for coaches [7]. This is not the case regarding the effect on balance performance. The current training program did not target certain balance determinants specifically. The applied movement variations were expected to affect the dynamics around the ankle joints and thus induce neuromuscular stimuli for ankle stabilization. Therefore, it can be concluded that these nonspecific stimuli are the essential factor to generate the observed adaptations in postural control. This makes the program practical for a range of coaches, given that neuromuscular stimuli are delivered. It may be presumed that the great coordinative challenge in ballistic balance during the jumping variations has a positive effect on the static balance performance.

A longer intervention period (8–10 weeks) may result in even larger effects [5]. Preventive effects were not directly measured in this study but can be expected based on the observed effect on postural control and the associated injury risk [6], especially for interventions conducted immediately after sprains [5] and in high-risk individuals. Due to its low physiological loads and complementary effects in jump height and postural control, the program is feasible during the competitive season for the whole team. It is also recommended for individuals who cannot fully participate in regular training after an ankle sprain.

5. Conclusions

The current program was a differential jump training program that successfully provided complementary improvements in sport-specific jump performance and postural control, which is an indicator of injury risk and especially relevant for high-risk target groups (e.g., volleyball players). The program adds no severe physiological loads and requires no compromises in regular training. This suggests its potential for implementation during the competitive season to enhance performance and injury prevention without the risk of overtraining.

Author Contributions: Conceptualization, P.X.F., A.F., C.C. and H.W.; methodology, P.X.F., A.F., C.C. and H.W.; validation, P.X.F., A.F., C.C. and H.W.; formal analysis, P.X.F. and A.F.; investigation, P.X.F. and A.F.; resources, C.C. and H.W.; writing—original draft preparation, P.X.F.; writing—review and editing, P.X.F., A.F., C.C. and H.W.; visualization, P.X.F. and A.F.; supervision, C.C. and H.W.; project administration, P.X.F.; All authors have read and agreed to the published version of the manuscript.

Acknowledgments: We want to thank the players and the coaches of the PSV Salzburg for participation in this training intervention study. Special thanks also to Kathryn A. Hill for technical support allowing us to advance the analytical measures used in this study.

References

1. Ziv, G.; Lidor, R. Vertical jump in female and male volleyball players: A review of observational and experimental studies. *Scand. J. Med. Sci. Sports* **2010**, *20*, 556–567. [CrossRef] [PubMed]
2. Powers, M.E. Vertical Jump Training for Volleyball. *Strength Cond. J.* **1996**, *18*, 18–23. [CrossRef]
3. Sheppard, J.M.; Cronin, J.B.; Gabbett, T.J.; McGuigan, M.R.; Etxebarria, N.; Newton, R.U. Relative importance of strength, power, and anthropometric measures to jump performance of elite volleyball players. *J. Strength Cond. Res.* **2008**, *22*, 758–765. [CrossRef] [PubMed]

4. Bahr, R.; Bahr, I. Incidence of acute volleyball injuries: A prospective cohort study of injury mechanisms and risk factors. *Scand. J. Med. Sci. Sports* **1997**, *7*, 166–171. [CrossRef] [PubMed]
5. Verhagen, E.; Bay, K. Optimising ankle sprain prevention: A critical review and practical appraisal of the literature. *Br. J. Sport Med.* **2010**, *44*, 1082–1088. [CrossRef]
6. Hübscher, M.; Zech, A.; Pfeifer, K.; Hänsel, F.; Vogt, L.; Banzer, W. Neuromuscular Training for Sports Injury Prevention: A Systematic Review. *Med. Sci. Sports Exer.* **2010**, *42*, 413–421. [CrossRef]
7. Fuchs, P.X.; Fusco, A.; Bell, J.W.; von Duvillard, S.P.; Cortis, C.; Wagner, H. Effect of Differential Training on female volleyball spike jump technique and performance. *Int. J. Sports Physiol.* **2020**, *15*, 1019–1025. [CrossRef]
8. Schöllhorn, W.I. Applications of systems dynamic principles to technique and strength training. *Acta Acad. Olymp. Est.* **2000**, *8*, 67–85.
9. Schöllhorn, W.I.; Hegen, P.; Davids, K. The Nonlinear Nature of Learning—A Differential Learning Approach. *Open Sports Sci. J.* **2012**, *5*, 100–112. [CrossRef]
10. Haudum, A.; Birklbauer, J.; Kröll, J.; Müller, E. Constraint-led changes in internal variability in running. *J. Sports Sci. Med.* **2012**, *11*, 8–15.
11. Pfeiffer, M.; Jaitner, T. Sprungkraft im Nachwuchstraining Handball: Training und Diagnose. *Z. Angew. Train.* **2003**, *10*, 86–95.
12. Fuchs, P.X.; Fusco, A.; Bell, J.W.; von Duvillard, S.P.; Cortis, C.; Wagner, H. Movement characteristics of volleyball spike jump performance in females. *J. Sci. Med. Sports* **2019**, *22*, 833–837. [CrossRef] [PubMed]
13. Fuchs, P.X.; Menzel, H.-J.K.; Guidotti, F.; Bell, J.; von Duvillard, S.P.; Wagner, H. Spike jump biomechanics in male versus female elite volleyball players. *J. Sports Sci.* **2019**, *37*, 2411–2419. [CrossRef] [PubMed]
14. Brown, C.N.; Mynark, R. Balance deficits in recreational athletes with chronic ankle instability. *J. Athl. Train.* **2007**, *42*, 367–373. [PubMed]
15. Horak, F.B. Postural orientation and equilibrium: What do we need to know about neural control of balance to prevent falls? *Age Ageing* **2006**, *35*, ii7–ii11. [CrossRef]
16. Fusco, A.; Giancotti, G.F.; Fuchs, P.X.; Wagner, H.; Varalda, C.; Cortis, C. Wobble board balance assessment in subjects with chronic ankle instability. *Gait Posture* **2019**, *68*, 352–356. [CrossRef]
17. Mancini, M.; Horak, F.B. The relevance of clinical balance assessment tools to differentiate balance deficits. *Eur. J. Phys. Rehab. Med.* **2010**, *46*, 239–248.
18. Crétual, A. Which biomechanical models are currently used in standing posture analysis? *Neurophysiol. Clin.* **2015**, *45*, 285–295. [CrossRef]
19. Ruhe, A.; Fejer, R.; Walker, B. The test–retest reliability of centre of pressure measures in bipedal static task conditions—A systematic review of the literature. *Gait Posture* **2010**, *32*, 436–445. [CrossRef]
20. Fusco, A.; Giancotti, G.F.; Fuchs, P.X.; Wagner, H.; Varalda, C.; Capranica, L.; Cortis, C. Dynamic balance evaluation: Reliability and validity of a computerized wobble board. *J. Strength Cond. Res.* **2020**, *34*, 1709–1715. [CrossRef]
21. Janura, M.; Bizovska, L.; Svoboda, Z.; Cerny, M.; Zemkova, E. Assessment of postural stability in stable and unstable conditions. *Acta Bioeng. Biomech.* **2017**, *19*, 89–94. [CrossRef]
22. Newton, R.U.; Rogers, R.A.; Volek, J.S.; Häkkinen, K.; Kraemer, W.J. Four weeks of optimal load ballistic resistance training at the end of season attenuates declining jump performance of women volleyball players. *J. Strength Cond. Res.* **2006**, *20*, 955–961.
23. Coutinho, D.; Santos, S.; Conçalves, B.; Travassos, B.; Wong, D.P.; Schöllhorn, W.; Sampaio, J. The effects of an enrichment training program for youth football attackers. *PLoS ONE* **2018**, *13*, e0199008. [CrossRef]
24. Savelsbergh, G.J.; Kamper, W.J.; Rabius, J.; De Koning, J.J.; Schöllhorn, W. A new method to learn to start in speed skating: A differencial learning approach. *Int. J. Sports Psychol.* **2010**, *41*, 415–427.
25. Wagner, H.; Müller, E. The effects of differential and variable training on the quality parameters of a handball throw. *Sports Biomech.* **2008**, *7*, 54–71. [CrossRef]
26. Schöllhorn, W.I.; Beckmann, H.; Davids, K. Exploiting system fluctuations. Differential training in physical prevention and rehabilitation programs for health and exercise. *Medicina* **2010**, *46*, 365–373. [CrossRef]
27. Sinclair, J.; Taylor, P.J.; Hobbs, S.J. Digital filtering of three-dimensional lower extremity kinematics: An assessment. *J. Hum. Kinet.* **2013**, *39*, 25–36. [CrossRef]
28. Bishop, C.; Read, P.; Lake, J.; Chavda, S.; Turner, A. Interlimb asymmetries: Understanding how to calculate differences from bilateral and unilateral tests. *Strength Cond. J.* **2018**, *40*, 1–6. [CrossRef]

29. McCulloch, C.; Searle, S. *Generalized, Linear, and Mixed Models*; John Wiley and Sons: New York, NY, USA, 2000. [CrossRef]
30. Linear Mixed-Effects Modeling in SPSS. Available online: https://www.spss.ch/upload/1126184451_Linear%20Mixed%20Effects%20Modeling%20in%20SPSS.pdf (accessed on 30 June 2020).
31. Van Dongen, H.P.A.; Olofsen, E.; Dinges, D.F.; Maislin, G. Mixed-Model Regression Analysis and Dealing with Interindividual Differences. *Method Enzymol.* **2004**, *384*, 139–171. [CrossRef]

4

Validation and Application of Two New Core Stability Tests in Professional Football

Saioa Etxaleku [1], Mikel Izquierdo [2,*], Eder Bikandi [3], Jaime García Arroyo [4], Iñigo Sarriegi [5], Iosu Sesma [1] and Igor Setuain [1,2,*]

1 TDN, Orthopedic Surgery and Advanced Rehabilitation Center, Clinical Research Department, Pol Mutilva C/V nave 3, 31192 Mutilva, Spain; setxaleku@tdnclinica.es (S.E.); sesmanoble@hotmail.com (I.S.)
2 Navarrabiomed, Complejo Hospitalario de Navarra (CHN)-Universidad Pública de Navarra (UPNA), Navarra Institute for Health Research (IdiSNA), 31008 Pamplona, Spain
3 Athletic Club, Mazarredo Zumarkalea, 23. 48009 Bilbao, Bizkaia, Spain; ederbikandi@gmail.com
4 TEN Centre, C/San Julian nº 8 Majadahonda, 28220 Madrid, Spain; jaimegarroyo@gmail.com
5 Southampton FC, Staplewood Football Development & Support Centre, Marchwood, Southampton SO40 4WR, UK; isarriegui@saintsfc.co.uk
* Correspondence: mikel.izquierdo@gmail.com (M.I.); igorsetuain@gmail.com (I.S.);

Abstract: The purpose of the first study was to validate two newly proposed core stability tests; Prone Plank test (PPT) and Closed Kinetic Chain test (CCT), for evaluating the strength of the body core. Subsequently, these tests were employed in a longitudinal prospective study implementing a core stability training program with a professional Spanish football team. For the validation study, 22 physically active men (*Tegner Scale 6–7*) performed three trials of the PPT and CCT tests in two different testing sessions separated by one week. In the longitudinal study, 13 male professional football players were equally evaluated (PPT and CCT) before and after the competitive session in which they completed a core training program. Intra-/intersession, and intertester, reliability was analyzed. PPT and CCT demonstrated excellent to good test–retest reliability and acceptable error measurement (ICCs for intratester and intrasession reliability ranged from 0.77 to 0.94 for the PPT, and 0.8–0.9 for the CCT) in all but one of the testing conditions (female tester for CCT test; ICC = 0.38). Significant improvements on core strength were found from pre to post evaluation in both the PPT ($p < 0.01$) and CCT ($p < 0.01$) after the implementation of a core training program in professional football players.

Keywords: core function; football; field test; reliability

1. Introduction

The "Core musculature" term refers to the combination of muscles that surround and comprise the lumbopelvic region, and act synergistically to stabilize the trunk and hip, contributing to the movement control and stability of more distal joints [1]. On the other hand, core stability, defined as the ability to control the position and motion of the trunk over the pelvis, governs optimal force production, transfer and application to more distal segments in many functional athletic activities [2].

The core muscles are considered to play a key role in sport performance as they seem to provide "proximal stability for distal mobility" [1,3] throughout the entire kinetic chain. Moreover, core stabilization precedes gross motor movement, as the central nervous system activates the trunk musculature before limb movement to provide the stability and stiffness of the trunk and pelvis in anticipation of the forces produced at this level [3].

"Core stability" is accomplished through a complex interaction of neuromuscular coordination, proprioception, strength and endurance of the trunk and hip musculature. This inherent complexity has been the focus of a wide range of studies employing different measurement techniques for core stability evaluation in recent years [3]. In this way, there is a lack in the literature of a gold standard for core stability evaluation in sports. Therefore, the assessment of trunk stability in the field setting could become even more complex because it requires the combination of different variable measurements, such as force, endurance, etc. [4,5].

Considering this multi-characteristic approach, a wide variety of testing methods have been described to evaluate core stability performance, both in laboratory and in clinical settings. In the laboratory, the most common testing method to measure core strength has been developed by the use of isokinetic dynamometers, whereas trunk stability tests have been performed through the employment of custom-designed devices [6,7]. Beside these expensive and time-consuming tests, "clinical tests" are the preferred choice for evaluating core stability for "in the field conditions".

No gold standard for core stability evaluation has been established, until recently. These tests have also involved vague or unclear scoring systems and require expensive instrumentations or the development of individually customized equipment. The definition of a gold standard test for core stability evaluation has become challenging, as there is not a widely accepted conclusive definition for core stability. In fact, there are numerous muscles that participate in the body core's dynamic stabilization. Several reliable and easy to use methods have been proposed to assess core musculature function. These include the prone bridging test, the Biering–Sørensen test, the double leg lowering test, prone plank stability], the side plank bridging test], the front abdominal power test (FAPT), the side abdominal power test (SAPT) [3,8–12] and the flexion-rotation test [13]. Some of the limitations of these tests are as follows: (a) they isolate one aspect of this complex interaction, such as core strength or endurance; (b) they are linked to a subjective scoring or evaluation system; and (c) they asses a more complete picture of this interaction, but not in a functionally relevant position, aligned with the sport-specific core region's biomechanical and or functional requirements [3]. Furthermore, these tests have also reported vague or unclear scoring systems and/or require expensive equipment, or they require the development of individually customized measurement devices which limit the extrapolation of the results obtained to other populations.

The interaction among the lumbopelvic and hip muscles makes it difficult for researchers to develop a single test that could encompass all muscles and structures [12]. Considering the abovementioned methodological limitations, there is a clear need to develop a quick, simple, valid and reliable test to accurately evaluate the core stability of an athlete, due to this capacity's proven strong relationship with sport performance as well as with low back and lower limb injury risk [2,14–17].

In the present research, we aimed to describe two functional core stability tests that aimed to evaluate the athlete's ability to produce isometric force, from two core stability-challenging positions, through the use of a hand-held dynamometer. Secondly, we evaluated a professional football team before and after a standardized core training program in order to elucidate if a motor control-based progression would have any effect on the player's ability to produce isometric force in the previously validated tests.

2. Methods

2.1. Experimental Approach to the Problem

This investigation consisted of two consecutively performed studies.

Study I: (Cross-sectional validation study)

A preliminary validation study of the two new core functional strength tests was performed. The core function testing positions were derived from traditional core-conditioning exercises that address both closed [2] (Closed Kinetic Chain test; CCT) and open kinetic chain efforts [12] (Prone Plank Test; PPT) (Figure 1A and 1B respectively). These two tests aimed to assess the force exertion capacity in those two positions with a hand-held dynamometry. The intra- and intertester reliability of the measurements was evaluated for both tests.

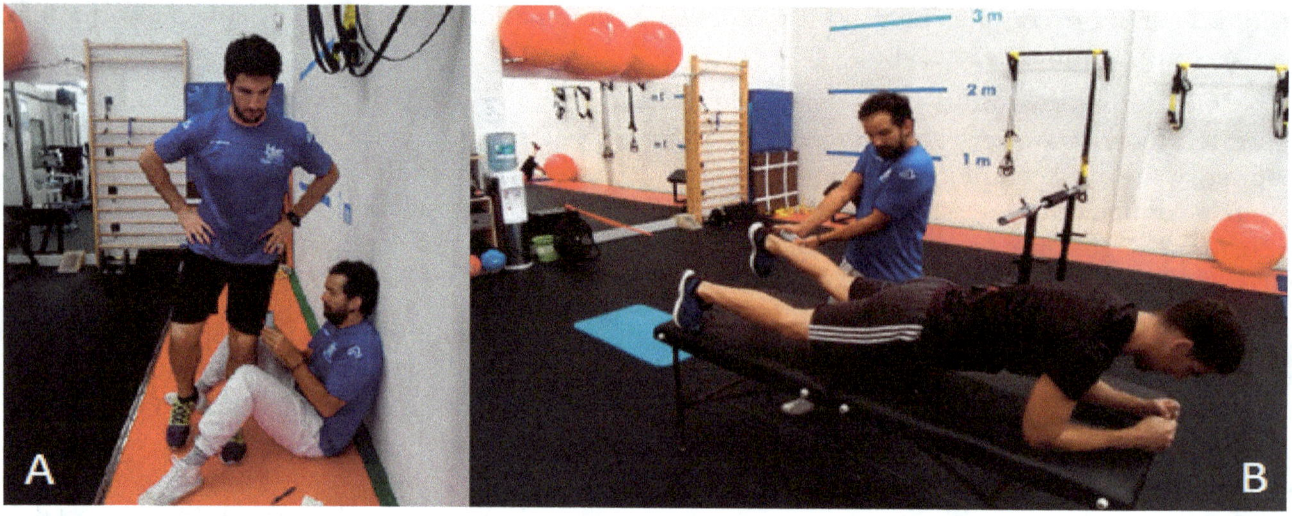

Figure 1. New proposed core functional strength field tests. (**A**) Closed Kinetic Chain Test (CCT). (**B**) Prone Plank Test (PPT).

Study II: (Longitudinal study)

Once the testing procedures were shown to be reliable, a prospective longitudinal study was performed aiming to analyze the core functional strength values in relation to the implementation of a core neuromuscular training program during the competitive season of a professional football team squad (Spanish league 2).

2.2. Participants

Study I: (Cross-sectional validation study)

Seven recreationally active males (6–7 on the Tegner scale) (mean ± standard deviation 19.23 ± 2.43 years old, 181.0 ± 6.23 cm, 75.42 ± 7.25 kg) were recruited for the between-session reliability study. Then, the sample was increased by adding 15 male junior football players competing in Spain's National Junior League (mean ± standard deviation 17.87 ± 1.13 years old, 181.20 ± 6.84 cm, 74.69 ± 6.63 kg). All participants were free from any previous spine or lower leg injury at the time of examination. Participants were instructed not to perform any kind of specific core stability training during the week between the two testing sessions.

Study II: (Longitudinal intervention study)

In total, 20 male professional football players competing in Spain's National Second League (mean ± standard deviation age 27.7 ± 5.1 years old, height 180.9 ± 6.9 cm, weight 76.5 ± 5.4 kg) were included in the longitudinal study.

2.3. Procedures

Two hand-held dynamometers (HOGGAN Health microFET3 Combo Manual Muscle Tester & Digital Inclinometer, United States) were used for data recording. Each tester employed the same device during the entire evaluation process.

Closed Kinetic Chain test (CCT)

The participant was placed in a standing position with the trunk positioned at 50° of flexion, knee positioned at 20° of flexion (0° of abduction/rotation of the knee) and with both hands placed at the iliac crest level. The tester was positioned ipsilateral to the testing leg and the HHD was placed just superior to the lateral femoral condyle. Then, the participant exerted a maximal isometric contraction toward hip abduction and external rotation, "squeezing their glutes" against the HHD which was firmly fixed by the examiner. The applied force had to be maintained for 3 s and 3 attempts were registered for each leg. (Figure 1A). No compensation at the trunk level was allowed during the execution of the test.

Prone Plank Test (PPT)

The participant was placed in a prone position with the ankles positioned at 0° of ankle dorsal flexion. They were instructed to hold their pelvis in a parallel position with respect to the stretcher and to move the testing leg into 20° of hip extension and abduction, with the knee in an extended position. The tester was positioned ipsilateral to the testing leg, and the dynamometer was placed superior to the external malleolus. Then, the participants exerted a maximal isometric contraction toward hip extension and hip abduction against the hand-held dynamometer (HHD) which was firmly fixed by the examiner. Participants had to maintain the generating force for 3 s and 3 attempts were registered for each leg. To ensure appropriate direction of force applied by the participant, they were asked to perform the task with the following instructions: "imagine you had a watch at the bottom of your feet at which you should have to tag the five or ten o'clock hours on it", when testing the right and left legs respectively (Figure 1B). No pelvis compensation was allowed during the execution of the test.

Study I: (Cross-sectional study)

Two test sessions were performed 1 week apart. No physical activity program focusing on the core muscles between the testing sessions was allowed for the participants.

All participants were evaluated by two testers (S.E. and E.B.) following the same testing protocol. Both testers were physical therapists and they had not been familiarized with the procedure of the new proposed core strength tests. Before each testing session, both testers were instructed about the testing procedure and were familiarized with the dynamometer by an expert instructor (I.S). One familiarization trial was followed by three testing measurements for each leg and test type. The two highest recordings were gathered for statistical analysis. If the difference between the trials was higher than 10%, another trial was performed.

Study II: (longitudinal study)

A 42 weeks standardized core stability training program was performed, divided into three different stages with progressively increasing stabilization demands (Figure 2). The difficulty was increased after every 14 weeks. The players performed 28 core program training sessions at each stage and were evaluated at the beginning and at the end of the whole standardized exercise program.

All participants were tested by the same evaluator (I.S) following the same testing protocol described in detail in the validation study. At the follow-up evaluation, 7 players missed the testing session due to either injury or national team recruitment for international call ups, hence the test–retest comparison was done with a sample of 13 football players.

The compliance with the core training program was recorded at every core training session by the athletic trainer of the football team (J.S), using a data log model generated by the authors.

All participants provided informed consent before participation. The football team's medical staff's permission was requested in study II. The study was approved by the ethic committee of the Public University of Navarra and was performed in accordance with the Declaration of Helsinki for longitudinal studies with human beings.

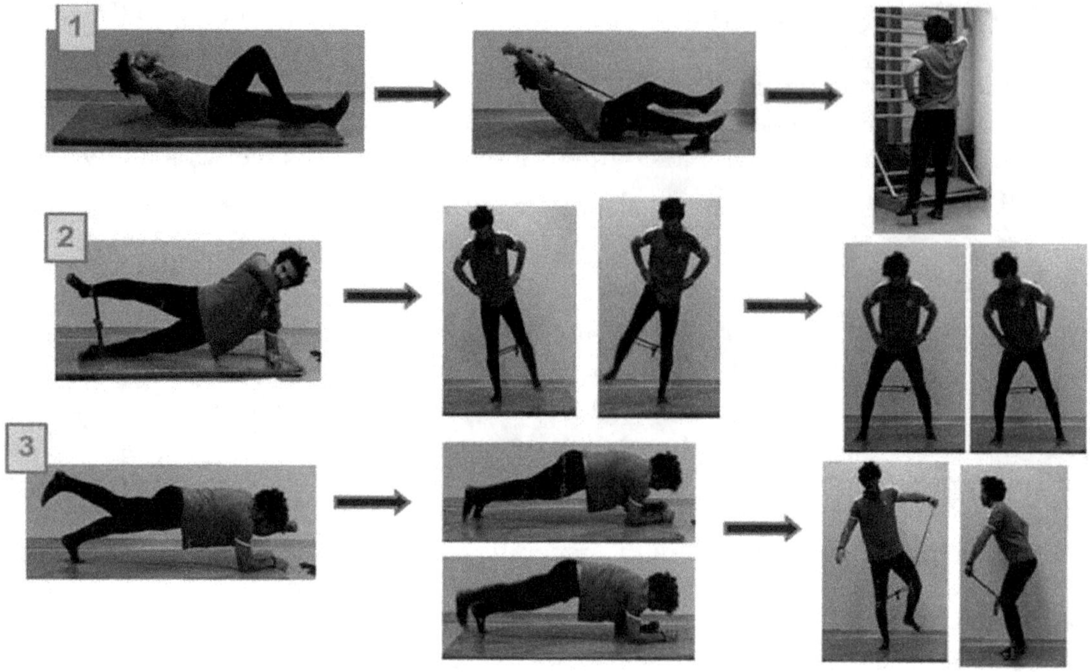

Figure 2. Core stability training program divided into 3 different training phases. The first column of the figure represents the 3 core exercises. The second and third columns exemplify the progression of each exercise, adding motor control difficulty, in ascending order.

2.4. *Statistical Analysis*

The SPSS statistical package (version 17.0.0.236; SPSS Inc. Chicago, IL, USA) was used to perform all the statistical analyses. All analyses assumed statistical significance at $p \leq 0.05$.

Study I: (Cross-sectional study)

A total of 22 participants were evaluated for the intrasession, and intra- and inter-rater reliability analysis. Furthermore, a subset of seven subjects was randomly selected from the initial cohort and they repeated the whole examination at seven days for the test–retest reliability calculations.

Descriptive statistics, including mean peak torque values with standard deviation, coefficient of variation (%) (expressed as the SD of the mean, multiplied by 100% and expressed as a percentage) and confidence intervals (95%), were calculated. The peak isometric force values obtained from each evaluator during the PPT and CCT were gathered for intra-rater (trial 1, trial 2), inter-rater (male tester, female tester) and intra-rater intersession (assessment day 1/day 2). Afterwards, a Paired *t*-test comparison and the corresponding non parametrical Wilcoxon Signed-rank test were run to primarily test whether the two sets of scores were significantly different from each other, before their test–retest reliability was analyzed [18].

The data was graphically examined using Bland and Altman [19] plots in, which the difference between test sessions was plotted against the mean of the two test sessions. Mean differences between test sessions with 95% CIs were calculated to determine whether there was any systematic bias. The relative reliability of the data was determined using a two-way random effect model intraclass correlation coefficient (2, k). Before calculating absolute reliability, Bland and Altman plots were generated to examine the correlation (R2) between the absolute differences and the mean values for each test, in order to detect the presence or absence of heteroscedasticity in the data [19]. If the random error increases as the measured values increase, the data is considered heteroscedastic. In contrast, when there is no relation between the error and the size of the measured value, the data is described as homoscedastic. With homoscedastic errors, providing that they are also normally distributed, the raw data can be analyzed with conventional parametric analyses, but heteroscedastic data should be transformed logarithmically before analysis, or investigated via an analysis based on ratio statistics. This comparison method is widely used to verify the reliability and reproducibility of the measurement, rather than the correlation coefficient (r) and regression techniques, which are inadequate and can be very misleading when assessing agreement, as they evaluate only the linear association of two sets of observations. With this graph, evaluation of the magnitude of the disagreement, identification of outliers and the observation of any bias are easily achieved [20]. Due to the simplicity and potential for the identification of pairs of observations whose differences reach beyond clinical tolerances, the Bland and Altman approach is currently the preferred approach to evaluate agreement between two measurements [19].

If R2 was between 0 and 0.1, the data were considered homoscedastic; consequently, the absolute reliability was assessed by determining the SEM, which was calculated using the square root of the mean square error from the analysis of variance model, as recommended by Atkinson and Nevill [21]. If R2 was greater than 0.1, the data was considered heteroscedastic; consequently, absolute reliability was determined by calculating the CV. When applicable, the CV was calculated for each subject by dividing the standard deviation of the two testing sessions by the mean of the two testing sessions ×100 (for intersession CV calculation), and the standard deviation of two testers by the mean of the two testers ×100 (for intrasession CV calculation).

Both the intra-rater (rater 1 and 2, between 2 days) and the inter-rater reliability (between rater 1 and 2, the same testing day) peak isometric force values were assessed using intraclass correlation coefficients (ICC) with 95% confidence intervals (CI) in order to assess relative reliability by utilizing a two-way random effects model with single measure reliability (ICC (2,1)). The mean value from each participant was used for the analysis. Values < 0.50 represented poor reliability, values > 0.50 and < 0.75 indicated fair to good reliability, and values > 0.75 marked excellent reliability [20]. Given that ICC values may be influenced by the inter-subject variability of scores, the standard error of measurement (SEM) was reported in conjunction with the ICCs. A large ICC may represent poor trial-to-trial consistency if the inter-participant variability is too high [18], in contrast to SEM, which is not affected by inter-subject variability [18]. SEM was calculated using the equation $SEM = SD \times (\sqrt{1} - ICC)$, where SD corresponds to the sample standard deviation [17,20–22] for intra- and inter-rater reliability analysis. In the case of the intersession reliability analysis, the SD of the T2 data set class was utilized, assuming that between the two assessment sessions, T2 generated lower SD [21]. The error in an individual's score at one point in time was estimated by multiplying the SEM by the z value for the 90% confidence level (z value = 1.65) [23–29]. This value was then multiplied by the square root of 2 (to account for the measurement error in two test sessions) in order to estimate the minimum detectable change (MDC) at the 90% confidence level.

Study II: (Longitudinal study)

A preliminary effect size calculation was performed to determine the adequate sample size required to account for a random error of 0.8. A total of 27 participants would have been necessary, but finally 20 participants were recruited (an entire second Spanish league football club). After that, only 13 players were included in the statistical analysis, because 7 players did not complete the testing session after the core training program due to either injury or national team recruitment for international match play. The compliance of the core training program was 82%, corresponding to 69 core training sessions accomplished out of the 84 total sessions established at the beginning of the intervention.

After checking the assumptions of parametric statistics, the mean comparisons before and after the implementation of the core training program were analyzed using a Paired Sample *t*-test. The estimation of MDC at a 90% confidence level was also calculated to determine whether the observed change in score between the pre- and post-testing evaluations was truly a change in patient status, or was merely associated with an error (noise) in the measurement process [17].

3. Results

Study I: (Cross-sectional study)

Bland and Altman plots for intrasession intratester and intratester intersession reliability (Figure 3) demonstrated no systematic biases between trials and testing days. In relation to intrasession and intertester reliability, the PPT test values were grouped together. Alternatively, in the case of the CCT test values, a systematic bias seemed to occur, given the fact that the higher the force values reported from the participants, the greater the differences encountered between testers.

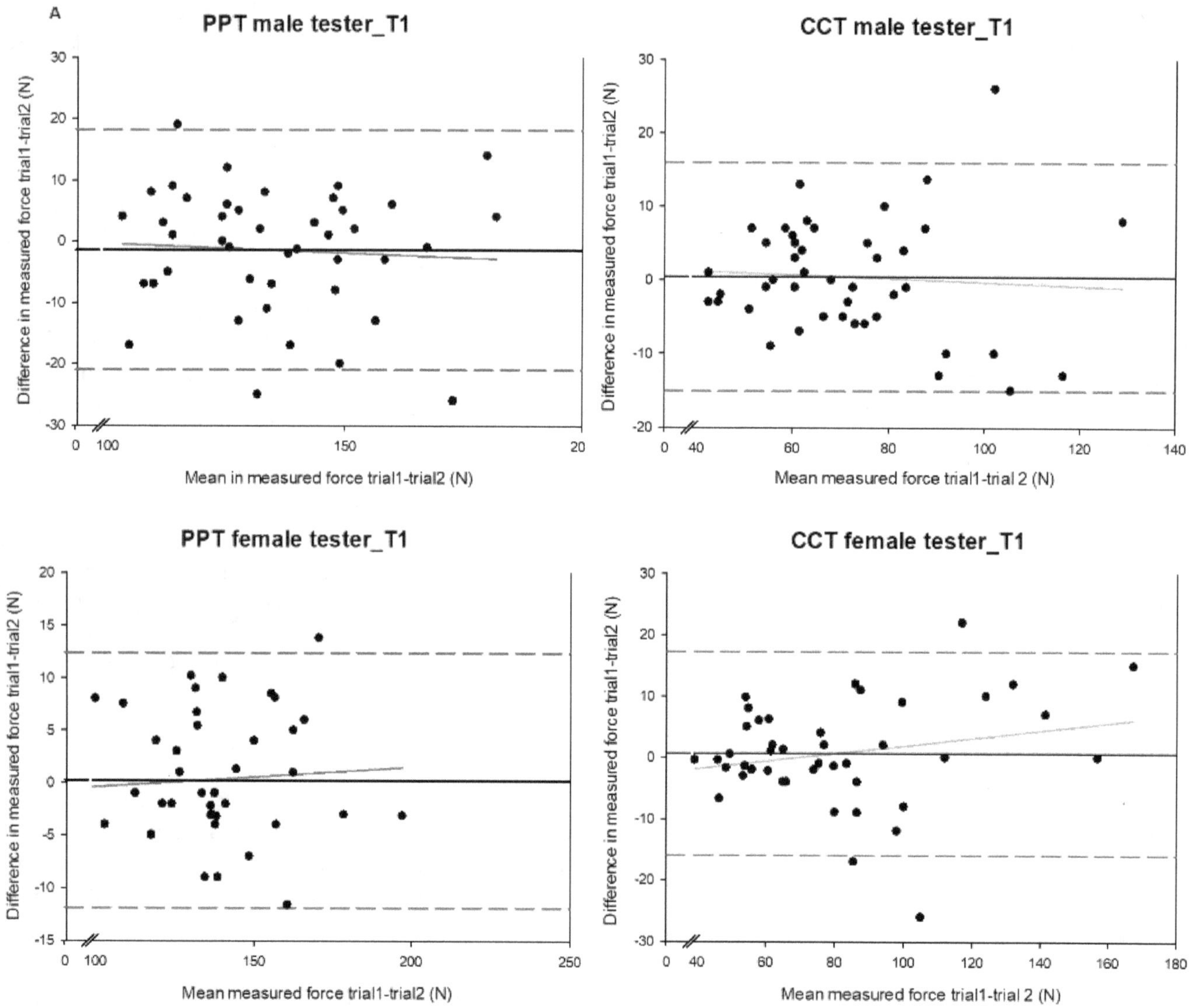

Figure 3. *Cont.*

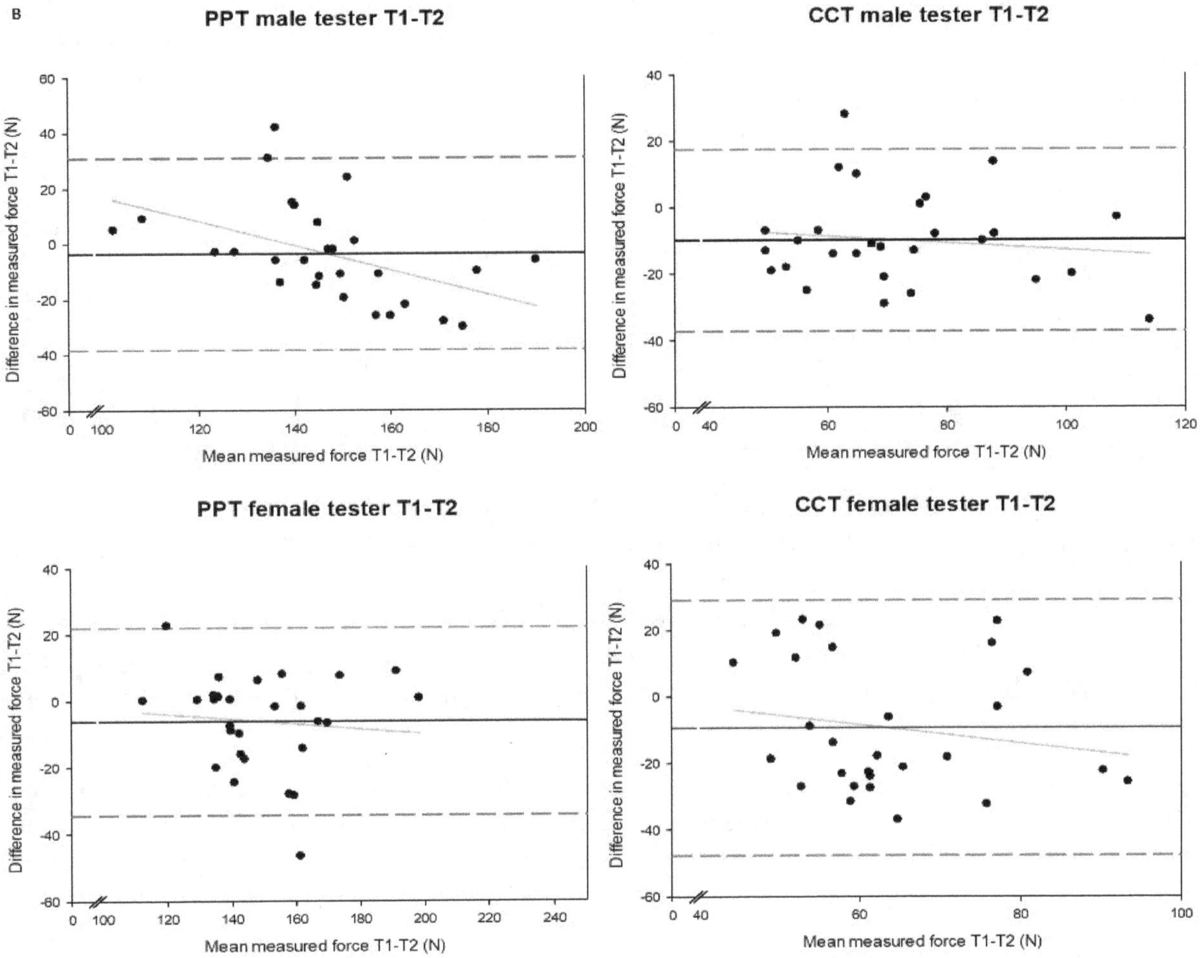

Figure 3. Bland and Altman plots representing mean differences and 95% limits of agreement. (**A**) Between trial 1 and trial 2 for both testers in the first testing session (T1). (**B**) Between first (T1) and second (T2) testing sessions for both testers.

Descriptive data from both testers for the intrasession analysis of the first testing session (T1) are presented in Table 1. Looking at between-trial variability, the mean CV (%) values for both core strength tests for the male tester (PPT = 4.11%; CCT = 5.79%) and the female tester (PPT = 2.73%; CCT = 5.05%) were below 10%, indicating low test–retest variation[22].

Table 1. Descriptive data PPT and CCC test (T1). N = Newton; Δ = mean difference; CV = coefficient of variation; CI = confidence intervals.

	PRONE PLANK TEST					CLOSED KINETIC CHAIN TEST				
	Mean Peak Torque N Trial 1 (±SD)	Mean Peak Torque N Trial 2 (±SD)	Δ (N)	CV (%)	95% CI	Mean Peak Torque N Trial 1 (±SD)	Mean Peak Torque N Trial 2 (±SD)	Δ (N)	CV (%)	95% CI
Tester Male	133.91 (±20.89)	135.31 (±21.49)	+1.4	4.1	128.52–140.69	71.56 (±16.67)	71.14 (±20.16)	−0.42	+5.8	65.58–77.12
Tester Female	133.87 (±26.86)	133.61 (±26.36)	−0.26	2.7	125.93–141.55	80.50 (±31.74)	79.84 (±29.86)	−0.66	+5.0	71.15–89.19

Regarding the intratester and intrasession reliability analysis, the data showed excellent reliability for both the core strength tests for the male tester (PPT = 0.94; CCT = 0.96) and the female tester (PPT = 0.99; CCT = 0.81) (Table 2).

Table 2. Reliability results (N = 22). N = Newton; SD = standard deviation; ICC = intraclass correlation coefficient; SEM = standard error of measurement; MDC_{90} = minimal detectable change 90% confidence level.

	PRONE PLANK TEST				CLOSED KINETIC CHAIN TEST			
	Mean Peak Torque N (±SD)	ICC (95% CI)	SEM (N)	MDC90 (N)	Mean Peak Torque N (±SD)	ICC (95% CI)	SEM (N)	MDC90 (N)
Tester Male	134.61 (±20.59)	0.94 (0.89–0.97)	5.12	11.95	71.35 (±19.52)	0.96 (0.93–0.98)	4.0	9.4
Tester Female	133.74 (±26.43)	0.99	3.02	7.04	80.17 (±30.52)	0.81 (0.68–0.89)	13.5	31.5

In relation to intratester and intersession reliability analysis, the data exhibited excellent reliability for both core strength tests for the male tester (PPT = 0.77; CCT = 0.94) and the female tester for PPT (ICC = 0.84), but poor reliability for the female tester in the case of the CCT (ICC = 0.38). These results are shown in Table 3. The intertester and intrasession reliability analysis is represented in Table 4. For the PPT test, the data exhibit fair to good reliability (ICC = 0.62) and poor reliability for the CCT test (ICC = 0.47). The SEMs and MDC_{90} for each reliability analysis are expressed in conjunction with the ICCs in Tables 2–4.

Table 3. Intratester intersession reliability results (T1) for both tester (N = 22). N = Newton; SD = standard deviation; ICC = intraclass correlation coefficient; SEM = standard error of measurement; MDC_{90} = minimal detectable change 90% confidence level.

	Mean Peak Torque N T1 (±SD)		Mean Peak Torque N T2 (±SD)		Δ T2-T1 (N)		ICC (95% CI)		SEM (N)		MDC_{90} (N)	
	Male Tester	Female Tester	Male Tester	Female Tester	Male Tester	Female Tester	Male Tester	Female Tester	Male Tester	Female Tester	Male Tester	Female Tester
Prone plank test	144.20 (±17.01)	145.44 (±21.48)	147.79 (±25.67)	150.34 (±21.00)	+3.59	+4.9	0.77 (0.28–0.93)	0.94 (0.79–0.98)	12.4	5.4	28.9	16.69
Closed kinetic chain test	66.13 (±18.05)	58.36 (±14.68)	73.89 (±17.83)	67.90 (±17.03)	−7.77	+9.54	0.84 (0.44–0.95)	0.38 (−0.59–0.78)	7.2	13.5	12.5	31.39

Table 4. Intertester intrasession reliability results (T1) for both test (N = 22). N = Newton; SD = standard deviation; ICC = intraclass correlation coefficient; SEM = standard error of measurement; MDC_{90} = minimal detectable change 90% confidence level.

	Rater Male Mean Peak Torque N (±SD)	Rater Female Mean Peak Torque N (±SD)	ICC (95% CI)	SEM (N)	MDC_{90} (N)
Prone plank test	134.61 (±20.59)	71.35 (±19.52)	0.62 (0.30–0.8)	14.47	33.76
Closed kinetic chain test	133.74 (±26.43)	80.17 (±30.52)	0.47 (0.06–0.70)	18.8	43.88

Study II: (Longitudinal study)

There was a statistically significant increase with respect to peak muscle force exertion between the two testing sessions, for both the PPT ($p < 0.00$) and CCT ($p < 0.00$) (Figure 4). Furthermore, large effect size values (Cohen's D), of 0.9 and 1.0, were reported for PPT and CCT, respectively (Table 5).

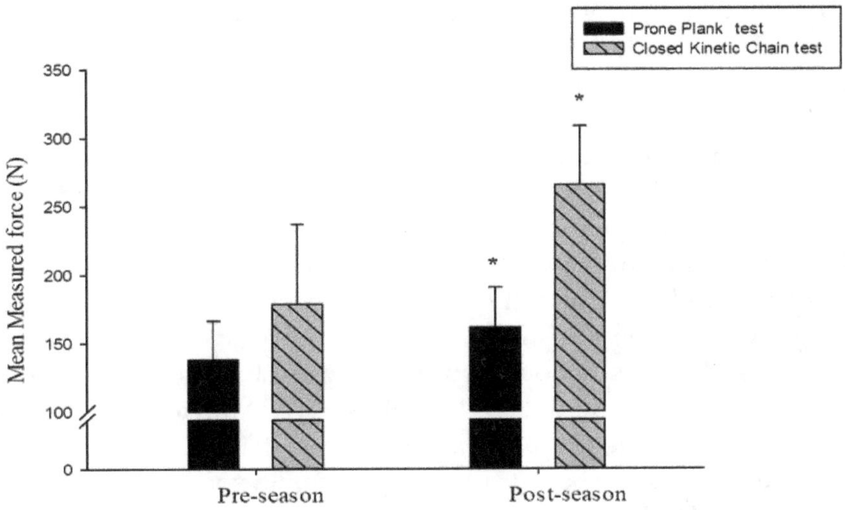

Figure 4. Pre-/post HHD values for PPT and CCT tests. $p < 0.05$. (*) denotes statistically significance between pre to post evaluations.

Table 5. Compared means for pre-season (T1) and post-season (T2) values for the two core strength test (N = 13). N = Newton; SD = standard deviation; Cohen's d = effect size; MDC_{90} = minimal detectable change 90% confidence level.

	Mean Peak Torque N (±SD)		Δ T2-T1 (%)	*D*	*t*-Test (*p*)	MDC_{90} (N)
	Pre-Season (T1)	Post-Season (T2)				
Prone plank test	137.87 (±28.13)	160.73 (±27.85)	+22.86	0.9	0.00	47.71
Closed kinetic chain test	184.64 (±56.10)	260.92 (±43.61)	+76.28	1.0	0.00	93.29

4. Discussion

Study I: (validation study)

The purpose of the validation study was to determine the validity and reliability of two new proposed core strength field tests, using an HHD to evaluate the ability to produce force in challenging positions, representing core stability. The observed ICCs in this study suggest the excellent test–retest reliability of the Prone Plank Test (PPT) and the Closed Kinetic Chain Test (CCT) (see Tables 3 and 4). The ICC is a measure of relative reliability indicating a measure's ability to discriminate between existing differences among two sets of data. It is calculated by dividing the between-patient variance by the total variance [17] (between-patient and within-patient variance). The present findings therefore suggest that the PPT and CCT demonstrated appropriate reliability for their use in the training field setting as a core strength functional evaluation.

The SEM provides an absolute measure of reliability with regard to the original test units, and can be used to estimate the error associated with an individual patient's test score [17,26]. The smaller the SEM value, the more reliable the measurements [17,20]. In our study, the SEM ranged from 4.01 N to 13.50 N for intratester intrasession and intersession reliability analyses. The results found in our study correlate with a similar study accomplished by De Blaiser et al. [10], in relation to intratester and intrasession reliability, who evaluated maximal isometric trunk flexion and extension strength tests using HHD on a healthy athletic population. They reported excellent intratester and intertester reliability values (ICC = 0.76–0.93) for all tests, except for the intratester reliability of the maximal isometric trunk flexion test starting at 0°, which was good (ICC = 0.67). The ICCs for the intertester and intrasession analysis in our study were lower than what they had found, probably because the testers from their study had similar physical characteristics, in order to counteract the participant's force exertion. Another study conducted by Moreland et al. [30] determined the intertester reliability of six tests of trunk muscle strength evaluation using practical measurement methods which could be applied in most clinical or work settings. For abdominal and back extensor isometric force tests using HHD, they reported poor (0.24 and 0.25, respectively) ICC values. These results contrast with those reported in our study, maybe because the rater's ability to apply force could have been limited, as they argued. In a more recent study conducted by Recio et al. [7], a flexion–extension isokinetic protocol was used to asses trunk muscle strength and endurance in a healthy and physically active population (1–3 h of moderate physical activity in recreational sports, 1–3 days a week). The ICC values obtained for the strength variables in this study ranged from 0.57 to 0.77 in extension, and from 0.62 to 0.84 in flexion, with low SEM values. Another study designed by Essendrop et al. [31] evaluated the intratester reliability of isometric strength tests by using a HHD device in a workplace environment, and found excellent ICCs for back flexion and extension tests (0.97–0.93, respectively).

Two distinct methodologies have been traditionally used in sport science for strength evaluation: isokinetic testing or isometric HHD [19]. Isokinetic dynamometers are computerized machines able to provide different variables of muscle strength (i.e., peak force, endurance, power, optimum angle of torque production, etc.). Isokinetic dynamometry is considered the "gold standard" for trunk muscle strength evaluation, mainly because it allows a controlled and accurate assessment of a large number of muscle force parameters, but the high technology requirements, as well as the time consumption, of these isokinetic protocols, along with their substantial economic cost, could limit the generalization of its use.

Alternatively, hand-held dynamometry (HHD) strength evaluation has been shown to be a reliable, objective way to obtain strength measurements [23–26]. HHD is a tool that can be placed between the practitioner's hand and the tested body part of the athlete. Stark et al. [22] recently demonstrated, in a systematic review, the moderate-to-good reliability and validity scores between the HHD vs. isokinetic testing procedures. Considering the cost of isokinetic testing devices and their logistical limitations for routine clinical testing purposes, the HHD could be considered a practical standard for muscle strength assessment in the training field or clinical setting. These results support those from our study, and enlarge the scientific verification of the use of HHD-based core strength evaluations in the field training arena, or the clinical setting itself, enabling clinicians to routinely perform quantitative and objective core body region strength evaluations on a science-based foundation. In the authors opinion, the employment of previously analyzed and validated tests, with adequate reliability and reproducibility, guarantees the internal methodological quality standards that this kind of in-the-field performed test have to demonstrate in order to ensure the appropriate extrapolation of these evaluation methodologies. Moreover, a robust validation process can also enable different researchers in the development of these routines and result interpretations.

Study II: (longitudinal study)

The purpose of the study was to determine whether these preliminary validated tests (PPT and CCT) would be able to detect changes in the force application capacities of professional football players after the implementation of a motor control-based core stability training program.

We found a significant improvement in the measured core strength values (PPT and CCT tests) after the core stability training program was implemented. The original result obtained from this longitudinal study was that participants were able to produce higher strength values in spite of the fact that the progression criteria were core neuromuscular control challenge-based, instead of being based on traditional resistance progression criteria. In fact, neuromuscular control training for athletes has traditionally been focused on resistance exercises for trunk musculature. However, these types of core training programs could not only lead to excessive applications of mechanical loads to the spine, but they can also fail to satisfy the biomechanical stabilization requirements necessary to counteract the acting internal and external forces during athletic maneuvers [30,31]. Even so, previous studies using non-elite or sub-elite instead of elite subjects have clearly demonstrated the effectiveness of core stabilization programs in improving core strength when compared with no or regular training only [32,33]. Regarding the literature available, it is difficult to find longitudinal studies recruiting elite professional football players due to the inability to have a control group and the high level competitive demand that often challenges this type of scientific effort.

A weak core body region has been linked with alterations in the transfer of energy throughout the whole kinetic chain, potentially resulting in reduced sport performance and increased injury risk [2,15,34]. As a result, the implementation of a core strength training program has become popular in sport and clinical settings as a means to improve performance and reduce injury risk. Several studies have examined the effects of improving core-related strength following a core training program, finding a wide variety of results. Similarly, few studies have analyzed the possible relationship between core strength and sport-performance, concluding that if founded, the correlations were weak to moderate [31,34–36]. One of the main sources that could explain the inconsistency of these results could involve the methodology used to measure the core strength. Most of the studies followed McGill testing protocol-derived methods. These studies, despite demonstrating excellent test–retest reliability, seem to be more related to trunk muscle endurance capacity, rather than being focused on the more functional and faster movements demands that most multi-directional sports seem to require [35].

Furthermore, in the present study, we found that those players displaying a limb symmetry index greater than 15% (described in the literature as the maximum physiological difference) displayed a trend toward the equalization of the observed deficit at the end of the season. In contrast, players reporting more symmetric limb-to-limb values at baseline significatively improved their performance in the tests at the end of the season. Whether this fact could be linked to both injury risk reduction and/or athletic performance enhancement should be appropriately addressed in future studies.

The present study had several limitations. The first is associated with the use of the HHD, which has been demonstrated to reproduce some tester bias as the evaluator has to produce sufficient force to ensure the actual isometric contraction of the participant. As such, inadequate force application by the evaluator may lead to decreased intertester reliability [23,24]. To avoid or diminish this bias, both testing sessions (test 1 and test 2) were conducted by the same tester in the longitudinal study [25]. Another limitation of HHD is that the force recorded by male and female testers is different. The female tester recorded lower values, as the subject could produce higher forces, and the force exerted by the same participant was different in the reports of different examiners [23]. This finding can be verified in the Bland and Altman plots. In relation to the longitudinal study, the a priori effect size calculation showed the necessity of obtaining 27 players for a random error of 0.8. This fact highlighted the fact that the study was slightly underpowered. Furthermore, seven dropouts were registered in the post-intervention evaluations. However, the statistically significant improvements, as well as the large to very large effect sizes achieved from pre- to post-evaluation, may serve as a starting point for future adequately powered studies targeting this issue. Another limitation of this study could be that there was not a control group, but the lack of a control group is common in interventions among professional players, because leaving a player out of an intervention that could be beneficial is not recommended due to potential ethical objections.

Despite these limitations, in the authors' opinion the HHD is easy to use, portable, inexpensive, and requires little training for proficient application. The present validation study revealed that the tester's experience has little or no bearing on intratester reliability measures. However, greater participant strength values could produce weaker intertester reliability measures [26,37]. To avoid this error, one solution could be to couple the HHD device to a rigid customized device. In this manner, the subject would exert the force against a structure that it is not possible to move, ensuring an actual isometric contraction [38].

5. Practical Applications

The Prone Plank Test (PPT) and Closed Kinetic Chain Test (CCT) both demonstrated good test–retest reliability and acceptable error measurement. This kind of easy-to-implement core region functional test could provide both athletic trainers and clinicians with a new and reliable tool for carrying out their core body region training routines in a more objective and standardized way.

The implementation of a core stability training program with a professional football team during the competitive season resulted in a significant core muscle force improvement, achieved with the PPT and CCT. This finding demonstrated that a progressive standardized core neuromuscular training program could be satisfactorily implemented in a professional football team environment, where competition pressure and results sometimes compromise the adequate implementation of an ideal training program.

Author Contributions: Data curation, S.E., E.B., I.S. (Iosu Sesma) and I.S. (Igor Setuain); Formal analysis, S.E., E.B. and I.S. (Igor Setuain); Investigation, M.I., E.B., J.G.A., I.S. (Iosu Sesma), I.S. (Iñigo Sarriegi) and I.S. (Igor Setuain); Methodology, S.E., M.I., J.G.A., I.S. (Iosu Sesma), I.S. (Iñigo Sarriegi) and I.S. (Igor Setuain); Project administration, M.I. and I.S. (Igor Setuain); Resources, M.I. and I.S. (Igor Setuain); Supervision, M.I., J.G.A., I.S. (Iñigo Sarriegi) and I.S. (Igor Setuain); Validation, M.I.; Writing—original draft, S.E. and E.B.; Writing—review & editing, M.I., I.S. (Iñigo Sarriegi) and I.S. (Igor Setuain). All authors have read and agreed to the published version of the manuscript.

Acknowledgments: The authors would like to express their great appreciation to the participants, as well as to the football club medical and technical stuff and to the players for their predisposition in taking part in the study.

References

1. Akuthota, V.; Ferreiro, A.; Moore, T.; Fredericson, M. Core Stability Exercise Principles. *Curr. Sports Med. Rep.* **2008**, *7*, 39–44. [CrossRef] [PubMed]
2. Kibler, W.B.; Press, J.; Sciascia, A. The role of core stability in athletic function. *Sports Med.* **2006**, *36*, 189–198. [CrossRef] [PubMed]
3. Mendiguchia, J.; Ford, K.R.; Quatman, C.E.; Alentorn-Geli, E.; Hewett, T.E. Sex differences in proximal control of the knee joint. *Sports Med.* **2011**, *41*, 541–557. [CrossRef] [PubMed]
4. Hodges, P.W.; A Richardson, C. Contraction of the Abdominal Muscles Associated With Movement of the Lower Limb. *Phys. Ther.* **1997**, *77*, 132–142. [CrossRef]
5. Ohnson, C.D.; Whitehead, P.N.; Pletcher, E.R.; Faherty, M.S.; Lovalekar, M.; Eagle, S.R.; Keenan, K.A. The Relationship of Core Strength and Activation and Performance on Three Functional Movement Screens. *J. Strength Cond. Res.* **2018**, *32*, 1166–1173. [CrossRef]
6. De Blaiser, C.; De Ridder, R.; Willems, T.; Danneels, L.; Roosen, P. Reliability and validity of trunk flexor and trunk extensor strength measurements using handheld dynamometry in a healthy athletic population. *Phys. Ther. Sport* **2018**, *34*, 180–186. [CrossRef]
7. Juan-Recio, C.; López-Plaza, D.; Murillo, D.B.; García-Vaquero, M.P.; Vera-Garcia, F.J. Reliability assessment and correlation analysis of 3 protocols to measure trunk muscle strength and endurance. *J. Sports Sci.* **2017**, *14*, 1–8. [CrossRef]
8. Reeves, N.P.; Popovich, J.M.; Priess, M.C.; Cholewicki, J.; Choi, J.; Radcliffe, C.J. Reliability of assessing trunk motor control using position and force tracking and stabilization tasks. *J. Biomech.* **2013**, *47*, 44–49. [CrossRef]
9. Barbado, D.; Barbado, L.C.; Elvira, J.L.L.; Van Dieën, J.H.; Vera-Garcia, F.J. Sports-related testing protocols are required to reveal trunk stability adaptations in high-level athletes. *Gait Posture* **2016**, *49*, 90–96. [CrossRef]
10. De Blaiser, C.; De Ridder, R.; Willems, T.; Danneels, L.; Bossche, L.V.; Palmans, T.; Roosen, P. Evaluating abdominal core muscle fatigue: Assessment of the validity and reliability of the prone bridging test. *Scand. J. Med. Sci. Sports* **2017**, *28*, 391–399. [CrossRef] [PubMed]
11. Sorensen, F.B. Physical measurements as risk indicators for low-back trouble over a one-year period. *Spine* **1984**, *9*, 106–119.
12. Krause, D.A.; Youdas, J.W.; Hollman, J.H.; Smith, J. Abdominal Muscle Performance as Measured by the Double Leg-Lowering Test. *Arch. Phys. Med. Rehabilit.* **2005**, *86*, 1345–1348. [CrossRef] [PubMed]

13. McGill, S.M. Low Back Stability: From Formal Description to Issues for Performance and Rehabilitation. *Exerc. Sport Sci. Rev.* **2001**, *29*, 26–31. [CrossRef]
14. Cowley, P.M.; Swensen, T.C. Development and Reliability of Two Core Stability Field Tests. *J. Strength Cond. Res.* **2008**, *22*, 619–624. [CrossRef]
15. Peco, N.; Vera-garcia, F.J. Flexion-Rotation Trunk Test to Assess Abdominal Muscle Endurance. *J. Strength Cond. Res.* **2013**, *27*, 1602–1608.
16. Bliven, K.C.H.; Anderson, B.E. Core Stability Training for Injury Prevention. *Sports Health* **2013**, *5*, 514–522. [CrossRef]
17. Leetun, D.T.; Ireland, M.L.; Willson, J.D.; Ballantyne, B.T.; Davis, I.M. Core Stability Measures as Risk Factors for Lower Extremity Injury in Athletes. *Med. Sci. Sports Exerc.* **2004**, *36*, 926–934. [CrossRef]
18. Hernaez, R. Reliability and agreement studies: A guide for clinical investigators. *Gut* **2015**, *64*, 1018–1027. [CrossRef]
19. Bland, J.M.; Altman, D.G. Measuring agreement in method comparison studies. *Stat. Methods Med. Res.* **1999**, *8*, 135–160. [CrossRef]
20. Weir, J.P. Quantifying test-retest reliability using the intraclass correlation coefficient and the SEM. *J. Strength Cond. Res.* **2005**, *19*, 231–240. [PubMed]
21. Atkinson, G.; Nevill, A. Statistical Methods for Assssing Measurement Error (Reliability) in Variables Relevant to Sports Medicine. *Sports Med.* **1998**, *26*, 217–238. [CrossRef] [PubMed]
22. Stark, T.; Walker, B.F.; Phillips, J.K.; Fejer, R.; Beck, R. Hand-held Dynamometry Correlation With the Gold Standard Isokinetic Dynamometry: A Systematic Review. *PM&R* **2011**, *3*, 472–479.
23. Denegar, C.R.; Ball, D.W. Assessing Reliability and Precision of Measurement: An Introduction to Intraclass Correlation and Standard Error of Measurement. *J. Sport Rehabilit.* **1993**, *2*, 35–42. [CrossRef]
24. De Vet, H.C.; Terwee, C.B.; Knol, D.L.; Bouter, L.M. When to use agreement versus reliability measures. *J. Clin. Epidemiol.* **2006**, *59*, 1033–1039. [CrossRef]
25. Kelln, B.M.; McKeon, P.; Gontkof, L.M.; Hertel, J. Hand-held dynamometry: Reliability of lower extremity muscle testing in healthy, physically active, young adults. *J. Sport Rehabilit.* **2008**, *17*, 160–170. [CrossRef]
26. Lu, T.-W.; Hsu, H.; Chang, L.; Chen, H.-L. Enhancing the examiner's resisting force improves the reliability of manual muscle strength measurements: Comparison of a new device with hand-held dynamometry. *Acta Derm. Venereol.* **2007**, *39*, 679–684. [CrossRef]
27. Celik, D.; Dirican, A.; Baltaci, G. Intrarater Reliability of Assessing Strength of the Shoulder and Scapular Muscles. *J. Sport Rehabilit.* **2017**, *3*, 1–5. [CrossRef]
28. Bohannon, R.W.; Andrews, A.W. Interrater Reliability of Hand-Held Dynamometry. *Phys. Ther.* **1987**, *67*, 931–933. [CrossRef]
29. Stratford, P.W.; Goldsmith, C.H. Use of the standard error as a reliability index of interest: An applied example using elbow flexor strength data. *Phys. Ther.* **1997**, *77*, 745–750. [CrossRef]
30. Moreland, J.; Finch, E.; Stratford, P.; Balsor, B.; Gill, C. Interrater Reliability of Six Tests of Trunk Muscle Function and Endurance. *J. Orthop. Sports Phys. Ther.* **1997**, *26*, 200–208. [CrossRef] [PubMed]
31. Essendrop, M.; Schibye, B.; Hansen, K. Reliability of isometric muscle strength tests for the trunk, hands and shoulders. *Int. J. Ind. Ergon.* **2001**, *28*, 379–387. [CrossRef]
32. Zazulak, B.T.; Hewett, T.E.; Reeves, N.P.; Goldberg, B.; Cholewicki, J. Deficits in Neuromuscular Control of the Trunk Predict Knee Injury Risk. *Am. J. Sports Med.* **2007**, *35*, 1123–1130. [CrossRef] [PubMed]
33. Prieske, O.; Muehlbauer, T.; Borde, R.; Gube, M.; Bruhn, S.; Behm, D.G.; Granacher, U. Neuromuscular and athletic performance following core strength training in elite youth soccer: Role of instability. *Scand. J. Med. Sci. Sports* **2015**, *26*, 48–56. [CrossRef] [PubMed]
34. Sharma, A.; Geovinson, S.G.; Sandhu, J.S. Effects of a nine-week core strengthening exercise program on vertical jump performances and static balance in volleyball players with trunk instability. *J. Sports Med. Phys. Fit.* **2012**, *52*, 606–615.
35. Hoshikawa, Y.; Iida, T.; Muramatsu, M.; Ii, N.; Nakajima, Y.; Chumank, K.; Kanehisa, H. Effects of Stabilization Training on Trunk Muscularity and Physical Performances in Youth Soccer Players. *J. Strength Cond. Res.* **2013**, *27*, 3142–3149. [CrossRef]
36. Nesser, T.W.; Huxel, K.C.; Tincher, J.L.; Okada, T. The Relationship Between Core Stability and Performance in Division I Football Players. *J. Strength Cond. Res.* **2008**, *22*, 1750–1754. [CrossRef]

37. Roth, R.; Donath, L.; Zahner, L.; Faude, O. Muscle Activation and Performance During Trunk Strength Testing in High-Level Female and Male Football Players. *J. Appl. Biomech.* **2016**, *32*, 241–247. [CrossRef]
38. Hölmich, P.; Larsen, K.; Krogsgaard, K.; Gluud, C. Exercise program for prevention of groin pain in football players: A cluster-randomized trial. *Scand. J. Med. Sci. Sports* **2009**, *20*, 814–821. [CrossRef]

5

The Acute Effect of Match-Play on Hip Isometric Strength and Flexibility in Female Field Hockey Players

Violeta Sánchez-Migallón [1], Alvaro López-Samanes [1,*], Pablo Terrón-Manrique [1], Esther Morencos [2], Vicente Fernández-Ruiz [1], Archit Navandar [3] and Victor Moreno-Pérez [4]

1 Exercise Physiology Group, School of Physiotherapy, Faculty of Health Sciences, Universidad Francisco de Vitoria, Pozuelo de Alarcón, 28049 Madrid, Spain; violeta.smigallon@ufv.es (V.S.-M.); p.terron.prof@ufv.es (P.T.-M.); vicente.fernandez@ufv.es (V.F.-R.)

2 School of Exercise and Sports Sciences, School of Health Sciences, Universidad Francisco de Vitoria, Pozuelo de Alarcón, 28049 Madrid, Spain; esther.morencos@ufv.es

3 Faculty of Sport Sciences, Europea de Madrid University, Villaviciosa de Odón, 28670 Madrid, Spain; archit.navandar@universidadeuropea.es

4 Center for Translational Research in Physiotherapy, Department of Pathology and Surgery, Miguel Hernández University, 03202 Elche, Alicante, Spain; vmoreno@goumh.umh.es

* Correspondence: alvaro.lopez@ufv.es;

Abstract: The aim of this study was to determine the acute effect of simulated field hockey match-play on isometric knee flexion, adductor (ADD) and abductor (ABD) strength, adductor/abductor (ADD/ABD) strength ratio, countermovement jump height (CMJ), hip flexion and ankle dorsiflexion range of motion (ROM). Thirty competitive female field hockey players (23.0 ± 3.9 years old) participated in the study. Apart from the afore-mentioned variables, external (through GPS) and internal load (through RPE) were measured before (pre-match) and immediately after simulated hockey match-play (post-match) in both limbs. Isometric knee flexion strength (+7.0%, $p = 0.047$) and hip flexion ROM (+4.4%, $p = 0.022$) were higher post-match in the non-dominant limb, while CMJ values reduced (−11.33%, $p = 0.008$) when comparing from pre-match data. In addition, no differences were observed for isometric hip ADD, ABD, ADD/ABD strength ratio, passive hip flexion ROM and ankle dorsiflexion ROM test. A simulated field-hockey match produces an increment in hip isometric strength and hip flexion ROM values in the non-dominant limb and a decrease in jump height capacity. As a result, CMJ assessment should be considered post-match in order to identify players who would require further rest before returning to training.

Keywords: risk factors; performance; team sport; fatigue; groin; hamstring

1. Introduction

Field hockey is an intermittent sport where hockey players perform repeated actions such as changes of direction, dribbles, sprints, accelerations, decelerations and body impacts alternating high and moderate with low intensity efforts [1]. During an official field hockey match, consisting of four quarters of fifteen minutes each, hockey players cover around 6000–8000 m [2,3] primarily at low and medium intensities, with high-intensity efforts (>19 km/h^{-1}) making up around 6% of the total playing time [2]. Previous studies have reported an average of 14 to 48 injuries per 1000 h attributed to the high physical demands of this sport [4,5]. Specifically, most of these field hockey injuries have been reported in the lower limbs, especially in the thigh and groin [6], with the hamstring strain injury being the most frequent muscle injury (32%) [4], followed by the groin injury (10%) [6]. Consequently, identification of the risk factors associated with groin and/or hamstring injury occurrence is essential.

In this sense, previous studies in different intermittent sports such as football [7], tennis [8] and ice hockey [9], have identified several modifiable intrinsic risk factors as causing an increased likelihood of developing groin and hamstring injuries. Among them, a weakness in the isometric adductor strength (ADD) [7,10] and lower adduction/abduction strength ratio (ADD/ABD) [9] have been associated with a higher risk of sustained groin injuries, while a lower hamstring strength [11–13], decreased range of hip flexion [14] and ankle dorsiflexion range of motion (ROM) have been associated with hamstring strain injuries [15]. However, some conflicting results have been found in literature regarding these factors [16–18]. Notably, most researches have investigated these risk factors before the commencement of the season or in off-season situations [19]. However, the ability to capture fluctuations in ROM and/or strength profile in-season, specifically in response to match-play, has not been studied [19].

Similar to other intermittent sports, field hockey players reported a higher incidence of injuries during matches compared to training [6] probably due to the higher intensity reported in matches versus training, and the appearance of fatigue [20,21]. It is well known that there is a decrement of lower limbs' power performance after match-play, and this measure is one of the potential factors in injury causation in intermittent sport [22]. Appearance of fatigue is known to reduce sports performance through reduced muscle strength, neuromuscular control and ROM [22]. In this line, the impact of match-play on ADD, ABD, hamstring strength and ROM during hip flexion and ankle dorsiflexion has been studied recently in several sports such as tennis, football and basketball [19,23–25]; however, to the best of the authors' knowledge, there is no information regarding this effect in field hockey. Therefore, the aim of this study was to examine the acute effect of hockey match-play on several risk factors such as isometric knee flexion and hip ADD and ABD strength, ADD/ABD strength ratio, passive hip flexion ROM and ankle dorsiflexion ROM and countermovement jump (CMJ) in elite female hockey players.

2. Materials and Methods

2.1. Subjects

Thirty highly competitive female hockey players (age, 23.0 ± 3.9 years; body mass, 60.0 ± 7.5 kg; height, 1.60 ± 0.09 m; body mass index, 22.0 ± 2.1 kg·m^2; hours per week, 9.4 ± 4.4; playing experience, 14.3 ± 4.9 years) volunteered to participate in this investigation. The players were recruited from two different professional teams. The inclusion criteria were: (a) To be healthy and able to complete a full game of field hockey; (b) to be uninjured and declared match-fit by the medical and coaching staff at the time of the experiment and not to have taken any type of medication to treat pain or musculoskeletal injuries at the time of the study; and (c) to have an absence of late onset muscle pain during the training session [26]. All players were informed of the tests they were to perform and signed the consent form. The experimental procedure of this study was conducted in accordance with the Declaration of Helsinki and the approval by the Ethics Committee of the University Francisco de Vitoria, number 45/2018.

2.2. Experimental Protocol

Following their arrival, female hockey players filled out a questionnaire which included personal information such as body mass, height, medical history, training frequency and experience (practice hours per week and playing experience in field hockey). Testing (i.e., ROM, isometric strength, and countermovement jump) was performed in the clinical area of each field hockey club. Testing was conducted by two sports physiotherapists: a senior physiotherapist with over nineteen years of experience and a junior physiotherapist with two years of experience, to ensure participants' positioning during measurements. Considering recommendations by Wollin, Thorborg and Pizzari [19], the testing order of the players and the selection of the leg tested were randomly chosen prior to the pre-match test. Pre-match testing was performed 60 min prior to match-play, and the post-match re-testing was performed immediately after the match. At the beginning of the pre-match testing, participants carried out a standardized warm-up that consisted of 5 min of jogging at 10 km·h^{-1} and 5 min of static stretches and joint mobility exercises [27]. Subsequently, participants played the simulated field hockey match according to the International Hockey Federation rules on a rectangular surface, 91.40 m long and 55.00 m wide. The external load of the simulated matches were estimated using a global positioning system (GPS) (Wimu ProTM, RealTrack Systems, Spain) placed in specific vests worn by the players, these devices operated at a sampling frequency of 10 Hz and its validity and reliability have been reported previously [28]. In addition, subjective internal load of the game was obtained using the modified RPE scale (i.e., 0–10 points) within 30 min of match termination [29]. The following variables were used to assess the external load during match-play, total distance covered per minute at different velocities ranges during a 60 min match as previously reported [3]. To reduce the interference of uncontrolled variables, all subjects were instructed to maintain their habitual lifestyle and normal dietary intake before and during the study, and refrain from caffeine ingestion 24 h before the experiment [30].

2.3. Isometric Strength of Abductors (ABD) Adductors (ADD) and Knee Flexion

Hip isometric ADD and ABD strength were measured according to the methodology previously reported [31] using a portable handheld dynamometer (Nicholas Manual Muscle Tester; Lafayette Indiana Instruments, Lafayette, IN, USA). Participants were placed in a supine position with their hips in a neutral position and told to stabilize themselves by holding onto the sides of the table. Examiner 1 applied a resistance on a fixed position (ABD: At 5 cm proximal to the lateral malleolus; ADD: At 5 cm proximal to the medial malleolus). The hockey players were instructed to exert a voluntary contraction for a maximum of 5 s against the dynamometer [31]. Two attempts were registered for each contraction of each limb and a 30 s rest period between attempts. Regarding the isometric knee flexion, the strength test was evaluated by placing the subject in the prone position, with 15 degrees of knee flexion and with their hips in a neutral position [32]. Examiner 1 placed the dynamometer on the distal portion of the sural triceps, three centimeters above the bimalleolar line. Examiner 2 clamped the subject's pelvis over the sacrum, to prevent elevation during the test. Examiner 1 requested the participant to flex their knee with the intention of bringing the heel of the foot to the gluteus. Similarly, two repetitions were recorded for each limb with a 30 s rest between attempts. Isometric hip ADD, ABD and knee flexion strength was expressed as the maximal hip and knee torque per kilogram of body weight ($Nm{\cdot}kg^{-1}$) using the external lever arm and body weight of each participant. The mean value out of two attempts was recorded and selected for further analysis.

2.4. Ankle Dorsiflexion ROM

Unilateral ankle dorsiflexion ROM was measured with LegMotion System (LegMotion, Check your Motion, Albacete, Spain). The testing was carried out following the methodology previously described by Calatayud et al. [33]; participants were in a standing position on the LegMotion System with the tested foot on the measurement platform and the contralateral foot out of the platform with the toes at the edge of it. Each player performed the test with their hands on the hips and the assigned foot in the middle of the longitudinal line behind the transversal line of the platform. From this position, subjects were instructed to flex the knee forwards, placing it in contact with the metal stick. When the subject was able to maintain heel and knee contact, the metal stick was progressively moved away from the knee, and the following achieved distance was recorded. Two attempts were allowed for each limb (i.e., left and right), with 15 s of passive recovery between trials. The mean value of the two attempts was selected for further analysis.

2.5. Hip Flexion ROM

Passive hip flexion ROM values with the knee extended were evaluated with the Straight Leg Elevation Test (SLET). Participants made two maximum passive attempts for the dominant and non-dominant leg, when the difference between one attempt and another was greater than 5%, a third attempt was made, selecting the mean value of the two attempts whose results were similar for further statistical analysis [34]. A unilevel inclinometer ISOMED (Portland, OR, USA) with a telescopic was used for the measurement. The test ended with one or more of the following criteria: (a) The examiner was unable to continue the joint movement evaluated due to the high resistance developed by the stretched muscle group; (b) The participant reported an important sensation of discomfort; or (c) The examiners noted compensations that could increase the ROM [35]. The inclinometer was placed approximately on the external malleolus and the distal arm was aligned parallel to an imaginary bisecting line of the extremity [35]. The mean value out of two attempts was recorded and selected for further analysis.

2.6. Countermovement Jump (CMJ)

Participants carried out three repetitions of CMJ using a contact mat jump system (Chronojump Boscosystem, Barcelona, Spain) with their arms on hips [36]. They were instructed to jump and land in the same place, with the body in an erect position during the jump until landing. Each participant performed two maximal CMJs interspersed with 45 s of passive recovery. In addition, the mean value out of two attempts was recorded and selected for further analysis.

2.7. Statistical Analysis

Data were calculated as means/standard deviation. The Shapiro–Wilk test was selected to assess the normal distribution. All study variables were compared using a t test (pre- vs. post-match). The statistical significance level was set at $p < 0.05$. Cohen's effect sizes were calculated and presented with their respective 95% confidence intervals (C.I.) based on the following criteria: Trivial effect (0–0.19), small effect (0.20–0.49), medium effect (0.50–0.79) and large effect (0.80 and greater) [37]. All the statistical analyses were completed using the SPSS software version 25 (SPSS Inc., Chicago, IL, USA).

3. Results

3.1. Match-Play Workload

The internal match-play workload was 6.83 ± 0.80 units (RPE). In addition, female hockey players covered a mean distance of 5456.50 ± 699.09 m across different velocity profiles (Table 1).

Table 1. Mean distances and % of total distance covered during the match at different velocity ranges.

Velocity Range	Distance Covered (m)	Total Distance (%)
0.0–6.0 km·h^{-1}	2692.04 ± 614.70	49.36 ± 9.71
6.1–12.0 km·h^{-1}	1781.15 ± 380.97	32.47 ± 4.53
12.1–18.0 km·h^{-1}	851.66 ± 282.16	15.74 ± 5.48
18.1–21.0 km·h^{-1}	107.59 ± 75.87	1.98 ± 1.40
21.1–24.0 km·h^{-1}	21.59 ± 23.66	0.40 ± 0.44
>24.1 km·h^{-1}	2.47 ± 6.19	0.05 ± 0.12

Abbreviations: km·h^{-1} = kilometers/hour; m = meters.

3.2. Isometric Strength and Countermovement Jump

No statistical differences were seen in relative isometric hip ABD strength in the dominant (+2.42%, $p = 0.864$, ES [C.I.] = 0.01 [−0.08, 0.11]) (Figure 1a) and non-dominant limb (−1.46%, $p = 0.834$, ES [C.I.] = −0.02 [−0.12, 0.07]) (Figure 1b); nor in the relative isometric hip ADD strength in the dominant(−2.10%, $p = 0.399$, ES [C.I.] = 0.10 [0.00, 0.19]) (Figure 1c) and non-dominant limb (+3.38%, $p = 0.349$, ES [C.I.] = 0.11 [0.02, 0.21]) (Figure 1d). In addition, no differences were obtained in ADD/ABD strength ratios in dominant (1.14 vs. 1.19, $p = 0.220$, ES [C.I.] = 0.28 [0.19–0.37]) and non-dominant limbs (0.98 vs. 0.96, $p = 0.600$, ES [C.I.] = 0.14 [0.05–0.24]) when comparing them pre and post-match. However, for isometric knee flexion strength, statistical differences were obtained in the non-dominant limb (7.0%, $p = 0.047$; ES [C.I.] = 0.29 [0.20, 0.38]) (Figure 1f) but no differences were reported in the dominant limb (0.1%, $p = 0.983$; ES [C.I.] = 0.11 [0.02, 0.21]) (Figure 1f). Finally, neuromuscular fatigue was measured by a countermovement jump test after match-play (23.0 ± 4.9 vs. 20.5 ± 6.6 cm, $p = 0.008$, ES [C.I.] = 0.44 [0.34, 0.53]).

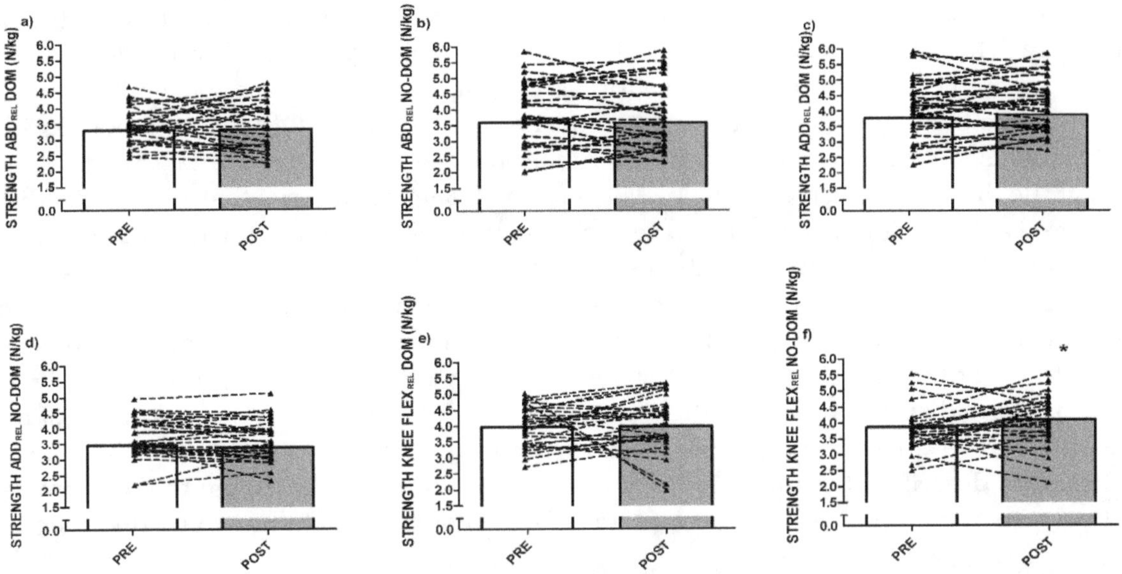

Abbreviations: DOM = dominant; NO-DOM = non-dominant; ADD = Adductor; ABD = Abductor; FLEX = flexion; REL = relative. * Significant differences compared to the PRE values at p < 0.05.

Figure 1. Hip and knee isometric hip abduction (ABD), adduction (ADD) and knee flexion strength values. (**a**) Relative isometric hip ABD strength in the dominant limb; (**b**) relative hip abductor strength in the non-dominant limb; (**c**) relative hip adductor strength in the dominant limb; (**d**) relative hip adductor strength in the non-dominant limb; (**e**) relative knee flexion strength in the dominant limb; (**f**) relative knee flexion strength in the non-dominant limb.

3.3. Hip Flexion and Ankle ROM

A significant increase was found when comparing the ROM in the hip flexion (straight leg elevation raise test) for the non-dominant limb (+4.38% $p = 0.022$). However, no differences were found in the dominant limb (+1.19%, $p = 0.753$) (Table 2). In addition, no differences were obtained for ankle dorsiflexion ROM values after field hockey match in the dominant limb (−3.77%; $p = 0.316$) and non-dominant limb (−2.34%; $p = 0.362$) (Table 2).

Table 2. Hip and ankle range of motion (ROM).

Variables	Pre-Match	Post-Match	*p*-Value	ES [95%CI]
Straight Leg Elevation Test DOM (°)	81.1 ± 12.3	82 0 ± 9.1	0.753	0.09 [0.00–0.18]
Straight Leg Elevation Test NO-DOM (°)	81.4 ± 10.3	84.9 ± 9.9	0.022 *	0.35 [0.26–0.45]
Ankle dorsiflexion DOM (cm)	10.9 ± 2.5	10.4 ± 2.7	0.316	0.16 [0.06–0.25]
Ankle dorsiflexion NO-DOM (cm)	11.1 ± 2.7	10.8 ± 2.7	0.362	0.10 [0.00–0.19]

Abbreviations: DOM = dominant-side; NO-DOM = non-dominant side; ° = degrees; cm = centimeters; * Significant differences compared to the PRE values at $p < 0.05$.

4. Discussion

The aim of this study was to determine the acute effect of hockey match-play on several risk factors such as isometric knee flexion, hip ADD and ABD strength, ADD/ABD strength ratio, passive hip flexion ROM, ankle dorsiflexion ROM and CMJ in competitive female hockey players. To the best of the authors' knowledge, this is the first study that analyzed the acute effects of hockey match-play on several risk factors in female athletes. The main results showed that hockey match-play acutely produced a decrease in CMJ performance, and an increase in isometric knee flexion strength and hip flexion ROM with knee extension in the non-dominant limb. However, no significant differences were found in isometric hip ADD, ABD strength and ADD/ABD strength ratio and ankle dorsiflexion ROM in both limbs.

The CMJ is one of the most important tests used to evaluate the lower-limb muscles fatigue [38,39]. The results in this study showed a significant reduction in levels of performance in CMJ (−11.33%) after match-play which was in agreement with previous studies conducted in other intermittent sports [40,41]. Recent research from Kim and Kipp [42] has shown that the gastrocnemius, soleus and vastus muscles have the largest contribution to vertical center of mass (COM) acceleration during the CMJ, and the soleus and gastrocnemius muscles function closest to their maximal capacities. If one were to look at the distances covered by the players (Table 1), one can observe that most of the distance had been covered at lower intensities. Here, the production of the horizontal force has been attributed to the muscles of the lower limb: namely tibialis anterior, gastrocnemius and soleus [2]. This indicates that a greater fatigue caused by distances ran at these intensities appears to have increased the neuromuscular fatigue associated with the CMJ, leading to a decrease in performance. In addition, albeit speculative, another possible reason for the decrease values in the CMJ test after match-play has been attributed to disruptions within the muscular fibers [41], increasing some markers of muscle damage (e.g., creatine-kinase, myoglobin) after a match in intermittent sports [41,43]. Moreover, previous literature described the inflammatory responses and fibrillar damage to the muscles and showed a decrease in metabolic indices in athletes after playing a match; however, this speculation requires further investigation.

Muscle strength in the lower limbs is essential to produce explosive actions in hockey (e.g., accelerations, changes of direction). The results obtained in the present study showed improvements in the isometric knee flexion strength (+7.0%) immediately post-match in the non-dominant limb. While no previous study has reported knee flexion strength values in field hockey players, these results differ from previous studies conducted in other intermittent sports, which revealed a lower knee flexion strength post-match-play [19,44]. The lack of agreement between studies could be related to the different match-play demands of the participants (e.g., total distance covered, duration of match, etc.). While in the current study hockey players reported an average of 5456.50 ± 699.09 m total distance covered and 21.59 ± 23.66 m at high speeds over 21 km·h^{-1}, previous studies in female soccer players showed they covered distances over 10,000 m during a match (90 min duration), of which at least 600 m were at high speed running intensities [45]. The current results suggest that the effect provoked by field-hockey match-play did not decrease the isometric knee flexion strength in the dominant limb, which has been related to a higher hamstring injury risk in previous studies [46,47]. The absence of changes in the isometric knee flexion strength can be attributed to the lower distances covered at high running speeds. Extensive research [47] has shown that the hamstring muscles are most active in this phase, when their function is to increase stride frequency and produce a greater horizontal force as the contact time reduces. Given the distances covered in the different zones, it can be assumed that the hamstring muscles are not fatigued as in sports such as soccer, where a greater distance is covered at these intensities.

A reduced ROM during the straight leg raise test and dorsiflexion of the ankle ROM has been linked to the risk of hamstring injury [14,15]. Present results have shown an increase in the straight leg raise ROM levels for the non-dominant limb (+5.81%) and no significant differences in the dominant limb. No differences were seen for the ankle dorsiflexion ROM either for both legs after match-play. To the best of the authors' knowledge, only Wollin et al. (2017) analyzed the straight leg raise ROM after match-play on intermittent sports and report no significant differences after match-play [19]. Concerning ankle dorsiflexion ROM, some previous studies conducted in football [24], basketball [25] and Australian-rules football [44] showed different results. While Charlton et al. [44] reported reductions in ankle dorsiflexion ROM immediately after an Australian-rules football match, Wollin et al. [19] showed non-significant decrements in football players, and finally Moreno-Pérez et al. [24,25] in football and basketball observed increased ROM values post-match from pre-match in dominant and non-dominant limbs. While these sports involve the same multidirectional movements (e.g., accelerations, decelerations, changes of direction) during practice, they cannot be compared due to the differences in the characteristics of the sport; for example, the total duration is less in field hockey than other intermittent sports. Thus, increases in hip flexion ROM immediately post-match are likely due to the increase in tissue extensibility induced by temperature increment which leads to a reduction of the viscous resistance of muscle tissues and joints [48,49]. However, this is a speculation that needs to be elucidated in future studies.

As far as isometric hip ADD and ABD strength values and ADD/ABD strength ratio go, the results showed no significant differences between post-match from pre-match. While is difficult to establish comparisons, as no previous study has reported isometric hip ADD and ABD strength values in hockey players, the findings of the current study were similar to those of a previous study [50] conducted with 14 rugby players. However, the present results disagree with the results reported by a previous study in tennis players [23]. This lack of agreement between studies may be due to differences in physical demands and tactical aspects between the sports. In tennis, players are required to perform repetitive short high-intensity movements, which impose an elevated concentric and eccentric load on the ADD muscles, while hockey players perform multiple different movements at several intensities. One must also consider that hockey, like in rugby, permits rolling substitutions.

This study contains limitations that require acknowledgment. Firstly, as the current study was conducted with a specific sample of female field hockey players, conducted during a simulated match, the characteristics of the players do not permit a generalization of the results found. In addition, the selected measures in this study in response to hockey match-play were performed immediately post-match; future studies should evaluate these variables using several time-points to understand the recovery fatigue induces, for example registering data 48 h after the match. This study looked at the effect following a single simulated match; more data collected over a series of official matches, or even, over an entire season could provide more conclusive results about the effects of match-play on these potential risk factors.

5. Conclusions

A simulated field-hockey match increases hip isometric flexion strength and hip flexion ROM in the non-dominant limb and decreases jump height capacity. However, no differences were reported in isometric ADD and ABD strength and ADD/ABD strength ratio in the dominant and non-dominant limb, or in dominant hip flexion and ankle dorsiflexion ROM values between the pre- and post-match examinations. Finally, female hockey players who present a decrease in jump height capacity, may require additional rest between training and competitions.

Author Contributions: Conceptualization, V.S.-M., A.L.-S. and V.M.-P.; methodology, A.L.-S. and V.M.-P.; software, A.N.; validation, V.S.-M., A.L.-S., A.N. and V.M.-P.; formal analysis, V.S.-M., A.L.-S., A.N. and V.M.-P.; investigation, V.S.-M., A.L.-S., P.T.-M., E.M., V.F.-R., A.N. and V.M.-P.; resources, V.S.-M., A.L.-S., P.T.-M. and V.M.-P.; data curation, V.S.-M., A.L.-S., A.N. and V.M.-P.; writing-original draft preparation, V.S.-M., A.L.-S., A.N. and V.M.-P.; writing-review and editing, V.S.-M., A.L.-S., P.T.-M., E.M., V.F.-R., A.N. and V.M.-P.; visualization, A.L.-S. and V.M.-P.; supervision, A.L.-S. and V.M.-P.; project administration, A.L.-S. and V.M.-P.; funding acquisition, P.T.-M.; All authors have read and agreed to the published version of the manuscript.

Acknowledgments: We would like to thank the participants for their uninterested participation in this project.

References

1. Reilly, T.; Borrie, A. Physiology applied to field hockey. *Sports Med.* **1992**, *14*, 10–26. [CrossRef] [PubMed]
2. Lythe, J.; Kilding, A.E. Physical demands and physiological responses during elite field hockey. *Int. J. Sports Med.* **2011**, *32*, 523–528. [CrossRef] [PubMed]

3. White, A.D.; MacFarlane, N. Time-on-pitch or full-game GPS analysis procedures for elite field hockey? *Int. J. Sports Physiol. Perform.* **2013**, *8*, 549–555. [CrossRef] [PubMed]
4. Rodas, G.; Pedret, C.; Yanguas, J.; Pruna, R.; Medina, D.; Hägglund, M.; Ekstrand, J. Male field hockey prospective injury study. Comparison with soccer. *Arch. Med. Deporte* **2009**, *129*, 22–30.
5. Theilen, T.M.; Mueller-Eising, W.; Wefers Bettink, P.; Rolle, U. Injury data of major international field hockey tournaments. *Br. J. Sports Med.* **2016**, *50*, 657–660. [CrossRef] [PubMed]
6. Barboza, S.D.; Joseph, C.; Nauta, J.; van Mechelen, W.; Verhagen, E. Injuries in Field Hockey Players: A Systematic Review. *Sports Med.* **2018**, *48*, 849–866. [CrossRef]
7. Engebretsen, A.H.; Myklebust, G.; Holme, I.; Engebretsen, L.; Bahr, R. Intrinsic risk factors for groin injuries among male soccer players: A prospective cohort study. *Am. J. Sports Med.* **2010**, *38*, 2051–2057. [CrossRef]
8. Moreno-Perez, V.; Lopez-Valenciano, A.; Barbado, D.; Moreside, J.; Elvira, J.L.L.; Vera-Garcia, F.J. Comparisons of hip strength and countermovement jump height in elite tennis players with and without acute history of groin injuries. *Musculoskelet Sci. Pract.* **2017**, *29*, 144–149. [CrossRef]
9. Tyler, T.F.; Nicholas, S.J.; Campbell, R.J.; McHugh, M.P. The association of hip strength and flexibility with the incidence of adductor muscle strains in professional ice hockey players. *Am. J. Sports Med.* **2001**, *29*, 124–128. [CrossRef]
10. Moreno-Perez, V.; Travassos, B.; Calado, A.; Gonzalo-Skok, O.; Del Coso, J.; Mendez-Villanueva, A. Adductor squeeze test and groin injuries in elite football players: A prospective study. *Phys. Ther. Sport Off. J. Assoc. Chart. Physiother. Sports Med.* **2019**, *37*, 54–59. [CrossRef]
11. Lee, J.W.Y.; Mok, K.M.; Chan, H.C.K.; Yung, P.S.H.; Chan, K.M. Eccentric hamstring strength deficit and poor hamstring-to-quadriceps ratio are risk factors for hamstring strain injury in football: A prospective study of 146 professional players. *J. Sci. Med. Sport* **2018**, *21*, 789–793. [CrossRef]
12. Ribeiro-Alvares, J.B.; Oliveira, G.D.S.; De Lima, E.S.F.X.; Baroni, B.M. Eccentric knee flexor strength of professional football players with and without hamstring injury in the prior season. *Eur. J. Sport Sci.* **2020**, 1–9. [CrossRef] [PubMed]
13. Tol, J.L.; Hamilton, B.; Eirale, C.; Muxart, P.; Jacobsen, P.; Whiteley, R. At return to play following hamstring injury the majority of professional football players have residual isokinetic deficits. *Br. J. Sports Med.* **2014**, *48*, 1364–1369. [CrossRef] [PubMed]
14. Witvrouw, E.; Danneels, L.; Asselman, P.; D'Have, T.; Cambier, D. Muscle flexibility as a risk factor for developing muscle injuries in male professional soccer players. A prospective study. *Am. J. Sports Med.* **2003**, *31*, 41–46. [CrossRef] [PubMed]
15. Gabbe, B.J.; Finch, C.F.; Bennell, K.L.; Wajswelner, H. Risk factors for hamstring injuries in community level Australian football. *Br. J. Sports Med.* **2005**, *39*, 106–110. [CrossRef]
16. Mosler, A.B.; Weir, A.; Serner, A.; Agricola, R.; Eirale, C.; Farooq, A.; Bakken, A.; Thorborg, K.; Whiteley, R.J.; Holmich, P.; et al. Musculoskeletal Screening Tests and Bony Hip Morphology Cannot Identify Male Professional Soccer Players at Risk of Groin Injuries: A 2-Year Prospective Cohort Study. *Am. J. Sports Med.* **2018**, *46*, 1294–1305. [CrossRef]
17. van Dyk, N.; Bahr, R.; Burnett, A.F.; Whiteley, R.; Bakken, A.; Mosler, A.; Farooq, A.; Witvrouw, E. A comprehensive strength testing protocol offers no clinical value in predicting risk of hamstring injury: A prospective cohort study of 413 professional football players. *Br. J. Sports Med.* **2017**, *51*, 1695–1702. [CrossRef]
18. van Dyk, N.; Farooq, A.; Bahr, R.; Witvrouw, E. Hamstring and Ankle Flexibility Deficits Are Weak Risk Factors for Hamstring Injury in Professional Soccer Players: A Prospective Cohort Study of 438 Players Including 78 Injuries. *Am. J. Sports Med.* **2018**, *46*, 2203–2210. [CrossRef]
19. Wollin, M.; Thorborg, K.; Pizzari, T. The acute effect of match play on hamstring strength and lower limb flexibility in elite youth football players. *Scand. J. Med. Sci. Sports* **2017**, *27*, 282–288. [CrossRef] [PubMed]
20. Morencos, E.; Romero-Moraleda, B.; Castagna, C.; Casamichana, D. Positional Comparisons in the Impact of Fatigue on Movement Patterns in Hockey. *Int. J. Sports Physiol. Perform.* **2018**, *13*, 1149–1157. [CrossRef]
21. Rishiraj, N.; Taunton, J.E.; Niven, B. Injury profile of elite under-21 age female field hockey players. *J. Sports Med. Phys. Fit.* **2009**, *49*, 71–77.
22. Small, K.; McNaughton, L.R.; Greig, M.; Lohkamp, M.; Lovell, R. Soccer fatigue, sprinting and hamstring injury risk. *Int. J. Sports Med.* **2009**, *30*, 573–578. [CrossRef] [PubMed]

23. Moreno-Perez, V.; Nakamura, F.Y.; Sanchez-Migallon, V.; Dominguez, R.; Fernandez-Elias, V.E.; Fernandez-Fernandez, J.; Perez-Lopez, A.; Lopez-Samanes, A. The acute effect of match-play on hip range of motion and isometric strength in elite tennis players. *PeerJ* **2019**, *7*, e7940. [CrossRef] [PubMed]
24. Moreno-Perez, V.; Soler, A.; Ansa, A.; Lopez-Samanes, A.; Madruga-Parera, M.; Beato, M.; Romero-Rodriguez, D. Acute and chronic effects of competition on ankle dorsiflexion ROM in professional football players. *Eur. J. Sport Sci.* **2020**, *20*, 51–60. [CrossRef]
25. Moreno-Perez, V.; Del Coso, J.; Raya-Gonzalez, J.; Nakamura, F.Y.; Castillo, D. Effects of basketball match-play on ankle dorsiflexion range of motion and vertical jump performance in semi-professional players. *J. Sports Med. Phys. Fit.* **2020**, *60*, 110–118. [CrossRef] [PubMed]
26. Navandar, A.; Veiga, S.; Torres, G.; Chorro, D.; Navarro, E. A previous hamstring injury affects kicking mechanics in soccer players. *J. Sports Med. Phys. Fit.* **2018**, *58*, 1815–1822. [CrossRef] [PubMed]
27. Mora-Rodriguez, R.; Garcia Pallares, J.; Lopez-Samanes, A.; Ortega, J.F.; Fernandez-Elias, V.E. Caffeine ingestion reverses the circadian rhythm effects on neuromuscular performance in highly resistance-trained men. *PLoS ONE* **2012**, *7*, e33807. [CrossRef]
28. Bastida-Castillo, A.; Gomez-Carmona, C.D.; De La Cruz Sanchez, E.; Pino-Ortega, J. Comparing accuracy between global positioning systems and ultra-wideband-based position tracking systems used for tactical analyses in soccer. *Eur. J. Sport Sci.* **2019**, *19*, 1157–1165. [CrossRef]
29. Foster, C.; Florhaug, J.A.; Franklin, J.; Gottschall, L.; Hrovatin, L.A.; Parker, S.; Doleshal, P.; Dodge, C. A new approach to monitoring exercise training. *J. Strength Cond. Res.* **2001**, *15*, 109–115.
30. Jodra, P.; Lago-Rodriguez, A.; Sanchez-Oliver, A.J.; Lopez-Samanes, A.; Perez-Lopez, A.; Veiga-Herreros, P.; San Juan, A.F.; Dominguez, R. Effects of caffeine supplementation on physical performance and mood dimensions in elite and trained-recreational athletes. *J. Int. Soc. Sports Nutr.* **2020**, *17*, 2. [CrossRef]
31. Thorborg, K.; Bandholm, T.; Petersen, J.; Weeke, K.M.; Weinold, C.; Andersen, B.; Serner, A.; Magnusson, S.P.; Holmich, P. Hip abduction strength training in the clinical setting: With or without external loading? *Scand. J. Med. Sci. Sports* **2010**, *20*, 70–77. [CrossRef] [PubMed]
32. Thorborg, K.; Petersen, J.; Magnusson, S.P.; Holmich, P. Clinical assessment of hip strength using a hand-held dynamometer is reliable. *Scand. J. Med. Sci. Sports* **2010**, *20*, 493–501. [CrossRef] [PubMed]
33. Calatayud, J.; Martin, F.; Gargallo, P.; Garcia-Redondo, J.; Colado, J.C.; Marin, P.J. The validity and reliability of a new instrumented device for measuring ankle dorsiflexion range of motion. *Int. J. Sports Phys. Ther.* **2015**, *10*, 197–202. [PubMed]
34. Cejudo, A.; Sainz de Baranda, P.; Ayala, F.; Santonja, F. Test-retest reliability of seven common clinical tests for assessing lower extremity muscle flexibility in futsal and handball players. *Phys. Ther. Sport Off. J. Assoc. Chart. Physiother. Sports Med.* **2015**, *16*, 107–113. [CrossRef] [PubMed]
35. Moreno-Perez, V.; Ayala, F.; Fernandez-Fernandez, J.; Vera-Garcia, F.J. Descriptive profile of hip range of motion in elite tennis players. *Phys. Ther. Sport Off. J. Assoc. Chart. Physiother. Sports Med.* **2016**, *19*, 43–48. [CrossRef]
36. Bosco, C.; Luhtanen, P.; Komi, P.V. A simple method for measurement of mechanical power in jumping. *Eur. J. Appl. Physiol. Occup. Physiol.* **1983**, *50*, 273–282. [CrossRef]
37. Cohen, J. A power primer. *Psychol. Bull.* **1992**, *112*, 155–159. [CrossRef]
38. Markovic, G.; Dizdar, D.; Jukic, I.; Cardinale, M. Reliability and factorial validity of squat and countermovement jump tests. *J. Strength Cond. Res.* **2004**, *18*, 551–555. [CrossRef]
39. Gathercole, R.J.; Sporer, B.C.; Stellingwerff, T.; Sleivert, G.G. Comparison of the Capacity of Different Jump and Sprint Field Tests to Detect Neuromuscular Fatigue. *J. Strength Cond. Res.* **2015**, *29*, 2522–2531. [CrossRef]
40. de Hoyo, M.; Cohen, D.D.; Sanudo, B.; Carrasco, L.; Alvarez-Mesa, A.; Del Ojo, J.J.; Dominguez-Cobo, S.; Manas, V.; Otero-Esquina, C. Influence of football match time-motion parameters on recovery time course of muscle damage and jump ability. *J. Sports Sci.* **2016**, *34*, 1363–1370. [CrossRef]
41. Andersson, H.; Raastad, T.; Nilsson, J.; Paulsen, G.; Garthe, I.; Kadi, F. Neuromuscular fatigue and recovery in elite female soccer: Effects of active recovery. *Med. Sci. Sports Exerc.* **2008**, *40*, 372–380. [CrossRef]
42. Kim, H.; Kipp, K. Number of Segments Within Musculoskeletal Foot Models Influences Ankle Kinematics and Strains of Ligaments and Muscles. *J. Orthop. Res. Off. Publ. Orthop. Res. Soc.* **2019**, *37*, 2231–2240. [CrossRef] [PubMed]

43. Magalhaes, J.; Rebelo, A.; Oliveira, E.; Silva, J.R.; Marques, F.; Ascensao, A. Impact of Loughborough Intermittent Shuttle Test versus soccer match on physiological, biochemical and neuromuscular parameters. *Eur. J. Appl. Physiol.* **2010**, *108*, 39–48. [CrossRef] [PubMed]
44. Charlton, P.C.; Raysmith, B.; Wollin, M.; Rice, S.; Purdam, C.; Clark, R.A.; Drew, M.K. Knee flexion strength is significantly reduced following competition in semi-professional Australian Rules football athletes: Implications for injury prevention programs. *Phys. Ther. Sport Off. J. Assoc. Chart. Physiother. Sports Med.* **2018**, *31*, 9–14. [CrossRef]
45. Datson, N.; Drust, B.; Weston, M.; Jarman, I.H.; Lisboa, P.J.; Gregson, W. Match Physical Performance of Elite Female Soccer Players During International Competition. *J. Strength Cond. Res.* **2017**, *31*, 2379–2387. [CrossRef] [PubMed]
46. Schache, A.G.; Dorn, T.W.; Williams, G.P.; Brown, N.A.; Pandy, M.G. Lower-limb muscular strategies for increasing running speed. *J. Orthop. Sports Phys. Ther.* **2014**, *44*, 813–824. [CrossRef]
47. Morin, J.B.; Gimenez, P.; Edouard, P.; Arnal, P.; Jimenez-Reyes, P.; Samozino, P.; Brughelli, M.; Mendiguchia, J. Sprint Acceleration Mechanics: The Major Role of Hamstrings in Horizontal Force Production. *Front. Physiol.* **2015**, *6*, 404. [CrossRef]
48. Bishop, D. Warm up I: Potential mechanisms and the effects of passive warm up on exercise performance. *Sports Med.* **2003**, *33*, 439–454. [CrossRef]
49. Opplert, J.; Babault, N. Acute Effects of Dynamic Stretching on Muscle Flexibility and Performance: An Analysis of the Current Literature. *Sports Med.* **2018**, *48*, 299–325. [CrossRef]
50. Roe, G.A.; Phibbs, P.J.; Till, K.; Jones, B.L.; Read, D.B.; Weakley, J.J.; Darrall-Jones, J.D. Changes in Adductor Strength After Competition in Academy Rugby Union Players. *J. Strength Cond. Res.* **2016**. [CrossRef]

6

Can We Rely on Flight Time to Measure Jumping Performance or Neuromuscular Fatigue-Overload in Professional Female Soccer Players?

Estrella Armada-Cortés [1,2], Javier Peláez Barrajón [1], José Antonio Benítez-Muñoz [3], Enrique Navarro [1] and Alejandro F. San Juan [1,*]

1 Department of Health and Human Performance, Sport Biomechanics Laboratory, Facultad de Ciencias Actividad Física y Deporte—INEF, Universidad Politécnica de Madrid, 28040 Madrid, Spain; cortesarmadaestrella@gmail.com (E.A.-C.); javi.pelaezb@gmail.com (J.P.B.); enrique.navarro@upm.es (E.N.)

2 Department of Physical Activity and Sports Science, Faculty of Sport Sciences, University of Castilla-La Mancha, 45071 Toledo, Spain

3 Department of Health and Human Performance, LFE Research Group, Facultad de Ciencias Actividad Física y Deporte—INEF, Universidad Politécnica de Madrid, 28040 Madrid, Spain; jbenitez020@gmail.com

* Correspondence: alejandro.sanjuan@upm.es

Featured Application: It is recommended that high-level sportswomen and men should be assessed with the force platform through the take-off velocity method in a vertical jump as gold standard technology to ensure correct performance and/or fatigue-overload control during the sport season.

Abstract: The main purpose of this study was to compare the validity of the take-off velocity method (TOV) measured with a force platform (FP) (gold standard) versus the flight time method (FT) in a vertical jump to measure jumping performance or neuromuscular fatigue-overload in professional female football players. For this purpose, we used a FP and a validated smartphone application (APP). A total of eight healthy professional female football players (aged 27.25 ± 6.48 years) participated in this study. All performed three valid trials of a countermovement jump and squat jump and were measured at the same time with the APP and the FP. The results show that there is a lack of validity and reliability between jump height (JH) calculated through the TOV method with the FP and the FT method with the FP ($r = 0.028$, $p > 0.84$, intraclass correlation coefficient (ICC) = −0.026) and between the JH measured with the FP through the TOV method and the APP with the FT method ($r = 0.116$, $p > 0.43$, ICC = −0.094 (−0.314–0.157)). A significant difference between the JH measured through the TOV with the FP versus the APP ($p < 0.05$), and a trend between the JH obtained with the FP through the TOV and the FT ($p = 0.052$) is also shown. Finally, the JH with the FP through the FT and the APP did not differ ($p > 0.05$). The eta-squared of the one-way ANOVA was $\eta 2 = 0.085$. It seems that only the TOV measured with a FP could guarantee the accuracy of the jump test in SJ+CMJ and SJ, so it is recommended that high-level sportswomen and men should be assessed with the FP through TOV as gold standard technology to ensure correct performance and/or fatigue-overload control during the sport season.

Keywords: vertical jump; flight time; take-off velocity; fatigue; muscle overload; performance; force platform; smartphone application; APP; female soccer

1. Introduction

The vertical jump (VJ) is one of the most widely used performance tests. Its popularity is due both to its simplicity and effectiveness [1], and to the similarity between its movement patterns and sports, explosiveness, speed, and intensity [2,3]. Moreover, it is a useful tool to assess physical fitness in a healthy population (i.e., children, adults, and elderly people) [4–6], and to control an adequate musculoskeletal injury recovery [7]. There are different jump protocols; two of the most frequently used are: (1) The squat jump (SJ), which provides a basic leg strength parameter and is described by some authors as pure concentric [3]; (2) the counter movement jump (CMJ) adds an elastic-reactive component of the subject. It is estimated that the CMJ value can be up to 25% higher than the SJ in athletes [8]. Their performance has been used to: (1) monitor the positive effects of strength, plyometric, resistance, and speed training; and (2) control mechanical and neuromuscular fatigue status in individual and team sports [9]. Several researchers have found that CMJ performance is an interesting objective marker of fatigue and overcompensation for athlete performance [9], being one of the factors related to the high incidence of injuries (e.g., muscle overload) in the lower limb muscles [10,11]. Thus, a relationship has been observed between height loss in the CMJ and metabolic markers such as lactate or ammonium in the sprint [12], and after a Wingate test [13]. This suggests that through decreases in the CMJ's mechanical variables such as jump height (JH), it should be possible to estimate the metabolic stress, neuromuscular fatigue, and overload of the subject [5,12,14].

Specific performance factors for both the CMJ and SJ include a number of different kinematic and kinetic variables. Some of these variables are more sensitive than others to determine an athlete's neuromuscular status and may depends of the age and level of the subjects: JH, power, velocity and force (peak, relative peak, and mean of the last three), rate of force development (RFD), and mean impulse [9]. In addition, it has been proven that it is better to average the number of jumps executed than to choose the one that obtained the maximum height [9].

To obtain the height value of the jump we can use two variables: the take-off velocity (TOV) or the flight time (FT) [15,16]:

1. The TOV is the vertical velocity of the center of mass at takeoff. The height value of the jump will be the result of velocity at takeoff squared divided by twice the gravity:

$$\left(h = \frac{V^2}{2g}\right) \tag{1}$$

2. The FT is the time period between takeoff and land contact (i.e., the subject is on the air, without land contact). The height value of the jump will be the result of the gravity value multiplied by FT squared, divided by eight:

$$\left(h = \frac{gt^2}{8}\right) \tag{2}$$

There are many tools used to evaluate the performance of the jump (e.g., force platforms (FP), contact mats, video analysis through a smartphone applications (APPs), accelerometers, infrared systems, *Vertec* Vertical Jump Measuring Device). Most devices use the FT to calculate the JH [17]. However, to measure it in an accurate manner, the height of the center of mass at takeoff and landing has to be the same. Any difference between the athlete's takeoff and landing center of mass position (e.g., different joint position of ankle, knee, or hip) could increase or decrease the FT, and then change the result of the JH estimation [15,17]. Considering these technical implications, TOV has been suggested as the more suitable method to evaluate the JH [18]. If the TOV can be measured easily by a FP, then it is considered the gold standard for measuring the height of the VJ [19,20]. A FP can measure and use either the FT or the TOV methodology, the latter being the most accurate method for determining the height of the VJ [19].

The need to quantitatively evaluate the performance of the athlete's JH has promoted the emergence of APPs for this purpose. Some authors have reported that these APPs have a high reliability and accuracy in their measures [21,22], while others qualify their results as equivocal, so it is not yet clear what is the ideal methodology to use [23].

Although the VJ and its performance can be extrapolated to any sport level, the greater the level the subjects have, the more correlation exists in its variables, so it is in high performance sport where it has more utility [24]. Moreover, the accuracy of the results is essential from a competitive point of view in high-level sports, for example in elite-cyclists improvements of around 0.6% are sufficient to make a difference [25].

Therefore, the main purpose of this study was to compare the validity of the TOV method using a FP versus the FT method using a FP and a smartphone application to measure jumping performance or neuromuscular fatigue-overload in professional female football players.

2. Materials and Methods

2.1. Participant Selection: Inclusion and Exclusion Criteria

A total of eight healthy professional female football players of the First and Second Spanish Football Divisions (Liga Iberdrola and Reto Iberbrola, respectively) (aged 27.25 ± 6.48 years; body mass 56.73 ± 4.86 kg; height 1.61 ± 0.06 m. Values expressed as mean ± standard deviation) participated in this study.

Inclusion criteria were: (1) playing in a female professional soccer league; (2) not having suffered a musculoskeletal injury one year prior to the date of the protocol (i.e., checked through a previous exclusion questionnaire); (3) not presenting any cardiovascular, musculoskeletal, and/or neurological disease, nor previous ones that could affect participation in the study. Exclusion criteria were: (1) aged younger than 18 years; (2) having consumed any narcotic and/or psychotropic agents or drugs during the test. We have selected this specific study population to homogenize the level of the sample and to deepen the knowledge of women's professional soccer.

At the study outset, participants were informed of the study protocol, schedule, and nature of the exercises and tests to be performed before signing an informed consent form. The study protocol adhered to the tenets of the Declaration of Helsinki and was approved by the Ethics Committee of the Technical University of Madrid (Madrid, Spain).

2.2. Experimental Design

This study consisted of a single evaluation session (see Figure 1) in a laboratory in the same time frame to avoid the detrimental performance effects associated with circadian rhythm [26]. Subjects were required to avoid physically demanding activity in the 24 h prior to the session.

Three valid trials of a CMJ and SJ were conducted with each subject, with 60 s recovery between trials, and three minutes between each jump test (see Figure 1). All jumps were measured at the same time with the mobile application and on the FP.

The sessions began with a 10-min general warm up consisting of continuous running, specific running, joint mobility, and ballistic stretching exercises, followed by a specific pre-test warm-up where participants performed five SJs and CMJs with 30 s between each jump. After three minutes of rest, the participants started the jumping test.

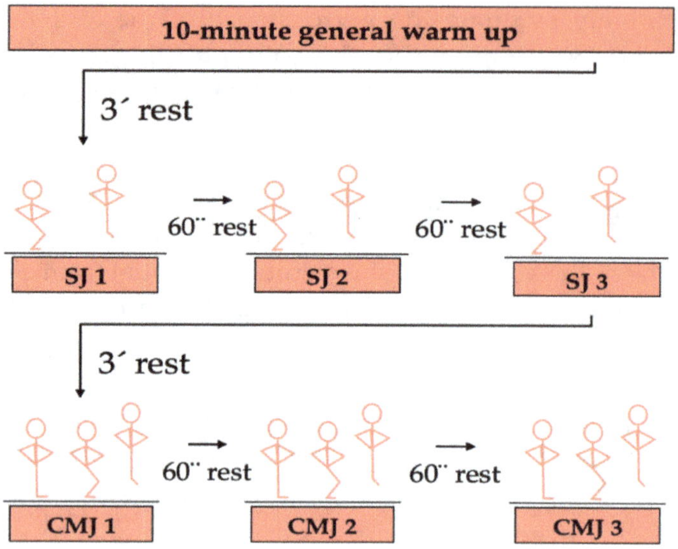

Figure 1. Experimental design. CMJ = countermovement jump test; SJ = squat jump.

2.3. Vertical Jump Test

The VJs included in the present study were the CMJ and SJ, which have been previously demonstrated to be reliable measures (intraclass correlation coefficient (ICC) = 0.97 and 0.96, respectively) [27]. All participants were completely familiarized with both techniques (i.e., they realized these tests during the soccer season). Moreover, they practice before the test during the specific warm-up (see warm-up description above). Participants were always instructed to jump as high as possible, keeping their hands on their hips and that their legs should remain straight during flight, making contact with the ground with the tips of their feet and knees extended [28]. In both modalities, the aim was to reach the maximum height by means of the jump; nevertheless, each modality of jump consists of different characteristics [29].

The CMJ (Figure 2a) initial position consists of a static standing position with hands on the hips. From this position, a continuous and fast triple hip, knee, and ankle flexion movement is executed until reaching ≈ 90° of knee flexion, followed by the triple extension of the same joints in a fluid, fast, and continuous way [29]. In this type of VJ, there is a stretching-shortening cycle (SSC), which takes place during the consecutive eccentric, isometric, and concentric phases [29].

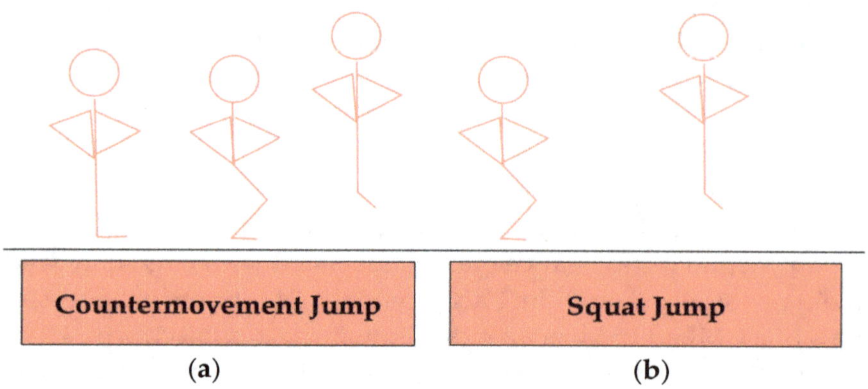

Figure 2. (**a**) Countermovement Jump; (**b**) Squat Jump.

The SJ (Figure 2b) only presents the concentric component. The initial position consists of maintaining the hips and knees flexed at ≈ 90° for approximately four seconds to avoid countermovement and the elastic component. From this position, the concentric phase of the jump with an explosive extension of the lower limb joints is performed. All participants were asked to jump as high as possible and without performing a SSC [29]. The SJ forces before takeoff were checked on the FP to ensure that the participant did not perform countermovement.

For both jumps, participants were asked to take off and land at the same place to avoid lateral or horizontal displacement. Only successful trials were considered. Participants were asked to repeat the trial if a jump was incorrectly performed.

2.4. Instruments

2.4.1. Force Platform

Two 600 mm × 400 mm piezoelectric platforms (Type 9286AA; Kistler Instruments AG, Winterthur, Switzerland) mounted together on the floor according to the manufacturer's instructions, were used in this experiment. The force sensors of these platforms were constituted by piezoelectric transducers 5 kN, total max 20 kN. Data were recorded at a sampling frequency of 1000 Hz. The FPs were connected to a portable computer with specific software, the Measurement, Analysis and Reporting Software "Kistler MARS" (Kistler Instruments AG, Winterthur, Switzerland).

2.4.2. Smartphone Application

The validated smartphone application used to measure the performance of the jump was My Jump2 (APP) [30] installed on a mobile phone (iPhone 6s Apple, Cupertino, CA, USA) at a sampling rate of 240 Hz. My Jump was designed for analyzing VJ measuring the time (in ms) between two frames selected by the user and subsequently to calculate the JH using the equation based on FT. The position of the camera was always at ~1.5 m from the middle line of the subject so that it was constantly aligned with the reference joint points.

After the recording, one researcher manually selected the frames in which the subject performed exactly the moments of take-off and landing. A second person was consulted in case of doubt when analyzing the jumps with the APP. The JH was calculated based on the FT between the selected take-off and landing frame, as previously described [30].

2.5. Statistical Analysis

The normality and homogeneity of the data were analyzed using the Shapiro–Wilk and Levene tests, respectively. The normality and homogeneity of the dependent variables was confirmed ($p > 0.05$); all of the data are provided as their means and standard deviations.

Various statistical analyses were used to prove the APP validity and reliability in comparison with the FP using FT and TOV to calculate JH. The Pearson correlation coefficient (r) was used to calculate the concurrent validity between the APP and the FP using different measurement methods.

To expound the magnitude of the relationship between height measurements by the APP and the FP, Cohen's convention was used. To measure reliability between the APP and the FP, the coefficient of variation (CV), an absolute agreement Intraclass Correlation Coefficient (ICC), and Cronbach's Alpha were used. The CV was used to observe the uniformity of the values with respect to the mean. A Bland–Altman plot was created to graphically represent the agreement between the APP's measured heights and FP FT measured heights.

The mean differences between the measurements for each jump (SJ and CMJ) and for both jumps together (CMJ + SJ) were calculated through a one-way ANOVA, and Tukey's post-hoc test was used to analyze pairwise comparisons between means. The standard error of estimate (SEE) was used to show the typical error in measurement. Significance was set at $p < 0.05$. All statistical analyses were performed using the software package SPSS® version 25 (IBM Co., USA).

3. Results

The coefficients of variation values were very small for the CMJs with the FP through the TOV, the FP through the FT and the APP (2.82%, 3.56%, and 3.55%, respectively), and for the SJ (12.44%, 5.24%, and 4.88%, respectively).

The Pearson's correlation showed a poor relationship and a small reliability between the JH measured through the FT and the TOV, both measured with the FP (r = 0.028, $p > 0.84$, ICC = −0.026, 95% CI = −0.276–0.24) (Figure 3), and between the JH measured with the FP through the TOV and the APP (r = −0.116, $p > 0.43$, ICC = −0.094, 95% CI = −0.314–0.157) (Figure 4).

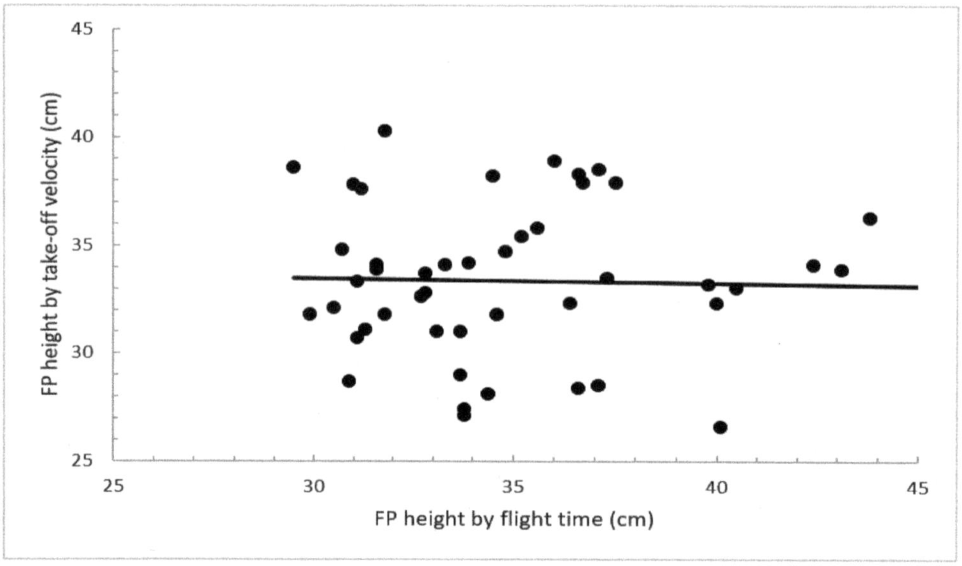

Figure 3. Pearson's correlation between jump heights measured by the FP using take-off velocity and the FP using flight time; FP, force platform; graph made by the authors.

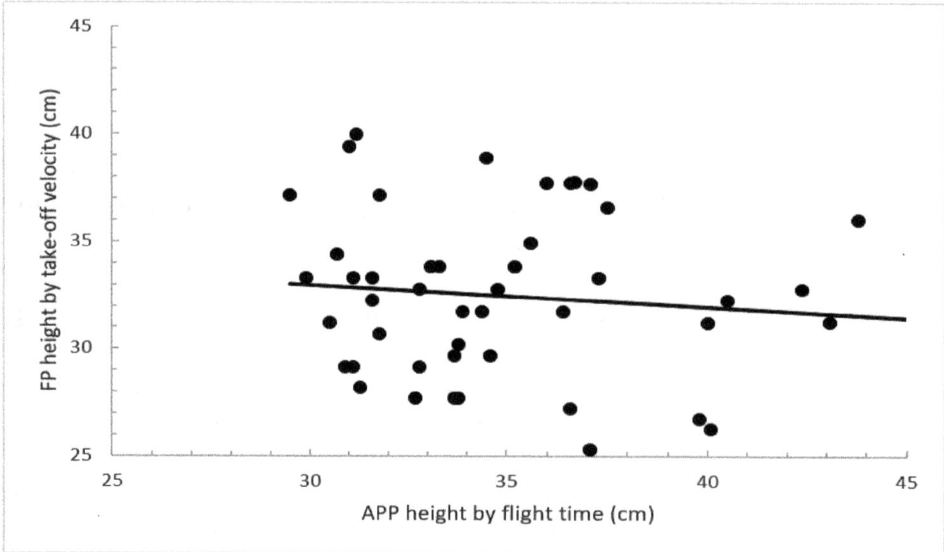

Figure 4. Pearson's correlation between jump heights measured by the FP using take-off velocity and the APP using flight time; FP, force platform; APP, My Jump App; graph made by the authors.

On the other hand, a high and significant relationship between the JH measured with the FP through the FT and the APP (r = 0.872, $p < 0.01$) was found (Figure 5). Moreover, there was a very high agreement between these two variables as revealed by the ICC = 0.843 (95% CI = 0.681–0.919) and Bland–Altman plots (Figure 6).

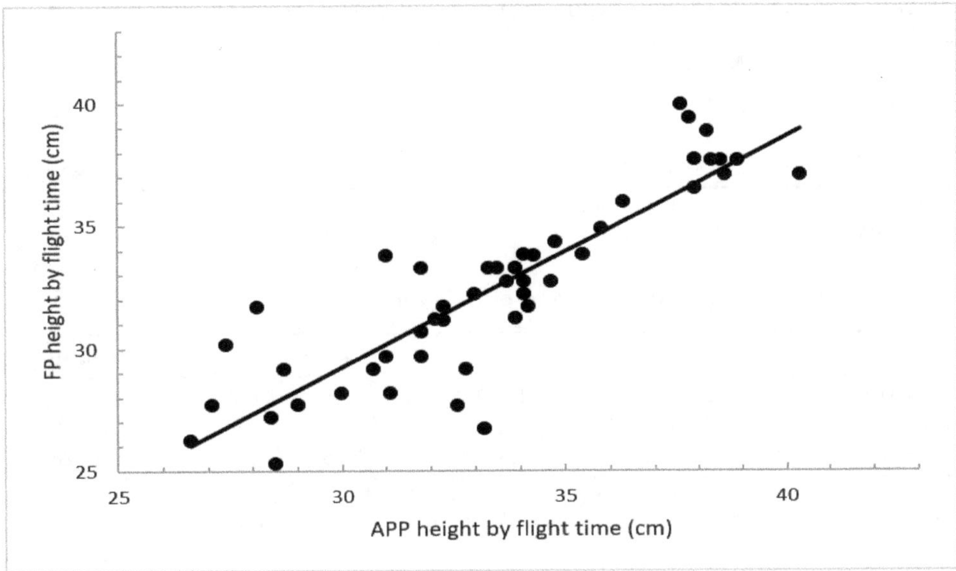

Figure 5. Pearson's correlation between jump heights measured by the FP using flight time and the APP using flight time; FP, force platform; APP, My Jump App; graph made by the authors.

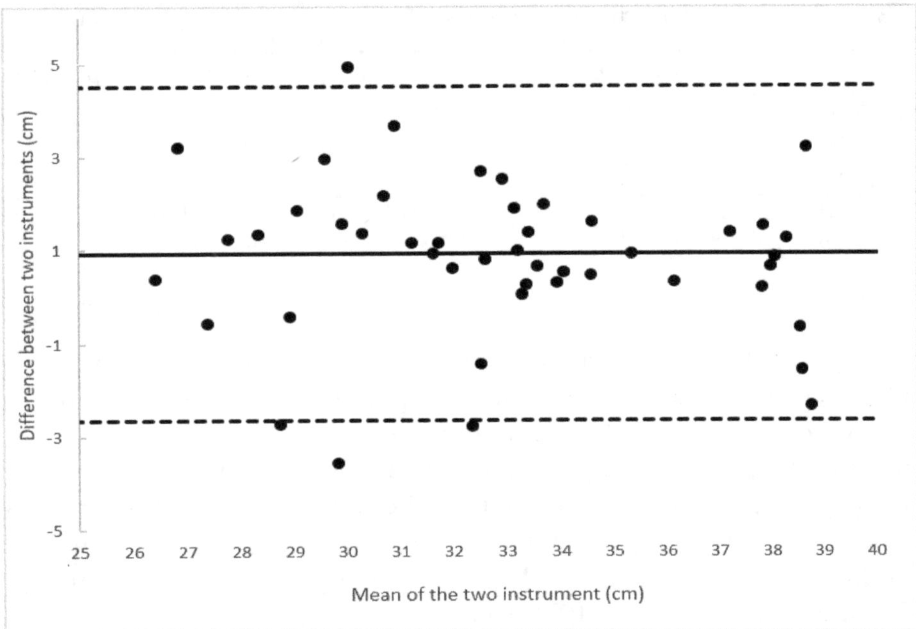

Figure 6. Bland–Altman plot between the FP using flight time and the APP using flight time to measure jump height. The central line represents the systematic bias between instruments, while the upper and the lower lines represent ± 1.96 SD; FP, force platform; APP, My Jump App; graph made by the authors.

The one-way ANOVA shows a significant difference between the JH measured with the FP through the TOV versus the APP ($p = 0.002$), and a trend versus the FP through the FT ($p = 0.052$). Finally, the JH analyzed with the FP through the FT and the APP did not differ ($p = 0.457$) (Table 1). The eta squared of the one-way ANOVA was $\eta 2 = 0.085$.

Specifically, in SJ, the one-way ANOVA shows a significant difference in JH measured with the FP through the TOV versus the FP and the APP both through the FT ($p < 0.01$). Finally, the JH analyzed with the FP through FT and the APP did not differ ($p = 0.826$) (Table 2). The eta squared of the one-way ANOVA used to compare SJ was $\eta 2 = 0.374$.

Table 1. Values of the different methods for measuring jump height combining CMJ and SJ.

	Mean ± SD		Mean ± SD	*p* Value
FP–TOV	35.21 ± 4.22	FP–FT	33.36 ± 3.48	0.052
FP–TOV	35.21 ± 4.22	APP	32.43 ± 3.77	0.002 *
FP–FT	33.36 ± 3.48	APP	32.43 ± 3.77	0.457

Data are presented as mean ± standard deviation. FP–TOV: Force Platform–Take-Off Velocity; FP–FT: Force Platform–Flight Time; APP: My Jump Application (flight time). * Significant difference.

Table 2. Values of the different methods for measuring SJ jump height.

	Mean ± SD		Mean ± SD	*p* Value
FP–TOV	37.23 ± 4.68	FP–FT	31.53 ± 3.09	0.000 *
FP–TOV	37.23 ± 4.68	APP	30.89 ± 3.33	0.000 *
FP–FT	31.53 ± 3.09	APP	30.89 ± 3.33	0.826

Data are presented as mean ± standard deviation. FP–TOV: Force Platform–Take-Off Velocity; FP–FT: Force Platform–Flight Time; APP: My Jump Application (flight time); SJ: squat jump. * Significant difference.

Lastly, in CMJ, the one-way ANOVA did not show significant differences between JH measured by the different methods ($p = 0.07$, η2 = 0.073) (Table 3).

Table 3. Values of the different methods for measuring CMJ jump height.

	Mean ± SD		Mean ± SD	*p* Value
FP–TOV	33.18 ± 2.44	FP–FT	35.19 ± 2.87	0.060
FP–TOV	33.18 ± 2.44	APP	33.96 ± 3.60	0.644
FP–FT	35.19 ± 2.87	APP	33.96 ± 3.60	0.336

Data are presented as mean ± standard deviation. FP–TOV: Force Platform–Take-Off Velocity; FP–FT: Force Platform–Flight Time; APP: My Jump Application (flight time); CMJ; countermovement jump.

4. Discussion

The main purpose of this study was to compare the validity of the TOV method using a FP versus the FT method using a FP and a smartphone application to measure jumping performance or neuromuscular fatigue-overload in professional female soccer players.

The major findings were the lack of reliability and validity between JH measured with the FP through the TOV and JH measured through the FT either by the FP (r = 0.028, $p > 0.84$, ICC = −0.026 (−0.276–0.24)) or the APP (r = 0.116, $p > 0.43$, ICC = −0.094 (−0.314–0.157)). To our knowledge, this is the first study that has researched the JH of SJ and CMJ together (SJ + CMJ) with these technologies: FP trough the TOV and trough FT, and APP through FT. Two previous studies [20,31] have analyzed the SJ, CMJ and CMJ with arms (CMJA), together comparing JH with FP vs. contact mat (both through FT method) [20], and with FP (TOV and FT methods) vs. contact mat (FT method) [31]. This latter study [31] concluded that the TOV must be used instead of the FT as a more valid and accurate way to calculate the VJ performance. It provides a more sensitive approach to scientifically establishing jump determinants, greater sensitivity in analyzing changes in performance factors after training (i.e., overcompensation, overload), and greater accuracy in monitoring performance within the session (i.e., fatigue) [18,19]. Further, the mean comparison shows a significant difference between the JH measured with the FP through the TOV versus the APP ($p = 0.002$), and a trend versus the FP through the FT ($p = 0.052$). To our knowledge, there is only one previous study that researched the differences between the FP through the TOV versus a smartphone application (FT method) [19], and it showed near perfect correlations (ICC = 0.996; $p < 0.001$). These differences with our results may be explain by some reasons: 1) In our study the subjects performed three different CMJs and SJs, while in the previous study the subjects performed five CMJs [19]; (2) The distance between the researcher and the subject was of 1 m in the previous study [19], while in our study it was of 1.5 m; (3) In addition, rest between jumps was not specified in the previous study [19], so it is not possible to know if fatigue could have affected their results through the FT method (i.e., Different joint position between take-off and landing), whilst our subjects rested 60 s between trials and three minutes between each jump test. Despite these methodological differences, their results comparing the FP through the TOV versus a smartphone application (FT method) regarding only CMJ did not differ with our CMJ results. Based on the present study and the literature [19,20], it seems that the flight time method, independent of the technology used (e.g., FP, contact mat, smartphone application), is an imprecise means of assessment.

On the other hand, there is a high correlation and good reliability between the JH SJ+CMJ measured through the FT with the FP and the APP (r = 0.872, $p < 0.01$, ICC = 0.843, CV = 4.88%). These results are in accordance with other studies that compare the SJ+CMJ+CMJA height using a FP and a contact mat (both through FT) (r = 0.99, $p < 0.001$, ICC = 0.985, CV% = 2.7) [21]. Additionally, the mean comparison of the present study shows that the JH analyzed with the FP through the FT and the APP did not differ ($p = 0.457$). Therefore, the APP and the contact mat seem to equal the accuracy of the FP with the FT method. However, it is important to highlight the fact that some studies compare the My Jump APP based on FT, with other instruments also based on FT (i.e., contact mat or FP through the FT) [21,30,31], instead of comparing it with the FP through the TOV (gold standard) [16]. Therefore, all these technologies that use the FT method are not as precise as the TOV method. Bearing in mind that the most accurate and considered the gold standard method to measure the height of the jump is the FP based on the TOV [19,20], these are the results that should be trusted.

Analyzing specifically the different jumps, it was found in SJ significant differences between the JH measured with the FP through the TOV and the FP and the APP through the FT ($p < 0.01$ in both cases). However, we found no significant difference comparing the JH measured with the FP and the APP (both through the FT) ($p = 0.826$). Further, CMJ data showed no significant differences among the three methods (i.e., FP through the TOV versus the FP and the APP through the FT) ($p > 0.05$ in both cases). Our results are in line with the only one previous study that researched the differences between the FP through the TOV versus a smartphone application (FT method) [19], and it showed near perfect correlations (ICC = 0.996; $p < 0.001$). Results of the reliability and validity obtained in the present study comparing the CMJ height through the FT with the FP and the APP (r = 0.872, $p < 0.01$, ICC = 0.843 and CV = 4.88%) are in accordance with the first validation study of My Jump App [30] that compare the CMJ height using a FP through FT (r = 0.995, $p < 0.001$, ICC = 0.997, CV% = 3.5), and other study that compare the CMJ height using a contact mat and the My Jump App (both through FT) (r = 0.999, $p < 0.001$, ICC = 0.948, CV% = 10.096) [21]. Despite the differences between the sampling frequency of the devices (i.e., FP $\approx$1000 Hz and the smartphone camera $\approx$ 240 Hz), the height values obtained were very similar between the two methods, as reflected by the ICC.

The literature that evaluates the smartphone applications in this area has analyzed the CMJ as the only vertical jump option discarding the SJ [19,21]. However, with this study it has been demonstrated that the results of the CMJ cannot be extrapolated to the SJ. The height of the SJ and CMJ is defended by several authors as a method to detect fatigue and individualize load prescriptions, so the reduction of the height of the VJ can be interpreted as evidence of the deterioration of neuromuscular function (i.e., fatigue, neuromuscular overload) [12]. Its measurement could provide a relatively simple and accessible tool for quantifying the degree of neuromuscular, mechanical, and metabolic fatigue [5,12,32]. This fatigue can remain for up to 48–72 h after a high-intensity session [33]. It could therefore provide useful feedback to coaches to determine the impact of training loads on player recovery and performance [12]. The neuromuscular factor is considered the most influential factor in training and is also an intrinsic risk factor of an athlete's injury [34]. The lack of strength and poor coordination capacity are part of it [35]. Several studies have observed that after a fatiguing exercise bout and during the landing phase of different jump types, there is a change in the neuromuscular control strategies used by these subjects [36,37]. These motor control alterations are associated with different injury risk factors, such as reduced knee and hip flexion, increased knee valgus, increased ground reaction force, and greater stabilization time [37]. In high-level sports, measurement accuracy is critical in the assessment of performance and in the control and assimilation of training loads to avoid muscle–tendon overloads [25]. In addition, some authors recommend the evaluation of jumping performance, especially at high and elite levels [24]. In this sense and referring to the exclusive sample of this study, as they are professional female soccer players, these small variations described above should be considered and limited as far as possible. In our study, the differences in JH between the FP through the TOV versus through the FT was 5.23% (1.84 cm) and the differences between the FP through the TOV versus the APP was 7.90% (2.78 cm). The only previous study that researched the differences between the FP (TOV method) versus a smartphone application (FT method) [19], found a small overestimated JH obtained from the APP of 0.78% compared to the FP based on TOV [19]. This small difference (0.78%) is more than ten times lower than the differences reported by us (7.90%), more than six times the difference between FP–TOV vs. FT methods (5.23%), and more than three times lower than the differences between the FP (FT method) and the APP (2.8%). This latter difference reported in the present study between the FP (FT method) and the APP agree with other studies comparing the My Jump application and a FP (FT method) [30], and an infrared contact mat and a FP (both through the FT method) [19]. More research regarding the issue is needed to clarify if smartphone applications may replace a FP (TOV method) in professional environments where accuracy is a key factor (i.e., high-level sport, medical clinic).

Furthermore, we observed that the difference of JH between the FP and the APP both through the FT was smaller, only 2.8% (0.94 cm). These latter results are in accordance with previous studies that observed differences in JH between an infrared contact mat and a FP, both through the FT of ≈ 2.5% (1.06 cm) [19], and between the My Jump application and a FP both through the FT (1.1 ± 0.5 cm) [30]. These concordances are produced because they use the FT method (i.e., less accurate) to compare different technologies. When the FT method is used with any technology, even the FP, there are many possibilities to produce measurement errors because the takeoff and the landing positions are different (e.g., different degree of lower limbs joint/s flexion) [38]. Then, it seems recommendable that high-level sportswomen and men should be assessed with this gold standard technology and method (i.e., FP and TOV method) to ensure correct performance and/or overload control during the sport season.

5. Conclusions

The results of the present study showed that in female professional soccer players, there is a lack of validity and reliability between JH in SJ + CMJ and SJ calculated with the TOV method versus the FT method. It seems that only the TOV measured with a FP could guarantee the accuracy of the jump test.

In order to be able to generalize our conclusions to different athlete populations, future research is needed, aiming at comparing the validity and reliability between JH of different kind of jumps calculated with the TOV method versus the FT method on high-level and recreationally trained athletes from different sport modalities and both sexes.

Author Contributions: Conceptualization, E.A.-C., J.A.B.-M. and A.F.S.J.; methodology, E.A.-C., J.P.B., J.A.B.-M., E.N. and A.F.S.J.; validation, E.A.-C. and A.F.S.J.; formal analysis, E.A.-C., J.P.B. and A.F.S.J.; investigation, E.A.-C., J.P.B., J.A.B.-M. and A.F.S.J.; resources, E.A.-C., E.N. and A.F.S.J.; supervision, E.N. and A.F.S.J.; project administration, E.N. and A.F.S.J. All authors have read and agreed to the published version of the manuscript.

References

1. Cronin, J.; Gill, N.D. Fatigue Monitoring in High Performance Sport: A Survey of Current Trends. *J. Aust. Strength Cond.* **2012**, *20*, 12–23.
2. Yamauchi, J.; Ishii, N. Relations Between Force-Velocity Characteristics of the Knee-Hip Extension Movement and Vertical Jump Performance. *J. Strength Cond. Res.* **2007**, *21*, 703–709. [PubMed]

3. Nagahara, R.; Naito, H.; Miyashiro, K.; Morin, J.B.; Zushi, K. Traditional and ankle-specific vertical jumps as strength-power indicators for maximal sprint acceleration. *J. Sports Med. Phys. Fitness* **2014**, *54*, 691–699. [PubMed]
4. Ramírez-Campillo, R.; Castillo, A.; de la Fuente, C.I.; Campos-Jara, C.; Andrade, D.C.; Álvarez, C.; Martinez, C.; Castro-Sepulveda, M.; Pereira, A.; Marques, M.C.; et al. High-speed resistance training is more effective than low-speed resistance training to increase functional capacity and muscle performance in older women. *Exp. Gerontol.* **2014**, *58*, 51–57. [CrossRef] [PubMed]
5. Maté-Muñoz, J.L.; Lougedo, J.H.; Garnacho-Castaño, M.V.; Veiga-Herreros, P.; Lozano-Estevan, M.D.C.; García-Fernández, P.; de Jesus, F.; Guodemar-Perez, J.; San Juan, A.F.; Dominguez, R. Effects of β-alanine supplementation during a 5-week strength training program: A randomized, controlled study. *J. Int. Soc. Sports Nutr.* **2018**, *15*, 19. [CrossRef]
6. Fernandez-Santos, J.R.; Ruiz, J.R.; Cohen, D.D.; Gonzalez-Montesinos, J.L.; Castro-Piñero, J. Reliability and Validity of Test to Assess Lower-Body Muscular Power in Children. *J. Strength Cond. Res.* **2015**, *29*, 2277–2285. [CrossRef]
7. Setuain, I.; Millor, N.; Alfaro, J.; Gorostiaga, E.; Izquierdo, M. Jumping performance differences among elite professional handball players with or without previous ACL reconstruction. *J. Sports Med. Phys. Fitness* **2015**, *55*, 1184–1192.
8. Sánchez, W.G.; Gómez, D.A.; Quiceno, H.B.; Alzate, S.J. Análisis comparativo intrasujeto en salto vertical 2d: Squat jump y counter-movement jump Resumen Introducción. *VIREF Rev. Educ. Fís.* **2016**, *5*, 1–17.
9. Gustavo, J.; Cronin, J.; Mezêncio, B.; Travis, D.; Mcguigan, M.; Tricoli, V.; Carlos Amadio, A.; Cerca Serrao, J. The countermovement jump to monitor neuromuscular status: A meta-analysis. *J. Sci. Med. Sport* **2017**, *20*, 397–402.
10. Greig, M.; Siegler, J.C. Soccer-specific fatigue and eccentric hamstrings muscle strength. *J. Athl. Train.* **2009**, *44*, 180–184. [CrossRef]
11. Science, E.; Kingdom, U.; Activity, P.; Kingdom, U. Effect of Timing of Eccentric Hamstring Strengthening Exercises During Soccer Training: Implications for Muscle Fatigability. *J. Strength Cond. Res.* **2009**, *23*, 1077–1083.
12. Jiménez-Reyes, P.; Pareja-Blanco, F.; Cuadrado-Peñafiel, V.; Ortega-Becerra, M.; Párraga, J.; González-Badillo, J.J. Jump height loss as an indicator of fatigue during sprint training. *J. Sports Sci.* **2018**, *37*, 414. [CrossRef] [PubMed]
13. Reeve, T.C.; Tyler, C.J. The validity of the smartjump contact mat. *J. Strength Cond. Res.* **2013**, *27*, 1597–1601. [CrossRef] [PubMed]
14. Aragón-Vargas, L. Evaluation of Four Vertical Jump Tests: Methodology, Reliability, Validity and accuracy. *Meas. Phys. Educ. Exerc. Sci.* **2000**, *4*, 215–228. [CrossRef]
15. Buckthorpe, M.; Morris, J.; Folland, J.P. Validity of vertical jump measurement devices. *J. Sports Sci.* **2012**, *30*, 63–69. [CrossRef] [PubMed]
16. Moir, G.L. Three different methods of calculating vertical jump height from force platform data in men and women. *Meas. Phys. Educ. Exerc. Sci.* **2008**, *12*, 207–218. [CrossRef]
17. Ferro, A.; Floría, P.; Villacieros, J.; Muñoz-lópez, A. Maximum velocity during loaded countermovement jumps obtained with an accelerometer, linear encoder and force platform: A comparison of technologies. *J. Biomech.* **2019**, *95*, 109281. [CrossRef]
18. Jiménez-Reyes, P.; Pareja-Blanco, F.; Rodríguez-Rosell, D.; Marques, M.C.; González-Badillo, J.J. Maximal velocity as a discriminating factor in the performance of loaded squat jumps. *Int. J. Sports Physiol. Perform.* **2016**, *11*, 227–234. [CrossRef]
19. Carlos-Vivas, J.; Martin-Martinez, J.P.; Hernandez-Mocholi, M.A.; Perez-Gomez, J. Validation of the iphone app using the force platform to estimate vertical jump height. *J. Sports Med. Phys. Fitness* **2018**, *58*, 227–232.
20. Glatthorn, J.F.; Gouge, S.; Nussbaumer, S.; Stauffacher, S.; Impellizzeri, F.M.; Maffiuletti, N.A. Validity and Reliability of Optojump Photoelectric Cells for Estimating Vertical Jump Height. *J. Strength Cond. Res.* **2011**, *25*, 556–560. [CrossRef]
21. Cruvinel-Cabral, R.M.; Oliveira-Silva, I.; Medeiros, A.R.; Claudino, J.G.; Jiménez-Reyes, P.; Boullosa, D.A. The validity and reliability of the "my Jump App" for measuring jump height of the elderly. *PeerJ* **2018**, *6*, e5804. [CrossRef] [PubMed]

22. Brooks, E.R.; Benson, A.C.; Bruce, L.M. Novel technologies found to be valid and reliable for the measurement of vertical jump height with jump-and-reach testing. *J. Strength Cond. Res.* **2018**, *32*, 2038–2845. [CrossRef] [PubMed]
23. Leard, J.S.; Cirillo, M.A.; Katsnelson, E.; Kimiatek, D.A.; Miller, T.W.; Trebincevic, K.; Garbalosa, J.C. Validity of Two Alternative Systems for Measuring Vertical Jump Height. *J. Strength Cond. Res.* **2007**, *21*, 1296–1299. [PubMed]
24. Jiménez-Reyes, P.; Samozino, P.; García-Ramos, A.; Cuadrado-Peñafiel, V.; Brughelli, M.; Morin, J.-B. Relationship between vertical and horizontal force-velocity-power profiles in various sports and levels of practice. *PeerJ* **2018**, *6*, e5937. [CrossRef]
25. Paton, C.D.; Hopkins, W.G. Variation in performance of elite cyclists from race to race. *Eur. J. Sport Sci.* **2006**, *6*, 25–31. [CrossRef]
26. Drust, B.; Waterhouse, J.; Atkinson, G.; Edwards, B.; Reilly, T. *Circadian Rhythms in Sports Performance—An Update*; Chronobiology International; Taylor and Francis Inc.: Abingdon, UK, 2005; Volume 22, pp. 21–44.
27. Markovic, G.; Dizdar, D.; Jukic, I.; Cardinale, M. Reliability and Factorial Validity of Squat and Countermovement Jump Tests. *J. Strength Cond. Res.* **2004**, *18*, 551–555.
28. Jiménez-Reyes, P.; Cuadrado-Peñafiel, V.; González-Badillo, J.; Alfonso El Sabio, U.X.; Jiménez Reyes Universidad Alfonso el Sabio, P.X. Analysis of Variables Measured in Vertical Jump Related to Athletic Performance and its Application to Training. *Cult. Cienc. Deport.* **2011**, *6*, 113–119.
29. Bosco, C. *La Fuerza Muscular. Aspectos Metodológicos*, 1st ed.; INDE, Ed.; INO Reproducciones, S.A.: Barcelona, Spain, 2000; pp. 177–187.
30. Balsalobre-Fernández, C.; Glaister, M.; Lockey, R.A. The validity and reliability of an iPhone app for measuring vertical jump performance. *J. Sports Sci.* **2015**, *33*, 1574–1579. [CrossRef]
31. Gallardo-Fuentes, F.; Gallardo-Fuentes, J.; Ramírez-Campillo, R.; Balsalobre-Fernández, C.; Martínez, C.; Caniuqueo, A.; Canas, R.; Banzer, W.; Loturco, I.; Nakamura, F.; et al. Intersession and intrasession reliability and validity of the my jump app for measuring different jump actions in trained male and female athletes. *J. Strength Cond. Res.* **2016**, *30*, 2049–2056. [CrossRef]
32. San Juan, A.F.; López-Samanes, Á.; Jodra, P.; Valenzuela, P.L.; Rueda, J.; Veiga-Herreros, P.; Perez-Lopez, A.; Dominguez, R. Caffeine supplementation improves anaerobic performance and neuromuscular effciency and fatigue in Olympic-level boxers. *Nutrients* **2019**, *11*, 2120. [CrossRef]
33. Hellsten-westing, Y.; Norman, B.; Balsom, P.D.; Sjodin, B. Decreased resting levels of adenine nucleotides in human skeletal muscle after high-intensity training. *J. Appl. Phys.* **1993**, *74*, 2523–2528. [CrossRef] [PubMed]
34. Griffin, L.Y.; Albohm, M.J.; Arendt, E.A.; Bahr, R.; Beynnon, B.D.; DeMaio, M.; Dick, R.W.; Engebretsen, L.; Garrett, W.E.; Hannafin, J.A.; et al. Understanding and preventing noncontact anterior cruciate ligament injuries: A review of the Hunt Valley II Meeting, January 2005. *Am. J. Sports Med.* **2006**, *34*, 1512–1532. [CrossRef] [PubMed]
35. Fort Vanmeerhaeghe, A.; Romero Rodriguez, D. Neuromuscular risk factors of sports injury. In *Apunts Medicina de l'Esport*; Elsevier España, S.L.: Cataluña, Spain, 2013; Volume 48, pp. 109–120.
36. Borotikar, B.S.; Newcomer, R.; Koppes, R.; McLean, S.G. Combined effects of fatigue and decision making on female lower limb landing postures: Central and peripheral contributions to ACL injury risk. *Clin. Biomech.* **2008**, *23*, 81–92. [CrossRef] [PubMed]
37. McLean, S.G.; Felin, R.E.; Suedekum, N.; Calabrese, G.; Passerallo, A.; Joy, S. Impact of fatigue on gender-based high-risk landing strategies. *Med. Sci. Sports Exerc.* **2007**, *39*, 502–514. [CrossRef] [PubMed]
38. Kibele, A. Possibilities and Limitations in the Biomechanical Analysis of Countermovement Jumps: A Methodological Study. *J. Appl. Biomech.* **1998**, *14*, 105–117. [CrossRef]

7

A Correlational Analysis of Shuttlecock Speed Kinematic Determinants in the Badminton Jump Smash

Mark King [1], Harley Towler [1,*], Romanda Dillon [1] and Stuart McErlain-Naylor [1,2]

1 School of Sport, Exercise, and Health Sciences, Loughborough University, Loughborough LE11 3TU, UK; M.A.King@lboro.ac.uk (M.K.); R.Dillon@lboro.ac.uk (R.D.); s.mcerlain-naylor@uos.ac.uk (S.M.-N.)

2 School of Health and Sports Sciences, University of Suffolk, Ipswich IP3 8AH, UK

* Correspondence: H.Towler@lboro.ac.uk;

Featured Application: The findings suggest that players and/or coaches should focus on proximal segment movements: specifically, producing greater pelvis-thorax separation during the retraction phase and greater shoulder internal rotation at shuttle contact to increase shuttlecock speed.

Abstract: The forehand jump smash is an essential attacking stroke within a badminton player's repertoire. A key determinate of the stroke's effectiveness is post-impact shuttlecock speed, and therefore awareness of critical technique factors that impact upon speed is important to players/coaches. Three-dimensional kinematic data of player, racket and shuttlecock were recorded for 18 experienced players performing maximal effort forehand jump smashes. Joint angles and X-factor (transverse plane pelvis-thorax separation) were calculated at key instants: preparation, end of retraction, racket lowest point, turning point and shuttlecock contact. Peak shoulder, elbow, and wrist joint centre linear velocities, phase durations and jump height were also calculated. Correlational analyses were performed with post-impact shuttlecock speed, revealing significant correlations to peak wrist joint centre linear velocity ($r = 0.767$), acceleration phase duration ($r = -0.543$), shoulder internal/external rotation angle at shuttlecock contact ($r = 0.508$) and X-factor at the end of retraction ($r = -0.484$). Multiple linear regression analysis revealed 43.7% of the variance in shuttlecock speed could be explained by acceleration phase duration and X-factor at the end of retraction, where shorter acceleration phase durations and more negative X-factor at end of retraction caused greater shuttlecock speeds. These results suggest that motions of the proximal segments (shoulder and pelvis–thorax separation) are critical to developing greater distal linear velocities, which subsequently lead to greater post-impact shuttlecock speed.

Keywords: velocity; technique; overhead; racket; swing; stroke

---

1. Introduction

The forehand smash is an effective attacking shot in badminton, accounting for 54% of "unconditional winner" and "forced failure" shots in international matches [1]. Success of the stroke is dependent upon two components: speed and direction, where speeds as high as 89.3 ± 7.2 m·s^{-1} have been reported in the literature for elite Malaysian players [2], whereas the competition world record is 118 m·s^{-1} [3]. A shuttlecock with a greater post-impact speed will give an opponent less reaction time, while directing the shuttlecock away from the opponent requires them to make fast reactive movements in order to return the shuttlecock.

Several studies have determined that both linear and angular velocities of distal segments (hand and racket) are strong positive correlates with shuttlecock speed [2,4], which is unsurprising due to higher velocities causing greater transfer of linear momentum to the shuttlecock. Explaining what kinematic parameters determine this greater distal velocities may be more useful for players, coaches and practitioners, as the greater joint powers associated with distal segments are not fully generated by the muscles associated with these segments, but transferred between segments through reaction forces of a proximal-to-distal nature, e.g., shoulder–elbow–wrist [5]. Varied experimental set-ups and methodologies of quantifying joint contributions have generated conflicting results, where Rambely et al. [4] suggested that a distal-to-proximal order of wrist, followed by the elbow and shoulder are the major contributors to racket head speed (26.5%, 9.4% and 7.4%, respectively). In contrast, Liu et al. [6] reported that a proximal-to-distal order of shoulder internal rotation, forearm pronation and wrist palmar flexion contribute 66%, 17% and 11%, respectively, towards racket head speed. Rambely et al. [5] captured video data at 50 Hz and calculated the resultant linear velocities of the shoulder, elbow and wrist joint centres at impact, and expressed the segment contributions as these velocities represented as percentages of the racket head centre resultant velocity at impact. Conversely, Liu et al. [6] used a three-dimensional kinematic method developed by Sprigings et al. [7] and calculated the relative angular velocities of distal segments by removing contributions from the adjacent proximal segment. Data were captured using high-speed video (200 Hz) and processed using direct linear transformation [8]. Teu et al. [9] found no specific proximity order using a dual Euler angles method with high-speed video (200 Hz), and reported torso rotation, shoulder internal rotation, forearm pronation and wrist abduction contributed 57%, 3%, 27% and 10% to resultant racket head velocity, respectively.

In summary, previous research has reported that linear velocities of the distal segments best explain variation in shuttlecock speed/racket head speed, however it is unclear how the distal segment velocities and subsequent racket head and shuttlecock speeds are generated. Additionally, use of low frame rates and unclear methodology for defining both shuttlecock speed and racket head speed mean that it is difficult to compare results. The present study therefore aims to identify full-body kinematic parameters that best explain the generation of post-impact shuttlecock velocities in the badminton jump smash, such that coaches/practitioners can advise players how best to increase smash speeds through technique and/or strength training. It is hypothesised that positions (joint angles) of proximal segments and linear velocities of more distal segments will best explain variation in post-impact shuttlecock speed.

2. Materials and Methods

2.1. Participants

Eighteen male badminton players (mean ± SD: age 24.3 ± 7.1 years, height 1.84 ± 0.08 m, mass 79.6 ± 8.8 kg) of regional (n = 9), national (n = 4) and international (n = 5) standards participated in this study, each performing a series of twelve forehand jump smashes from a racket-fed lift via an international coach/player, representative of match conditions. A range of abilities were used to provide a variety of maximal smash speeds, facilitating an investigation into causal factors associated with this variation. Testing procedures were explained to each participant, and informed written consent was obtained in accordance with the guidelines of the Loughborough University Ethical Advisory Committee (SSEHS-1959).

2.2. Data Collection

An eighteen-camera Vicon Motion Analysis System (400 Hz; OMG Plc, Oxford, UK) was used to collect three-dimensional kinematic data of the participant, racket and shuttlecock on a mock badminton court within a hall of sufficient height. Forty-seven 14 mm retroreflective markers were attached to the participant (Figure 1), where joint centres were calculated from a pair of markers placed across the joint so that their midpoint coincided with the joint centre [10]. Hip, thorax, neck and head joint centres were calculated according to Worthington et al. [11]. A further marker was placed on the bottom of the racket handle, seven pieces of 3M Scotchlite reflective tape were attached to the racket frame and a single piece of reflective tape was attached around the base of the cork of the shuttlecock (Figure 2). Participants used their own racket and new Yonex AS40 shuttlecocks throughout, where misshapen or broken shuttlecocks were removed.

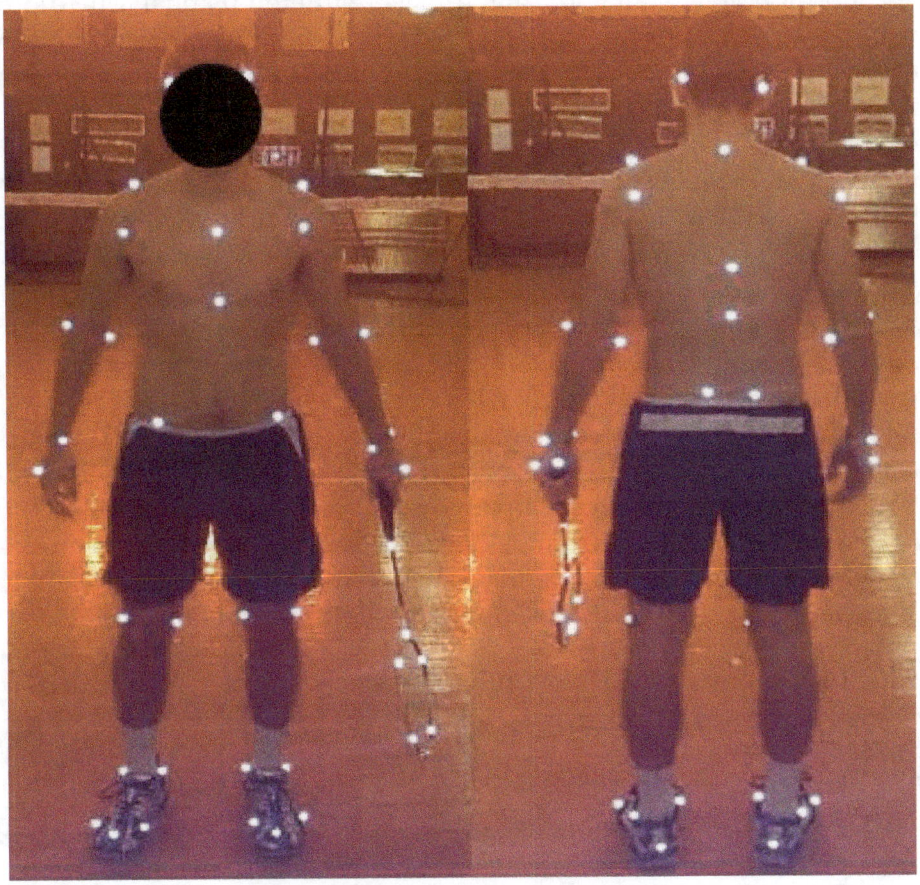

Figure 1. Participant marker locations.

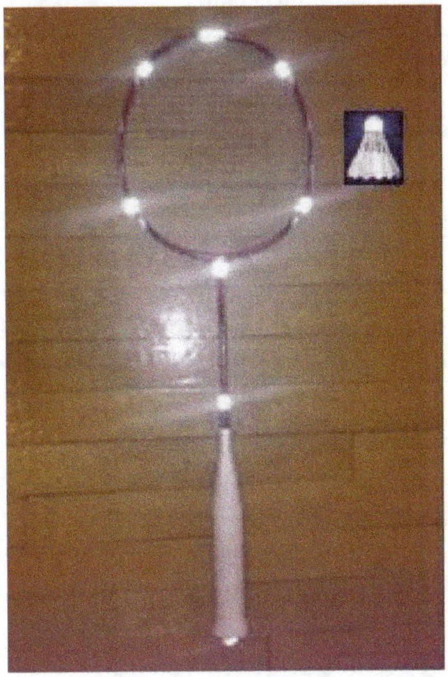

Figure 2. Racket and shuttlecock marker locations.

2.3. Data Reduction

Position data were labelled within Vicon Nexus 1.7.1 where gaps within marker trajectories were filled using the "pattern-filled" function where possible, and "spline-filled" function thereafter. All position data were then imported into Matlab v.2018b (The MathWorks Inc., Natick, MA, USA) for all further processing. Position data of all body markers were filtered using a fourth-order, zero-phase, low-pass Butterworth filter with a cut-off frequency of 30 Hz, determined through residual analysis [12]. Racket and shuttlecock markers remained unfiltered to avoid double-filtering during subsequent curve-fitting methodologies.

Joint angles were calculated using three-dimensional rotation matrices, defining the rotation applied to the proximal segment coordinate system to bring it into coincidence with the coordinate system of the distal segment [12]. An XYZ rotation sequence was used, representing flexion–extension, adduction–abduction and longitudinal axis rotation, respectively. When describing humerothoracic motion, a YZY rotation sequence was used as recommended by ISB [13], using a different coordinate system for the humerus segment where xyz represented adduction–abduction, longitudinal axis rotation and flexion–extension, respectively. Wrist angles were normalised based on the player adopting their normal grip within a static trial, which was considered the neutral position. The mean offset was 28.8 ± 8.4° and 7.1 ± 7.4° of palmar extension and ulnar deviation, respectively. X-factor referred to the separation angle between vectors connecting the right and left shoulder joint centres and, the right and left hip joint centres, respectively, in the transverse plane [14]. Centre of mass was calculated using segment inertial values from de Leva [15], where the body was modelled as fourteen segments. Jump height was defined as the difference between the maximum centre of mass height and the height of that during a static standing trial. Table 1 details the joint angles calculated.

Table 1. Calculated joint angles, with their relative zero positions and positive directions.

Joint	Motion	Anatomical Position (°)	Positive Direction
Shoulder	Internal/External Rotation	†	Internal Rotation
Elbow	Flexion/Extension	0	Extension
	Pronation/Supination	0	Supination
Wrist	Palmar Flexion/Extension	180	Extension
	Ulnar/Radial Deviation	0	Ulnar Deviation
Trunk	X-Factor (Transverse Plane)	0	‡

† For further details on motion of the shoulder joint as a result of the ISB rotation sequence recommendations, see Wu et al. [13]. ‡ Positive direction relates to the direction of rotation during the forward swing of the movement, i.e., anticlockwise for a right-handed player. Note transverse plane is viewed from above.

Instantaneous post-impact shuttlecock speed and racket–shuttlecock contact timing were determined using a logarithmic curve-fitting methodology [16] with minor adjustments for the application to the badminton smash. The time of impact was derived from the intersection of pre- and post-impact shuttlecock displacement curves in the global anterior–posterior direction (dominant direction of the smash), and an intermediate 1 ms contact period [17] was added between the pre- and post-impact shuttlecock curves, where the racket face and shuttlecock velocity were assumed equal. Post-impact shuttlecock speed was determined via differentiation of the post-impact logarithmic shuttlecock displacement curve. Racket head speed was the component of the linear racket head centre linear velocity acting perpendicular to the racket stringbed. The pre-impact racket head speed data was then interpolated to the calculated time of initial shuttlecock contact.

Based upon previous literature within badminton, the movement was defined around two phases, defined as backswing and acceleration phases [18]. Five discrete instants were identified such that trials could be compared appropriately: preparation (P) was defined as the point at which centre of mass height was minimal [2]; end of retraction (ER) was defined as the point at which the racket was most medio-laterally positioned towards the non-dominant side of the participant within the global coordinate system; racket lowest point (RLP) when the racket tip was at its lowest vertical point [19]; and turning point (TP) was defined as the point, after minimum (most negative), at which the racket head speed became positive [4] and shuttlecock contact (SC) was defined as the closest motion capture frame to the previously defined instant of racket-shuttlecock contact. The backswing phase (BSP) was defined as the time between PP and TP, whereas the acceleration phase (AP) was defined as the time between TP and SC.

Five joint angles (Table 1) were calculated for each trial, describing the elements of badminton smash technique which have previously been linked to shuttlecock velocity in literature or thought to be linked to shuttlecock velocity. Joint angles were defined at each key instant and their maximum range of motion through to SC calculated, e.g., maximum external rotation angle through to angle at contact. Furthermore, post-impact shuttlecock speed; racket head speed at impact; jump height; and peak shoulder, elbow and wrist joint centre linear velocities were calculated for each trial. Length of phases (BSP and AP), as well as total swing time, were also calculated for each trial. All kinematic variables for each player's trial with the greatest shuttlecock speed were entered into subsequent correlation analyses.

2.4. Statistical Analysis

All statistical correlational analyses were performed in Matlab v.2018b (The MathWorks Inc., Natick, MA, USA). Pearson product moment correlation analyses were performed between each kinematic (independent) variable and shuttlecock speed. Pearson product moment correlations (r) and their 95% confidence intervals (CI) were interpreted as negligible < 0.3; $0.3 \leq$ low < 0.5; $0.5 \leq$ moderate < 0.7; $0.7 \leq$ high < 0.9; very high ≥ 0.9 [20]. An alpha value of 0.05 was used to determine significance. Correlates were then entered as "candidate" variables into a forwards stepwise multiple linear regression model to identify key kinematic parameters that best explain variation in shuttlecock speed. Entry requirements for inclusion of a parameter were $p < 0.05$, with a removal coefficient of $p > 0.10$. The regression model was rejected if the 95% CI coefficients included zero, the residuals of the predictor were heteroscedastic or if the bivariate correlations, tolerance statistics or variance inflation factors showed any evidence of multicollinearity [21–25]. The normality of the standardised residuals in the regression model was also confirmed using the Shapiro–Wilk test. The percentage of variance in the dependent variable explained by the independent variables (predictors) within the regression equation was determined by Wherry's adjusted R^2 value [26]. Multiple linear regression analysis was performed in IBM SPSS Statistics 23 (IBM, Armonk, NY, USA).

3. Results

Maximal shuttlecock speeds for the cohort were 89.6 ± 5.3 m·s^{-1} (range: 80.1–99.8 m·s^{-1}). Racket head speeds at SC achieved during these trials were 56.3 ± 4.0 m·s^{-1} (range: 46.7–64.6 m·s^{-1}). Five kinematic variables were significantly correlated with shuttlecock speed, where a greater racket head speed, greater peak wrist joint centre linear velocity and shorter acceleration phase duration were associated with greater shuttlecock speeds. Likewise, greater shoulder internal rotation at SC and more negative X-factor at ER produced greater shuttlecock speeds. No other variables were significantly correlated to shuttlecock speed (Tables 2–4). Means and standard deviations, as well as a time-normalized comparison between the "fastest" and "slowest" participant for shoulder internal rotation angle, X-factor and racket head speed are shown in Figures 3–5, respectively.

Table 2. Pearson product moment correlation (r) between each of racket head speed, jump height, phase durations, joint centre linear velocities and ranges of motion, and shuttlecock speed.

Kinematic Variable	Key Instant/Phase	Mean (SD)	r	95% CI	p
Racket Head Speed ($m{\cdot}s^{-1}$)	SC	56.3 (4.0)	0.903	0.753, 0.964	<0.001 *
Jump Height (cm)		31.6 (9.2)	0.454	−0.017, 0.760	0.059
Phase duration (ms)	BSP	509.0 (94.8)	0.412	−0.067, 0.737	0.089
	AP	38.1 (5.2)	−0.543	−0.805, −0.101	0.020 *
	TS	547.1 (92.5)	0.392	−0.092, 0.726	0.108
Peak Shoulder JC LV ($m{\cdot}s^{-1}$)		3.5 (0.4)	0.177	−0.316, 0.595	0.482
Peak Elbow JC LV ($m{\cdot}s^{-1}$)		8.3 (0.8)	0.353	−0.136, 0.704	0.151
Peak Wrist JC LV ($m{\cdot}s^{-1}$)		14.2 (1.7)	0.767	0.467, 0.908	<0.001 *
Shoulder IR ROM (°)	Peak−SC	98.1 (20.7)	0.403	−0.079, 0.732	0.097
Elbow Flexion ROM (°)	Peak−SC	106.0 (7.9)	0.016	−0.454, 0.479	0.950
Elbow PRO ROM (°)	Peak−SC	21.2 (14.9)	0.298	−0.197, 0.671	0.230
Wrist Flexion ROM (°)	Peak−SC	40.4 (12.5)	−0.242	−0.254, 0.637	0.333
X−Factor ROM (°)	Peak−SC	46.0 (9.4)	0.208	−0.287, 0.615	0.408

Abbreviations: CI: confidence interval, BSP: backswing phase, AP: acceleration phase, TS: total swing, JC LV: joint centre linear velocity, IR: internal rotation, ROM: range of motion, PRO: pronation. * Significant ($p < 0.05$) .

Table 3. Pearson product moment correlation (r) between joint angles of the shoulder and elbow at key instants and shuttlecock speed.

Kinematic Variable	Key Instant/Phase	Mean (SD)	r	95% CI (Lower, Upper)	p
Shoulder INT/EXT Rotation Angle (°)	P	102.4 (29.8)	0.324	−0.168, 0.678	0.189
	ER	1.9 (8.8)	0.013	−0.457, 0.477	0.959
	RLP	−33.6 (8.2)	0.161	−0.331, 0.584	0.523
	TP	−29.2 (13.7)	0.299	−0.195, 0.672	0.228
	SC	58.7 (20.0)	0.508	0.054, 0.788	0.031 *
Elbow Flexion Angle (°)	P	88.4 (19.8)	0.329	−0.163, 0.690	0.183
	ER	64.9 (8.0)	−0.206	−0.614, 0.289	0.413
	RLP	74.2 (9.8)	0.161	−0.648, 0.236	0.298
	TP	120.6 (10.5)	0.225	−0.271, 0.626	0.370
	SC	166.1 (4.3)	0.243	−0.252, 0.638	0.331
Elbow Pronation Angle (°)	P	−61.6 (17.5)	0.398	−0.084, 0.730	0.102
	ER	−99.4 (20.0)	−0.180	−0.597, 0.313	0.475
	RLP	−84.0 (13.2)	0.120	−0.556, 0.368	0.636
	TP	−95.4 (15.4)	−0.376	−0.717, 0.111	0.125
	SC	−101.5 (19.0)	−0.420	−0.741, 0.059	0.083

Abbreviations: KI: key instant, CI: confidence interval, INT: internal, EXT: external, P: preparation, ER: end of retraction, RLP: racket lowest point, TP: turning point, SC: shuttlecock contact. * Significant ($p < 0.05$).

Table 4. Pearson product moment correlation (r) between joint angles of the wrist and X-factor at key instants and shuttlecock speed.

Kinematic Variable	Key Instant/Phase	Mean (SD)	*r*	95% CI (Lower, Upper)	*p*
Wrist Flexion Angle (°)	P	191.0 (13.0)	0.368	−0.120, 0.712	0.133
	ER	208.2 (10.6)	−0.134	−0.565, 0.356	0.598
	RLP	225.4 (9.9)	0.146	−0.344, 0.574	0.563
	TP	225.8 (9.3)	0.021	−0.451, 0.483	0.935
	SC	187.8 (8.9)	0.190	−0.304, 0.603	0.451
X−factor (°)	P	0.8 (8.6)	0.024	−0.448, 0.485	0.926
	ER	−33.3 (5.8)	−0.484	−0.775, −0.022	0.042 *
	RLP	−23.5 (7.1)	−0.362	−0.709, 0.126	0.140
	TP	−5.2 (7.6)	−0.175	−0.593, 0.318	0.489
	SC	7.9 (7.9)	−0.077	−0.525, 0.404	0.760

Abbreviations: KI: key instant, CI: confidence interval, P: preparation, ER: end of retraction, RLP: racket lowest point, TP: turning point, SC: shuttlecock contact. * Significant ($p < 0.05$).

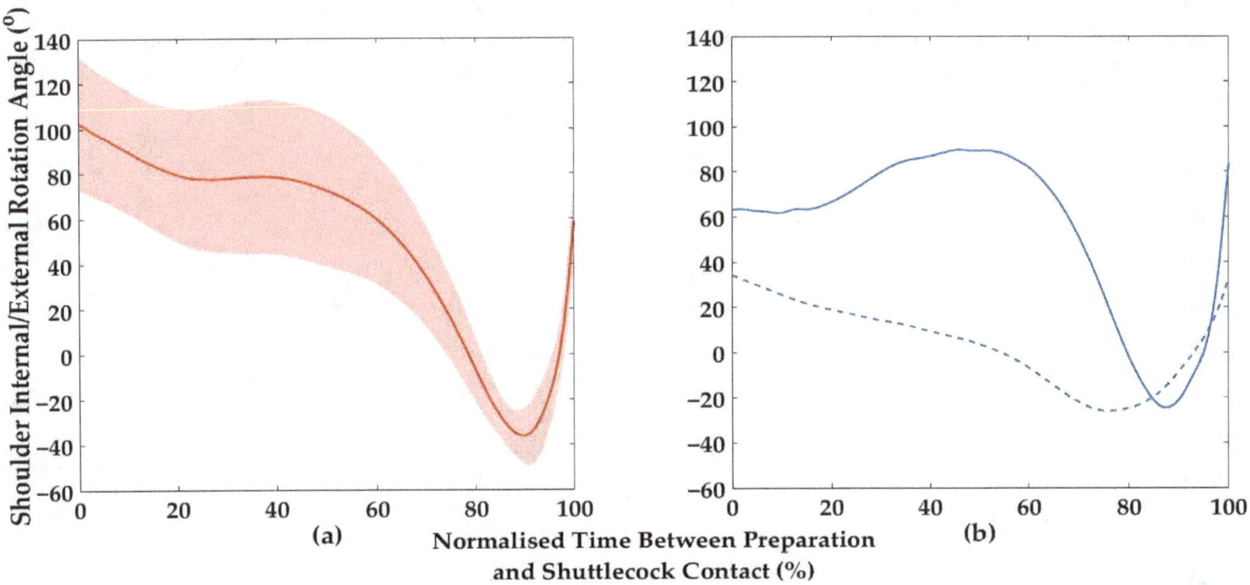

Figure 3. (**a**) Mean (solid line) ± SD (shaded area) for the normalised racket arm shoulder internal/external rotation angle between preparation and shuttlecock contact key instants. (**b**) Normalised racket arm shoulder internal/external rotation angle between preparation and shuttlecock contact key instants, for participants with the fastest (solid line) and slowest (dashed line) participant's smash. Internal rotation (positive); external rotation (negative). A significant correlation between shuttlecock speed and shoulder internal rotation angle was present at shuttlecock contact.

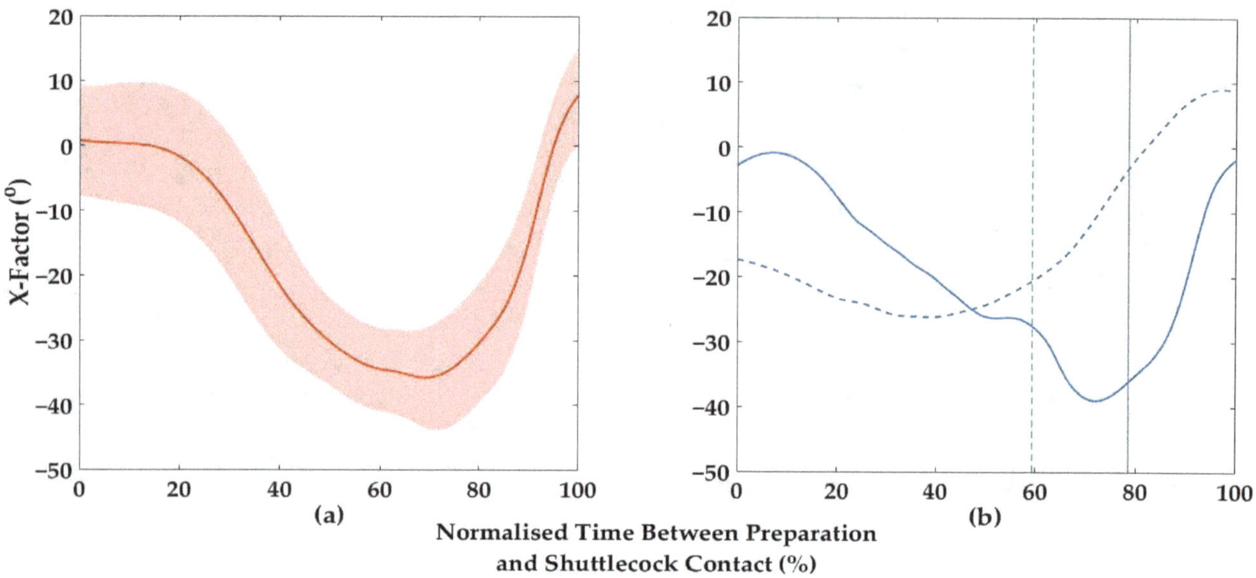

Figure 4. (**a**) Mean (solid line) ± SD (shaded area) for normalised X-factor between preparation and shuttlecock contact key instants for all participants; (**b**) Normalised X-factor between preparation and shuttlecock contact key instants for participants with the fastest (solid line) and slowest (dashed line) smash. The end of retraction (ER) key instant for each participant is represented by a vertical line. X-factor at ER was significantly correlated with shuttlecock speed.

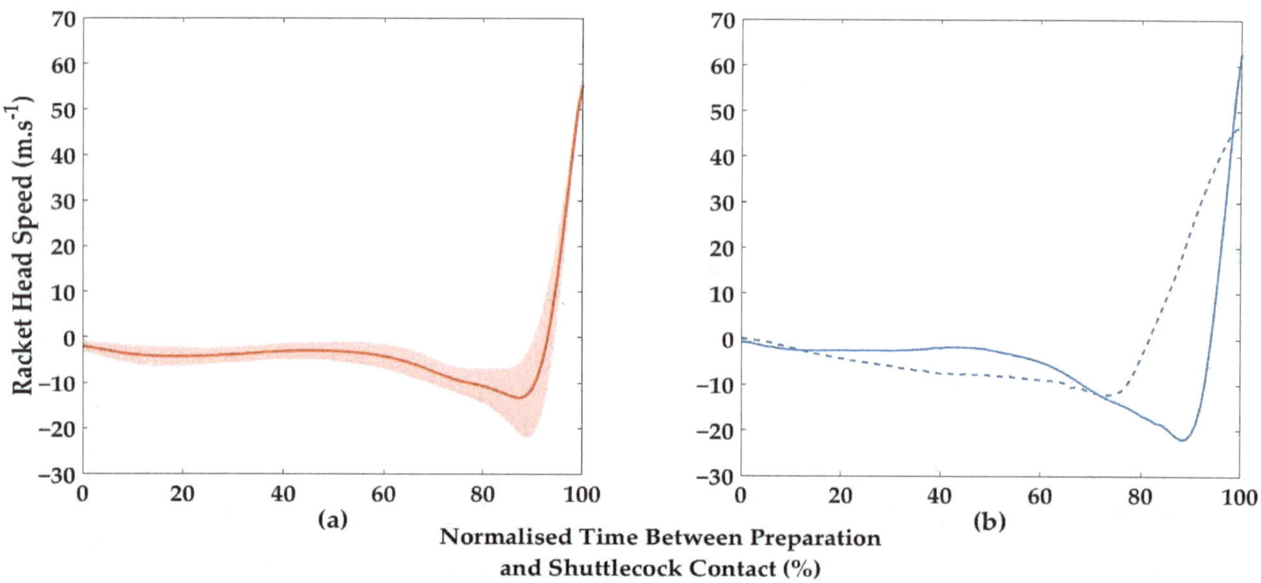

Figure 5. (**a**) Mean (solid line) ± SD (shaded area) for the normalised racket head speed between preparation and shuttlecock contact key instants for all participants; (**b**) Normalised racket head speed (normal to the stringbed plane) between preparation and shuttlecock contact key instants for participants with the fastest (solid line) and slowest (dashed line) smash. The acceleration phase begins at the point at which the racket head speed becomes positive, following the initial negative peak, and the duration between this turning point and shuttlecock contact was significantly negatively correlated with shuttlecock speed.

Multiple regression analysis revealed that the duration of AP alone explained 25.0% of the variation in shuttlecock speed, with a standard error of the estimate (SEE) of 4.4 m·s^{-1}. The addition of X-factor at ER explained 43.7% of the variance in post-impact shuttlecock speed (SEE = 3.8 m·s^{-1}), where a shorter acceleration phase and a more negative X-Factor at ER caused greater shuttlecock speeds (Table 5; Figure 6).

Table 5. Multiple regression equations explaining variance in shuttlecock speed.

Model	Kinematic Parameters	Coefficient	95% CI Lower Bound	95% CI Upper Bound	Variable, *p*	Model Percent Explained	Model *p*	Model SEE
a	(Constant)	110.1	93.2	127.0	<0.001	25.0	0.02	4.4
	AP Duration	−536.5	−976.8	−96.2	0.020			
b	(Constant)	95.8	76.7	114.9	<0.001	43.7	0.05	3.8
	AP Length	−514.0	−898.1	−129.9	0.012			
	X−Factor at ER	−0.4	−0.7	−0.1	0.024			

Abbreviations: CI: confidence intervals, SEE: standard error of the estimate, AP: acceleration phase, ER: end of retraction.

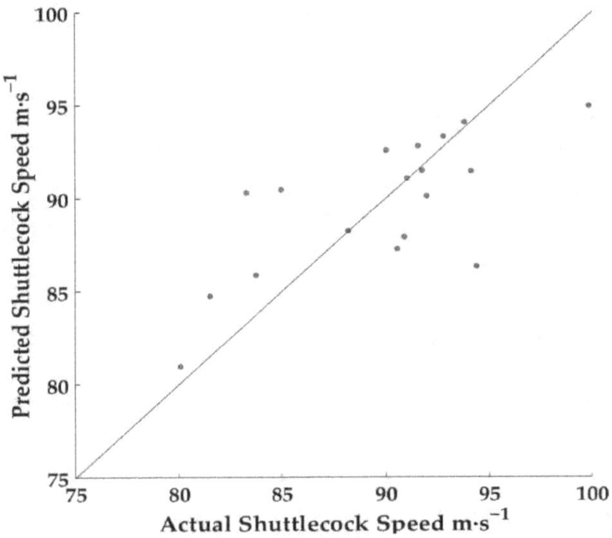

Figure 6. Predicted shuttlecock speed against actual shuttlecock speed for the two-parameter stepwise regression equation (Table 5; Model b). With a higher percentage of the variation in shuttlecock speed explained the closer the data points lie to the line y = x (predicted shuttlecock speed = actual shuttlecock speed).

4. Discussion

Racket head speeds and shuttlecock speeds achieved by the participants showed good agreement with previously reported values by elite players [2,27,28]. Shuttlecock speed was greatest in the international players (94.4 ± 3.2 m·s^{-1}), followed by national players (91.2 ± 2.6 m·s^{-1}) and then regional players (86.4 ± 4.6 m·s^{-1}), suggesting that the ability to achieve greater post-impact shuttlecock speeds is a good indication of playing level [29]. A one-way ANOVA revealed a significant difference in shuttlecock speed between groups ($F_{(2,15)} = 7.29$, $p = 0.006$). Bonferroni post-hoc tests revealed the international group smashed significantly faster than the regional group (mean difference = 8.06 m·s^{-1}, CI: 2.22, 13.90; $p = 0.006$). The national group were not significantly different to either the international or regional groups. Five kinematic variables correlated significantly with shuttlecock speed: racket head speed at impact, peak wrist joint centre linear velocity, length of the acceleration phase, shoulder internal rotation angle at SC and X-factor (transverse) at ER. These results are indicative of proximal joint motions (shoulder and trunk) causing greater linear velocities in the distal segments (wrist and racket).

Racket head speed at impact, normal to the stringbed plane, correlated very highly (r = 0.903; CI: 0.753, 0.964; $p < 0.001$) with instantaneous post-impact shuttlecock speed. This is a larger effect size than those previously reported [2,27], which may be due to the more accurate calculation of post-impact shuttlecock speed i.e., at a precise time of impact, and an appropriate racket head speed (normal to the stringbed plane) interpolated to the time of initial contact with the shuttlecock in the present study. The non-perfect relationship between racket head and shuttlecock speed may be due to differences in racket specifications used by each player, where impact efficiency (location and coefficient of restitution), as well as mass properties of the racket, will affect the amount of linear momentum transferred to the shuttlecock, for a given impact velocity. Longitudinal impact locations, calculated using the previously described methodology of Peploe et al. [16], ranged between −29.4 and 24.9 mm from the racket head centre, whereas medio-lateral impact locations ranged between −33.2 and 17.1 mm from the racket head centre (medial–negative, lateral–positive; relative to the player). Modelling the racket as two segments (handle and frame) and assuming a frame transverse angular velocity of 80 rad·s^{-1} at impact, consistent with experienced players [28], the difference in racket head speed at the most proximal and distal longitudinal impact locations would be 4.3 m·s^{-1}, suggesting that impact location can have a large effect on subsequent shuttlecock speed, even given identical input in terms of racket angular velocities.

As well as racket head speed, peak linear velocity of the wrist joint centre, was found to be a strong predictor of shuttlecock speed (r = 0.767; CI: 0.467, 0.908; $p < 0.001$), indicating that players should ultimately aim to achieve high linear velocities within distal components of the kinetic chain. This correlation was stronger than previous reported by Rambely et al. [4] in elite international players, who reported a low positive relationship (r = 0.454) despite mean values in the present study showing good agreement (14.2 vs. 11.7 m·s^{-1}) with differences attributable to the variety in player ability in the present study and differences in capture frequency (400 vs. 50 Hz), where 50 Hz may be inadequate for the badminton smash [28]. Greater shuttlecock speeds were also produced when AP was shorter in duration (r = -0.543; CI: -0.805, −0.101; $p = 0.020$), demonstrated in Figure 5b, where the racket head speed becomes positive much closer to impact, when comparing the "fastest" to the "slowest" participant.

Furthermore, two kinematic technique factors significantly correlated with shuttlecock speed. First, players who were in a position of greater shoulder internal rotation at impact produced greater shuttlecock speeds (r = 0.508, moderate; CI: 0.054, 0.788; $p = 0.031$), where a clear difference in position between the "fastest" and "slowest" player is shown in Figure 3b, despite very similar minimum positions. This suggests that greater shoulder internal rotation allows more work done by this joint rotation, which Liu et al. [6] found contributed 66% towards racket head velocity. However, correlational analysis revealed a non-significant relationship between shoulder internal rotation range of motion and shuttlecock speed (r = 0.403, low; CI: −0.079, 0.732; $p = 0.097$). When accounting for the time in which this range was completed, i.e., average angular velocity, the correlation came closer to significance (r = 0.444, low; CI: −0.029, 0.755; $p = 0.065$). Second, a low negative correlation was found between X-factor at ER and shuttlecock speed (r = 0.484; CI: −0.755, −0.022; $p = 0.042$), where players who produced a greater pelvis–thorax separation angle in the transverse plane at ER produced greater shuttlecock speeds. Again, a clear difference is seen between the "fastest" and "slowest" participants in Figure 4b. X-factor (maximum pelvis-thorax separation) has previously been found to be a strong correlate (r = 0.60, $p < 0.01$) with shuttlecock speed [12]. A greater rotational countermovement of the torso presumably allows greater trunk rotation contribution to racket head speed, which Teu et al. [9] found to contribute 57% to racket head speed.

It has been previously reported that both peak vertical ground reaction force and jump height significantly correlate with shuttlecock speed (r = 0.548 and 0.508, respectively) [2]. The present study found a non-significant correlation, with CI marginally crossing zero, between jump height and shuttlecock speed (r = 0.454; CI: −0.017, 0.760; p = 0.059); however, a similar effect size. Perhaps greater jump heights are a characteristic of more able players, who typically produce greater shuttlecock speeds [12,29], and serves as a tactical factor allowing players to produce steeper smash strokes as opposed to producing greater shuttlecock speeds. Note that jump height was significantly correlated with racket head speed in the present study (r = 0.494; CI: 0.035, 0.781; $p = 0.037$).

The fact that distal linear velocities (wrist and racket) best explain variation in shuttlecock speed, yet proximal angles of the trunk and shoulder best explain variation in shuttlecock speed, is suggestive of the kinetic link principle whereby movements of a proximal-to-distal nature generate and conserve angular momentum to produce high distal end-point velocities [5,30–32]. Important longitudinal axis rotations, typically difficult to measure and observe, may not always follow this strict sequence with regards to timing, however the proximal-to-distal nature of overhead strokes provides a good general understanding of how high distal end-point velocities can be generated [33,34]. A more negative X-factor at ER causing greater shuttlecock speed endorses the idea of the stretch–shortening cycle, whereby more elastic energy is stored and recovered to enhance the concentric phase when X-factor is more negative at ER. The stretch–shortening cycle has been linked to greater velocities in throwing actions due to enhancement of the concentric phase [35,36]. Finally, no ranges of motion were found to significantly correlate with shuttlecock speed. Lees et al. [32] previously suggested that increasing the range of motion can improve performance (racket head speed) by increasing the acceleration path of the racket, allowing more muscular force to be generated and applied to accelerate the racket.

A further relevant biomechanical principle, not explored in this study, is the velocity lever principle [32]. The angle between the forearm and racket longitudinal axes is of importance for generating racket head speed. For example, if the racket is held at 90° to the forearm, then the racket head will move through the greatest distance when the forearm pronates, increasing the racket head linear speed for any given angular velocity of pronation [31]. Likewise, if the elbow is flexed at 90°, the contribution from shoulder internal rotation is maximised [30]. This principle is difficult to analyse within a complex motion such as the badminton smash, as multiple segmental rotations are responsible for producing the racket motion, as well as ensuring racket head orientation is optimal at impact, which may make certain joint angles, such as a racket–forearm angle of 90°, undesirable. Tang et al. [37] reported that within their cohort of four elite players, the average racket–forearm angle was 147°, which may represent a suitable compromise between the height and the speed at contact in practical play.

The multiple linear regression analysis found that two predictor variables were able to explain 43.7% of the variance in shuttlecock speed (Table 5; Figure 6). Participants with the fastest smashes were found to have a shorter acceleration phase duration and more negative (greater separation) X-factor at ER. From a practical standpoint, this would suggest that players attempt to delay the onset of their forward swing (when the racket head velocity normal to the stringbed becomes positive) such that the forward swing can be completed in the shortest possible time. This would ultimately achieve a greater velocity of the racket, i.e., the same acceleration path of the racket for a given player but completed in a shorter time period [31]. Additionally, players should seek to utilise as much counter-rotation of the trunk as possible before reversing this rotation within the acceleration phase.

A potential limitation to the present study was use of each participant's own racket causing a lack of experimental control over the impact mechanics between racket and shuttlecock, including effective mass of the "racket particle" within the collision between racket and shuttlecock, and thus the momentum transferred [27]. The effect of racket properties on player kinematics is also a potential source of limitation, where Whiteside et al. [38] reported that increasing the "swingweight" of the racket caused a reduction in peak angular velocities of shoulder internal rotation and wrist flexion during the tennis serve, where both of these joint rotations have been reported to be the two greatest contributors to racket head speed at impact [39]. Conversely, players are accustomed to their own racket, and introducing a "control" racket may require a great amount of familiarization or cause suboptimal performances due to unfamiliarity with the racket. It must also be acknowledged that the present study relies on investigation of joint kinematics at discrete time points (i.e., key instants). Future studies may therefore extend the current work using methodologies to investigate the continuous time series of kinematic data, such as statistical parametric mapping [40], vector coding [41] or principal component analysis [42], as well as considering other biomechanical principles not explored within this study. Additionally, differences in anthropometric data were not accounted for, where the same angular velocities and joint angles may lead to different linear velocities. Retrospective power analysis revealed that for the lowest significant correlation coefficient ($r = 0.484$), with 80% power and a significance threshold ($p = 0.05$), a sample size of 31 would be required. The study was therefore underpowered; however, recruiting more participants meeting the minimum standard criteria was not achievable.

5. Conclusions

In conclusion, proximal kinematics explained the greatest proportion of variation in shuttlecock speed during the forehand jump smash stroke in a cohort of experienced male badminton players. From a practical standpoint, it is suggested that players and/or coaches attempt to produce high shuttlecock speeds by increasing racket and distal joint centre linear velocities. This should be achieved primarily by having a greater internal rotation angle at shuttlecock contact. Furthermore, greater pelvis–thorax separation during the backswing phase is likely to aid the concentric phase of the swing via the stretch–shortening cycle.

Author Contributions: Conceptualisation, methodology and data collection: all authors; data processing: H.T. and R.D.; formal analysis and writing—original draft preparation: H.T. and S.M.-N.; writing—review and editing: all authors; supervision, M.K. and S.M.-N. All authors have read and agreed to the published version of the manuscript.

References

1. Tong, Y.-M.; Hong, Y. The playing pattern of world's top single badminton players. In Proceedings of the 18th International Symposium on Biomechanics in Sports, Hong Kong, China, 25–30 June 2000; pp. 825–830.
2. Ramasamy, Y.; Osman, J.; Sundar, V.; Joseph, S. Ground reaction force and kinematics of forehand jumping smash among elite Malaysian badminton players. In Proceedings of the 37th International Society of Biomechanics in Sport Conference, Oxford, OH, USA, 21–25 July 2019.
3. Guinness World Records, Fastest Badminton Hit in Competition (Male). Available online: https://www.guinnessworldrecords.com/world-records/fastest-badminton-hit-in-competition-(male)/ (accessed on 19 June 2019).
4. Rambely, A.S.; Osman, N.A.A.; Usman, J.; Abas, W.A.B.W. The contribution of upper limb joints in the development of racket velocity in the badminton smash. In Proceedings of the 23rd International Symposium on Biomechanics in Sports, Beijing, China, 22–27 August 2005.
5. Rasmussen, J.; Kwan, M.; Andersen, M.S.; De Zee, M. Analysis of segment energy transfer using musculoskeletal models in a high speed badminton stroke. In Proceedings of the 9th International Symposium on Computer Methods in Biomechanics and Biomedical Engineering, Valencia, Spain, 24–27 February 2010.
6. Liu, X.; Kim, W.; Tan, J. An Analysis of the Biomechanics of Arm Movement during a Badminton Smash. Nanyang Technology University: Singapore, 2002.
7. Sprigings, E.; Marshall, R.; Elliott, B.; Jennings, L. A three-dimensional kinematic method for determining the effectiveness of arm segment rotations in producing racquet-head speed. *J. Biomech.* **1994**, *27*, 245–254. [CrossRef]
8. Abdel-Aziz, Y.I.; Karara, H.M. Direct linear transformation from comparator coordinates into object coordinates in close-range photogrammetry. In Proceedings of the ASP Symposium on Close-Range Photogrammetry, Urbana, IL, USA, 26–29 January 1971.
9. Teu, K.K.; Kim, W.; Tan, J.; Fuss, F.K. Using dual Euler angles for the analysis of arm movement during the badminton smash. *Sports Eng.* **2005**, *8*, 171–178. [CrossRef]
10. McErlain-Naylor, S.; King, M.; Pain, M.T.G. Determinants of countermovement jump performance: A kinetic and kinematic analysis. *J. Sports Sci.* **2014**, *32*, 1805–1812. [CrossRef] [PubMed]

11. Worthington, P.; King, M.; Ranson, C. The influence of cricket fast bowlers' front leg technique on peak ground reaction forces. *J. Sports Sci.* **2013**, *31*, 434–441. [CrossRef] [PubMed]
12. Winter, D.A. *Biomechanics and Motor Control of Human Movement*, 4th ed.; Wiley: New York, NY, USA, 2009; pp. 70–73.
13. Wu, G.; Van Der Helm, F.C.T.; Veeger, H.E.J.; Makhsous, M.; Van Roy, P.; Anglin, C.; Nagels, J.; Karduna, A.R.; McQuade, K.; Wang, X.; et al. ISM recommendation on definitions of joint coordinate systems of various joints for the reporting of human joint motion-Part II: Shoulder, elbow, wrist and hand. *J. Biomech.* **2005**, *36*, 981–992. [CrossRef]
14. Zhang, Z.; Li, S.; Wan, B.; Visentin, P.; Jiang, Q.; Dyck, M.; Shan, G. The influence of X-factor (trunk rotation) and experience on the quality of the badminton forehand smash. *J. Hum. Kinet.* **2016**, *53*, 9–22. [CrossRef]
15. De Leva, P. Adjustments to Zatsiorsky-Seluyanov's segment inertia parameters. *J. Biomech.* **1996**, *29*, 1223–1230. [CrossRef]
16. Peploe, C.; McErlain-Naylor, S.A.; Harland, A.R.; Yeadon, M.R.; King, M.A. A curve fitting methodology to determine impact location, timing, and instantaneous post-impact ball velocity in cricket batting. *J. Sports Eng. Technol.* **2018**, *232*, 185–196. [CrossRef]
17. Cohen, C.; Texier, B.D.; Quéré, D.; Clanet, C. The physics of badminton. *New J. Phys.* **2015**, *17*, 063001. [CrossRef]
18. Brahms, B.V. *Badminton Handbook: Training, Tactics, Competition*, 2nd ed.; Meyer & Meyer Sport: Maidenhead, UK, 2014.
19. Martin, C.; Kulpa, R.; Delamarche, P.; Bideau, B. Professional tennis players; serve: Correlation between segmental angular momentums and ball velocity. *Sports Biomech.* **2012**, *12*, 2–14. [CrossRef]
20. Hinkle, D.; Wiersma, W.; Jurs, S.G. *Applied Statistics for the Behavioural Sciences*, 5th ed.; Houghton Miffin: Boston, MA, USA, 2003.
21. Bowerman, B.L.; O'Connell, R.T. *Linear Statistical Models: An Applied Approach*; Duxbery Press: Belmont, CA, USA, 1990.
22. Draper, N.R.; Smith, H. *Fitting a Straight Line by Least Aquares, in Applied Regression Analysis*; John Wiley & Sons, Inc.: Hoboken, NJ, USA, 1998.
23. Field, A.P. *Discovering Statistics Using IBM SPSS Statistics*, 4th ed.; Sage: London, UK, 2013.
24. Menard, S. *Applied Logistic Regression Analysis: Sage University Series on Quantitative Applications in the Social Sciences*; Sage: Thousand Oaks, CA, USA, 1995.
25. Myers, R. *Classical and Modern Regression with Applications*, 2nd ed.; Duxbury Press: Boston, MA, USA, 1990.
26. Wherry, R. A new formula for predicting the shtrinkage of the coefficient of multiple correlation. *Ann. Math. Stat.* **1931**, *2*, 440–457. [CrossRef]
27. Kwan, M. Designing the World's Best Badminton Racket. Ph.D. Thesis, Aalborg University, Aalborg, Denmark, 2010.
28. Kwan, M.; Andersen, M.S.; Cheng, C.-L.; Tang, W.-T.; Rasmussen, J. Investigation of high-speed badminton racket kinematics by motion capture. *Sports Eng.* **2011**, *13*, 57–63. [CrossRef]
29. Phomsoupha, M.; Laffaye, G. Shuttlecock velocity during a smash stroke in badminton evolves linearly with skil level. *Comput. Methods Biomech. Biomed. Eng.* **2014**, *17* (Suppl. 1), 140–141. [CrossRef] [PubMed]
30. Waddell, D.B.; Gowitzke, B.A. Biomechanical principles applied to badminton power strokes. In Proceedings of the 18th International Symposium on Biomechanics in Sports, Hong Kong, China, 25–30 June 2000.
31. Lees, A. Technique analysis in sports: A critical review. *J. Sports Sci.* **2002**, *20*, 813–828. [CrossRef] [PubMed]
32. Lees, A.; Cabello, D.; Torres, G. *Science and Racket Sports IV*; Routledge: London, UK, 2008.
33. Marshall, R.N.; Elliott, B.C. Long axis rotation: The missing link in proximal-to-distal sequencing. *J. Sports Sci.* **2000**, *18*, 247–254. [CrossRef]
34. Fleisig, G.; Nicholls, R.; Elliott, B.; Escamilla, R. Kinematics used by world class tennis players to produce high-velocity serves. *Sports Biomech.* **2003**, *2*, 51–64. [CrossRef]
35. Elliott, B. Biomechanics and tennis. *Br. J. Sports Med.* **2006**, *40*, 392–396. [CrossRef]
36. Elliott, B.C.; Baxter, K.G.; Besier, T.F. Internal rotation of the upper-arm segment during a stretch-shorten cycle movement. *J. Appl. Biomech.* **1999**, *15*, 381–395. [CrossRef]
37. Tang, H.P.; Abe, K.; Ae, M.; Katoh, L. 3-D cinematographic analysis of the badminton forehand smash: Movement of the forearm and hand. In *Science & Racket Sports*; Reilly, T., Hughes, M., Lees, A., Eds.; E & FN SPON: Cambridge, UK, 1995; pp. 113–118.

38. Whiteside, D.; Elliott, B.; Lay, B.; Reid, M. The effect of racquet swing weight on serve kinematics in elite adolescent female tennis players. *J. Sci. Med. Sport* **2014**, *17*, 124–128. [CrossRef]
39. Elliott, B.C.; Marshall, R.N.; Noffal, G.J. Contributions of upper limb segment rotations during the power serve in tennis. *J. Appl. Biomech.* **1995**, *11*, 433–442. [CrossRef]
40. Serrien, B.; Coossens, M.; Baeyens, J.P. Statistical parametric mapping of biomechanical one-dimensional data with Bayesian inference. *Int. Biomech.* **2019**, *6*, 9–18. [CrossRef]
41. Floria, O.; Sánchez-Sixto, A.; Harrison, A.J.; Ferber, R. The effect of running speed on joint coupling coordination and its variability in recreational runners. *Hum. Mov. Sci.* **2019**, *66*, 449–458. [CrossRef] [PubMed]
42. Cushion, E.J.; Warmenhoven, J.; North, J.; Cleather, D.J. Principal component analysis reveals the proximal to distal pattern in vertical jumping is governed by two functional degrees of freedom. *Front. Bioeng. Biotechnol.* **2019**, *7*, 193. [CrossRef] [PubMed]

8

Effects of Soccer Training on Body Balance in Young Female Athletes Assessed Using Computerized Dynamic Posturography

Grażyna Olchowik and Agata Czwalik *

Department of Biophysics, Medical University of Lublin, K. Jaczewskiego 4, 20-090 Lublin, Poland; grazyna.olchowik@umlub.pl

* Correspondence: agata.czwalik@umlub.pl

Abstract: The aim of this study was to determine the effect of regular soccer training on the balance system for young women. Computerized dynamic posturography of female footballers (n = 25) and control group (n = 50) was assessed during three tests: Sensory Organization Test, Motor Control Test, and Adaptation Test. Statistically significant differences between the groups was found in Composite Equilibrium Score with higher values, indicating better postural stability, for footballers. Regular trainees also showed better usefulness of vestibular system while maintaining balance. Weight symmetry of the lower limbs during Motor Control Test also showed statistically significant differences between the groups. This study shows that female footballers have better postural stability than their inactive peers and that regular workouts may improve the balance system.

Keywords: posture stability; balance; football; exercise; training

1. Introduction

Football is the most popular sport discipline with around 200,000 professional players and 240 million amateur players. It is responsible for almost 10% of sports injuries requiring medical attention in adolescents [1,2]. This discipline requires players to have unprecedented coordination to cope with rapidly changing external conditions. With regular practice a player acquires precision in movement and more muscle mass. Frequent training helps the player acquire the ability to execute appropriate strategic movements to effectively target his/her opponent's goal and to prevent serious injuries. To evaluate motor coordination a test was adopted many years ago to measure maximum rotation to the left and right when jumping in the air with both feet [3]. In modern training it is necessary to constantly monitor the sportsperson's coordination and balance [4,5]. Presently there are many different methods to assess training progress, physical activity, and body postural stability, but the most important conditions in which football players should be assessed are dynamic conditions. Postural stability in athletes has been reported widely in several sports disciplines [6,7]. That suggest that the type of sport and repetitive training may affect the balance system control. Some researchers found that football players were better that other athletes [6,8] and that the level of playing experience influences postural control performance and adopted motor strategies [9].

The human body's static and dynamic balance is maintained by the posture control system, which coordinates the stimuli received by the vestibular system, the visual system, and proprioceptors, and also provides a selection of optimal postural responses aimed at preventing falls [10,11]. The posture control system tracks the position of the center of gravity (COG) over an area defined by the outline of the human feet, thus guaranteeing a stable posture [12]. The body's multi-segment construction, the height of the COG above the base of support (BOS), and a relatively small BOS, results in the human body being unstable when in an upright position. The balance control system therefore needs to constantly analyze and counterbalance all the destabilizing factors through proper stimulation of the relevant muscle groups [12,13]. The central nervous system watches over the appropriate choice of reaction and the stimulation of the appropriate muscle reflexes. To correct posture, it adapts a movement strategy based on its analysis of linear and angular accelerations of individual body segments. Stability control of body posture depends on many factors, which includes a range of movements in the joints, muscle strength, speed and precision of movement, and the ability to perceive body positioning in space ("body sense") [14].

Computerized Dynamic Posturography (CDP) allows the individual components of the human balance system to be evaluated. During CDP, signals from appropriate senses involved in maintaining balance are evaluated. The postural response time and the reaction time to unexpected support platform changes, with an appropriate motor response, is also determined as well as the efficiency of adaptive mechanisms [15]. CDP is the gold standard to differentiate between sensory, motor, and central adaptive impairments to postural control [16]. In football it can be an opportunity to track the rehabilitation of postural control impairment after anterior cruciate ligament injury, which is one of the most common in this sport [17].

The aim of this study was to compare the behavior of the balance system between two groups of young women and to determine the effect of regular practice. One group consisted of young female footballers who train regularly and the other, a group of peers who do not participate in any regular sporting activity. We hypothesize that football players would show better postural balance performance.

2. Materials and Methods

2.1. Participants

The study group consisted of 25 young (age = 18.9 ± 4.5 year) female footballers from AZS-PSW Biała Podlaska, a club in the Polish Women's Football League. Each footballer in this study group has been attending training sessions for at least 6 years with five training sessions per week of 90 min duration. The control group consisted of 50 students (age = 20.7 ± 1.2 year) from the Medical University of Lublin, who had declared a lack of sporting activity. Both groups were chosen such that there were no statistically significant differences between them in height, weight, or body mass index (BMI) (Table 1). All subjects participating in the study had the same functional preferences (right-sided handedness, footedness, and eyedness) and same postural lateral preferences (hand-clasping, arm-folding, leg-crossing, and stair climbing) [18].

Table 1. Characteristics of female footballers and the control group.

	Footballers (n = 25)		Control Group (n = 50)		*p*
	M	SD	M	SD	
Height [cm]	167.47	4.28	168.04	5.33	0.726
Body weight [kg]	62.00	5.17	61.72	5.55	0.873
BMI [kg/m^2]	22.06	1.65	21.86	1.51	0.672

M = mean, SD—standard deviation, *p*—probability value.

2.2. Procedure

The study was conducted with the approval of the Bioethics Committee at the Medical University of Lublin (KE 0254/195/2011). At the beginning, participants were informed about the purpose of the study and asked to complete a questionnaire and to sign the consent for the study. The questionnaire included questions about general health: all diseases or health problems, surgeries or hospitalizations, brain injuries, loss of consciousness episodes, bone/muscle/joint injuries as well as any medication or drugs (including alcohol) taken in the past month. Another part of the questionnaire was about physical activity: what sport or physical activity the participant undertakes, for how long, and how many times per week. Afterwards each participant was accurately weighed and measured, and a short lateralization preference test was performed (e.g., which hand the participant uses for drawing/throwing a small object, which leg for kicking a football or stepping onto a chair, and which eye for looking into a bottle or a door viewer). The final stage of the study was a posturographic examination during which the participant stood barefoot on the posturographic platform and was secured with a special harness.

2.3. Instruments

Posturographic tests were performed using an Equitest posturograph manufactured by NeuroCom International®. The device consists of a dynamic force plate, visual surround, and a computer with software. Both the force plate and visual surround are moveable (±10° rotation for both and a maximum angular velocity of 50°/s and 15°/s, respectively). The study protocol included the following tests: Sensory Organization Test, Motor Control Test, and the Adaptation Test.

The Sensory Organization Test (SOT) evaluates the usefulness of signals coming from the different senses involved in maintaining body balance. This test is performed using six sensory stimulation conditions, during which visual stimuli are changed and a rotation of the foot support platform, or movements of the visual surround, are introduced. During the first three tests (SOT1–SOT3) the foot support platform is stationary while the visual information is varied: SOT1—eyes open, SOT2—eyes closed, SOT3—moving visual surround. During these tests, analyzing postural stability determines the usefulness of the visual signal and the patient's ability to suppress visual stimuli which are contrary to reality. The next three tests (SOT4–SOT6) are performed with a moving foot support platform, which interferes with the information received by the proprioceptive system. As with the previous three tests, visual information is varied: SOT4—eyes open, SOT5—eyes closed, SOT6—moving visual surround. Two final trials evaluate the usefulness of the vestibular system, whose role increases significantly in the case of incorrect or missing stimuli from the remaining systems involved in posture control. During SOT, the Equilibrium Score (ES) that quantifies the COG sway or postural stability under each of the 3 trials of the 6 sensory conditions is evaluated. A score of 100 represents perfect balance (no sway) and a score of 0 indicates a fall. During SOT, Composite Equilibrium Score (CES)—a weighted average of all 6 individual scores ES—the body's COG displacement in the anterior–posterior direction, as well as the motor strategy (MS)—correctness of the selected postural strategy—is also assessed. A score near 100 indicates a full ankle strategy while a score near 0 indicates a full hip strategy with maximum shear force. In addition the Sensory Analysis (SRS) that determines a patient's ability to use input from the somatosensory (SOM), visual (VIS), vestibular (VES) system to maintain balance as well as the degree to which the patient relies on visual information whether it is correct or not (PREF) is assessed [19,20].

The Motor Control Test (MCT) is performed for 6 conditions using the foot support platform capable of forward and backward movements through small, medium, and large displacements. A series of three trials is performed for each condition during which the patient's ability to perform corrective movements is evaluated in response to unexpected changes in the foot support platform. The MCT analysis the Latency Response (L)—the time between start of platform movement and start of postural response—the Amplitude (A) of the postural response and the Weight Symmetry (WS)—a nondimensional quantity with a score of 100 indicating that weight is borne equally by the two legs. The WS score decreases to zero or increases to 200 when all the weight is borne by the left or right leg, respectively.

In the Adaptation Test (ADT), the patient is subjected to two series of sudden platform perturbations, one of which causes dorsiflexion (ATU) while the other causes plantarflexion (ATD) in the ankles. Each series consists of five trials. During subsequent trials, the patient should maintain a vertical posture, minimizing with every subsequent trial the amount of energy required to rebalance the body. This sway energy (SE) is determined after each platform perturbation and indicates the amount of COG displacement during each trial.

2.4. Data Analysis

Statistical analysis was performed using the STATISTICA 10 (StatSoft) computer program. To verify the normality of the data the Shapiro–Wilk test was used. Because normality tests failed to confirm that all the parameters variables studied had normal distribution (most probable reason for not normal distribution in footballers group was the small number of participants), all variables were analyzed with non-parametric statistics—the Mann–Whitney U-test—for differences between groups. Statistically significant changes were those with a statistical significance level of $p < 0.05$.

3. Results

The SOT results are shown in Figures 1–3. ES analysis (Figure 1) shows statistical significance ($p < 0.05$) for the CES, with higher values for footballers. Of the six SOT conditions, COG displacement differed significantly between the groups only for conditions ES5 and ES6 which provided conflicting information to the sense organs, carried out on a moving platform with eyes closed (ES5) or a moving visual surround (ES6). These results reflect significant differences in the use of vestibular stimuli (VES) between people training regularly and those not performing any regular sport.

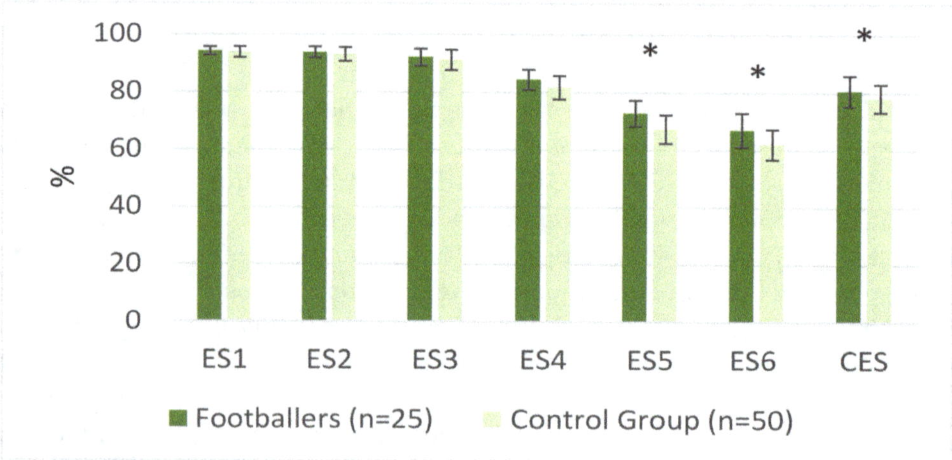

Figure 1. Sensory Organization Test—Composite Equilibrium Score (CES) and Equilibrium Score (ES) results (where the ES suffix refers to a particular SOT condition) for footballers and control group. The symbol * refers to a significant difference at $p < 0.05$.

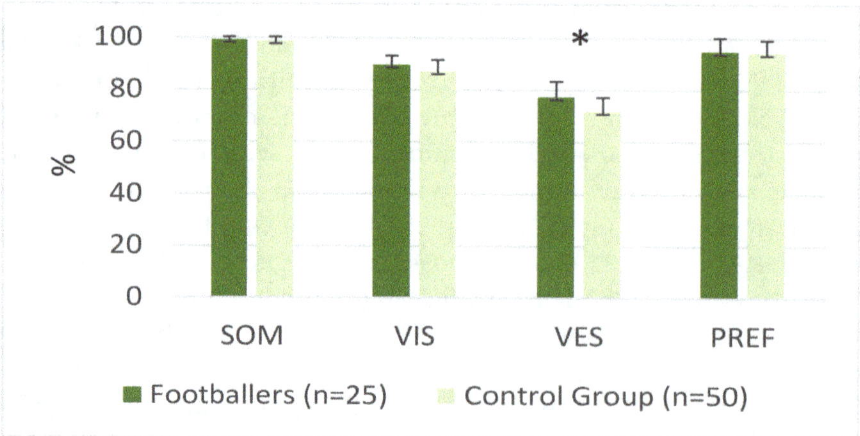

Figure 2. Sensory Organization Test—sensory analysis (SRS) results for the somatosensory system (SOM), the visual system (VIS), the vestibular system (VES), and visual preference (PREF) for footballers and control group. The symbol * refers to a significant difference at $p < 0.05$.

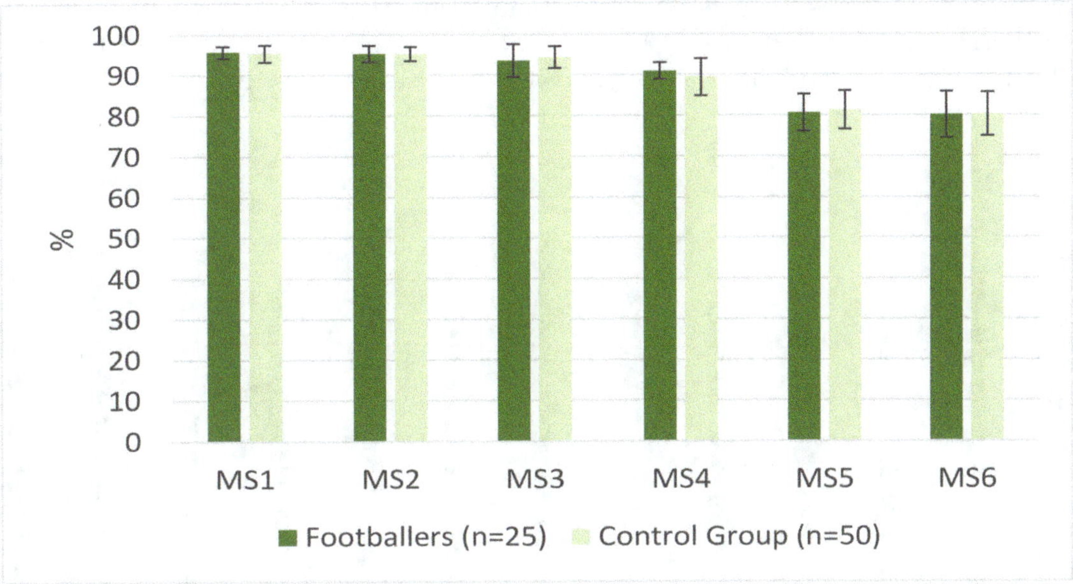

Figure 3. Sensory Organization Test—motor strategy (MS) for particular SOT conditions for footballers and control group.

The usefulness of the signals from the other sensory organs involved in the control of body balance (VIS, SOM, and PREF) did not highlight any significant differences between the two groups (Figure 2).

There was no impact on the selection of an appropriate motor strategy (MS1–MS6) by people playing football (Figure 3).

During MCT, statistically significant differences between the two groups were found in the symmetry of loading of the lower limbs during all the trials (Figure 4). Football players were characterized by disproportionate distribution of body weight with a predominance of left leg.

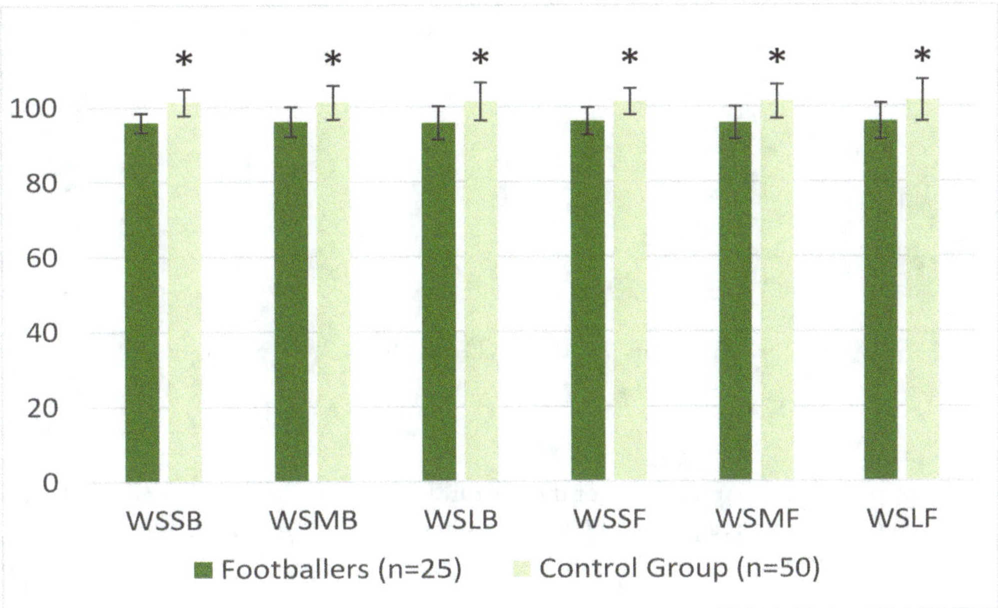

Figure 4. Motor Control Test—weight symmetry (WS) results for the lower limbs for small, medium and large platform transitions in backward (SB, MB, LB) and forward (SF, MF, LF) direction for footballers and control group. The symbol * refers to a significant difference at $p < 0.05$.

Postural response latencies (Figure 5) and their amplitudes (Figure 6) did not reveal any statistically significant differences between the two groups, which means that neither the reaction time nor the angular velocity of COG during the trials depends on the physical activity.

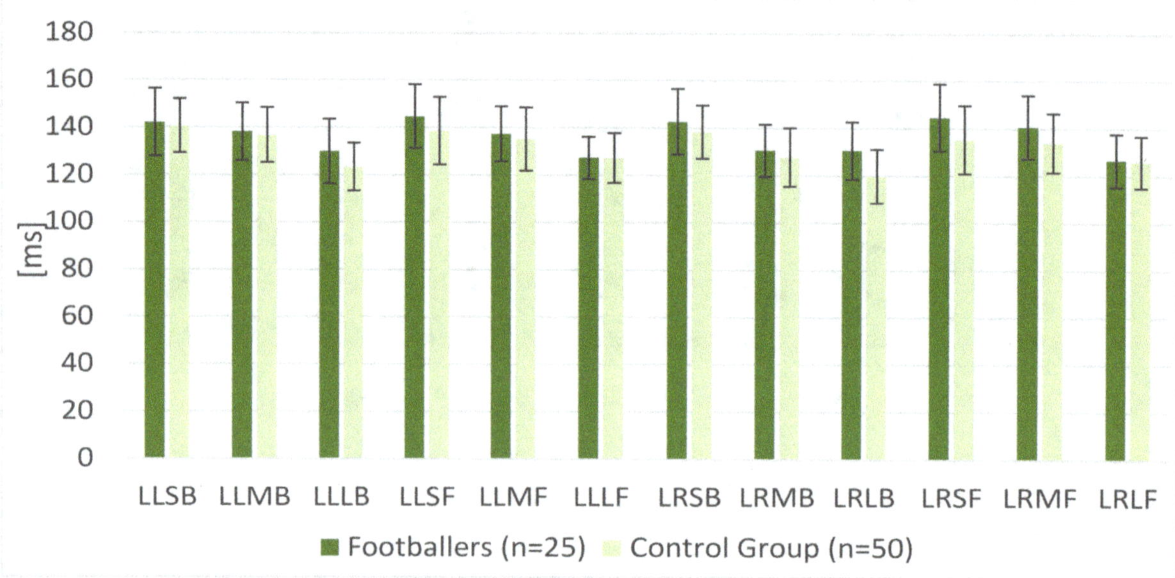

Figure 5. Motor Control Test—postural latencies for left (LL) and right (LR) lower limb for small, medium and large platform transitions in backward (SB, MB, LB) and forward (SF, MF, LF) direction for footballers and control group.

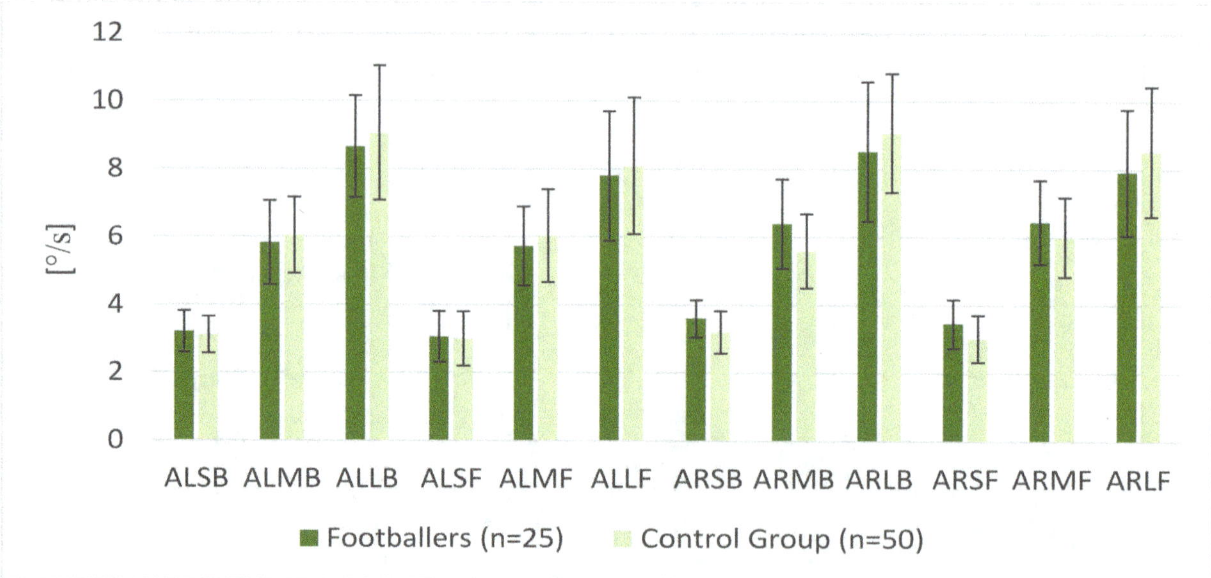

Figure 6. Motor Control Test—amplitudes of the postural responses for left (AL) and right (AR) lower limb for small, medium and large platform transitions in backward (SB, MB, LB) and forward (SF, MF, LF) direction for footballers and control group.

In the ADT there were no statistically significant differences between the measured parameters for both groups, which means that the adaptive postural response system is independent of physical activity. The results are shown in Figure 7.

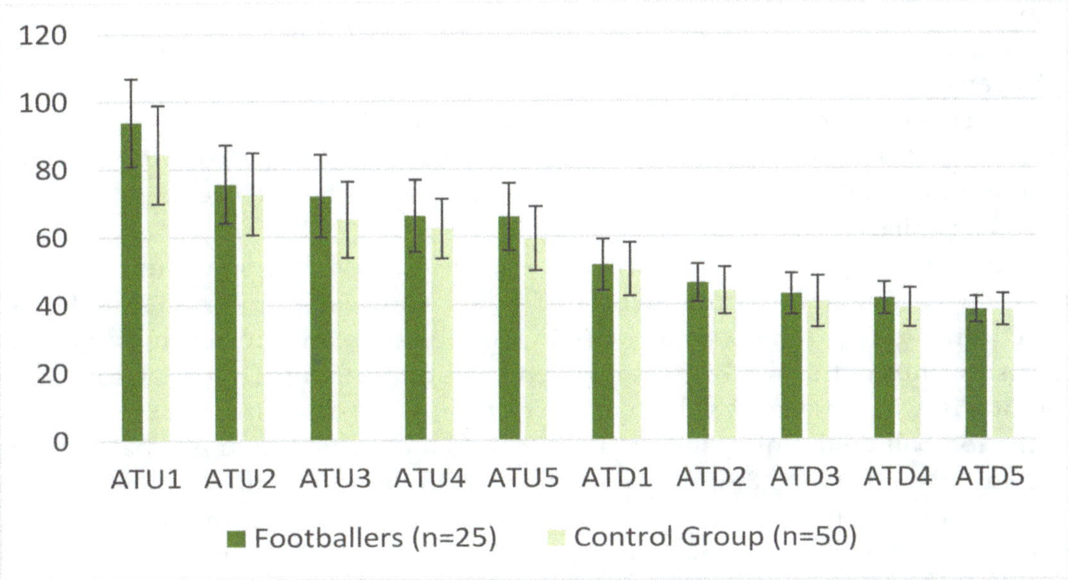

Figure 7. Adaptation Test—sway energy for 5 dorsiflexion (ATU) and 5 plantarflexion (ATD) condition for footballers and control group.

4. Discussion

Football is a sport discipline which, in addition to unprecedented coordination, requires exceptionally divided attention. The players must focus not only on the ball, but must also control their positions, the actions of the players in their team as well as those in the opposing team. They must analyze and foresee subsequent situations.

This study shows that professional footballers achieve significantly better results in the CES. The smaller COG displacements observed during all SOTs provides the evidence for the higher CES value for footballers who train regularly. The footballers also showed smaller COG displacements in the anterior–posterior direction for conditions which were inconsistent with the real signals from the somatosensory and visual systems. The footballers made better use of the signals from the vestibular system, which is the most reliable source of information regarding the positioning of the body's COG [15]. An analysis of the symmetry of the distribution of body weight gives a higher load asymmetry in the lower limbs in the footballers, which arises from using the dominant leg during the game. This is probably the result of more symmetrical actions performed during training and matches, which are due to unexpected situations arising during the game. For both male [21] and female footballers [22], in particular when shooting at goal, which is an important technical skill, there is a clear asymmetry with the right leg being dominant. Barone et al. [23] suspects that sportspeople prefer to use one leg (dominant), because they have better standing balance on non-dominant one.

The regularity of exercising in the context of improving balance has been written about repeatedly. One of the few studies relating to female footballers showed that doing dynamic exercises during warm-up improves both static and dynamic balance [24]. Jakobsen et al. [25] observed postural control improvement after 12 weeks of football training and high-intensity interval running. Paillard et al. [9] paid attention to the fact that the players with more frequent and intensive training sessions showed better postural control, which may be due to greater sensitivity of sensory receptors or better integration of information. Both the general muscular exercises (that mobilizes the whole body) and local muscular exercises (that concentrates on a particular muscle group) can disturb postural control. General muscular exercises (especially running and walking, which are a big part of a football training) contribute to changing the effectiveness of sensory inputs: vestibular—decreases the sensitivity of orthotic organs—and proprioceptive—disturbs the senses of the force and limb position [26]. Söderman et al. [27] Baghbaninaghadehi et al. [28] have drawn attention to the importance of maintaining proper body stability in team sports. This is an important issue, because footballers must have adequate stability, which is especially important when jumping up to head a ball. Brito et al. [29] found that the postural sway (represented by sway velocity) increased and the ankle proprioception decreased after a 45 min of a match. The authors suggest that prophylactic balance training should be performed following rather than before the practice session. Also, Gioftsidou et al. [30] observed improvement in the balance ability, especially in non-dominant lower limbs when the balance training was performed after the football training.

Mohammadi et al. [31] observed significant changes in both the static and dynamic balance parameters among young sportspeople who undertook a 6-week appropriately selected training schedule. According to the authors, an increase in the sportsperson's muscle mass was responsible for the changes. Results of this work also show better postural stability of young football players in dynamic conditions, which are more valuable than static ones, because they are the closest conditions to these on the football field. Interestingly, Pau et al. [32] observed dynamic balance impairment in young football players due to fatigue after the first half on football match. The impairment was observed in the increase in the time necessary to stabilize after landing from a single-leg jump.

On the basis of tracking professional players' COG trajectory while they were standing on one leg and then monitoring the time taken to stabilize their posture, Pau et al. [32] showed that they achieved significantly lower stabilization times while their center of pressure (COP) displacement surface area was significantly less than for their novice colleagues.

The assessment of the balance and dizziness following sports-related concussions is very important for making decisions about further training or removal from the team [33]. In addition, the study authors [34,35] have shown that the use of exercises to improve balance also has a positive effect on coping with stress and reduces the risk of injury during physical activity, which is extremely important in the effective use of a sportsperson during the game.

The findings of this study must be seen in light of some limitations. The first limitation is the sample size: because of the number of football players in the world it is difficult to deduce a general conclusion based on a small sample. The second limitation concerns the sample profile—using purely student sampling is also extremely limiting on the population. Another limit regarding the student population is the questionnaire and their truthfulness, especially in questions about alcohol, drugs, etc. Gribble et al. [36] observed that males were more adversely affected by fatigue than females. This may suggest that for future research the study group should consist of both sexes. In our research, only dynamic conditions were tested; however, Hrysomallis et al. [37] and Pau et al. [38] paid attention to the fact that assessment of balance in football players should be performed with both dynamic and static tests, because postural control performance is not related in these two cases.

5. Conclusions

In conclusion, postural stability in young female footballers was found to be better than their inactive peers. The study showed better usefulness of the vestibular system as well as asymmetrical weight-bearing in regularly trainees.

Further research to explore the possibilities of use CDP in assessing the progress of training is needed. The Sensory Organization Test assesses the quality of the human balance system, which could help with evaluation of training effects. Also, the results of the WS may be useful for determination of the dominant leg, which is important when selecting the role the player can play on the field. More studies are needed to specify which exercises contribute to improving the balance and perhaps apply them in rehabilitation techniques.

Author Contributions: Conceptualization, G.O.; methodology, G.O.; validation, G.O. and A.C.; formal analysis, A.C.; investigation, A.C..; resources, G.O.; writing—original draft preparation, G.O. and A.C.; writing—review and editing, G.O. and A.C. All authors have read and agreed to the published version of the manuscript.

Acknowledgments: We would like to pay our gratitude and our respects to our co-organizer Jozef Bergier, deceased March 2019.

References

1. Arliani, G.G.; Almeida, G.P.L.; dos Santos, C.V.; Venturini, A.M.; da Costa Astur, D.; Cohen, M. The effects of exertion on the postural stability in young soccer players. *Acta Ortop. Bras.* **2013**, *21*, 155–158. [CrossRef] [PubMed]
2. Gstöttner, M.; Neher, A.; Scholtz, A.; Millonig, M.; Lembert, S.; Raschner, C. Balance Ability and Muscle Response of the Preferred and Nonpreferred Leg in Soccer Players. *Mot. Control.* **2009**, *13*, 218–231. [CrossRef] [PubMed]
3. Starosta, W.; Karpińska, A.; Podciechowska, K. Lateral differentiation of global movement coordination results in girls and women depending in their age, kind of physical activity and dominant hand. *Pol. J. Sports Med.* **2011**, *27*, 289–298. [CrossRef]
4. Kraemer, W.J.; Adams, K.; Cafarelli, E.; Dudley, G.A.; Dooly, C.; Feigenbaum, M.S.; Fleck, S.J.; Franklin, B.; Fry, A.C.; Hoffman, J.R.; et al. American College of Sports Medicine position stand. Progression models in resistance training for healthy adults. *Med. Sci. Sports Exerc.* **2002**, *34*, 364–380. [PubMed]
5. Randers, M.B.; Nielsen, J.J.; Krustrup, B.R.; Sundstrup, E.; Jakobsen, M.D.; Nybo, L.; Dvorak, J.; Bangsbo, J.; Krustrup, P. Positive performance and health effects of a football training program over 12 weeks can be maintained over a 1-year period with reduced training frequency. *Scand. J. Med. Sci. Sports* **2010**, *20*, 80–89. [CrossRef] [PubMed]
6. Bressel, E.; Yonker, J.C.; Kras, J.; Heath, E.M. Comparison of Static and Dynamic Balance in Female Collegiate Soccer, Basketball, and Gymnastics Athletes. *J. Athl. Train.* **2007**, *42*, 42–46. [PubMed]
7. Liang, Y.; Hiley, M.; Kanosue, K. The effect of contact sport expertise on postural control. *PLoS ONE* **2019**, *14*, e0212334. [CrossRef]
8. Matsuda, S.; Demura, S.; Uchiyama, M. Centre of pressure sway characteristics during static one-legged stance of athletes from different sports. *J. Sports Sci.* **2008**, *26*, 775–779. [CrossRef]
9. Paillard, T.; Noé, F.; Rivière, T.; Marion, V.; Montoya, R.; Dupui, P. Postural Performance and Strategy in the Unipedal Stance of Soccer Players at Different Levels of Competition. *J. Athl. Train.* **2006**, *41*, 172–176.
10. Biegański, P.; Pyskir, M.; Pyskir, J.; Trela, E.; Hagner, W. Postural stability of young football players against their physically inactive peers. *J. Health Sci.* **2013**, *3*, 477–488.
11. Maranesi, E.; Merlo, A.; Fioretti, S.; Zemp, D.D.; Campanini, I.; Quadri, P. A statistical approach to discriminate between non-fallers, rare fallers and frequent fallers in older adults based on posturographic data. *Clin. Biomech.* **2016**, *32*, 8–13. [CrossRef] [PubMed]
12. Horak, F.B. Postural orientation and equilibrium: What do we need to know about neural control of balance to prevent falls? *Age Ageing* **2006**, *35*, ii7–ii11. [CrossRef] [PubMed]
13. Maranesi, E.; Fioretti, S.; Ghetti, G.G.; Rabini, R.A.; Burattini, L.; Mercante, O.; Di Nardo, F. The surface electromyographic evaluation of the Functional Reach in elderly subjects. *J. Electromyogr. Kinesiol.* **2016**, *26*, 102–110. [CrossRef]
14. Błaszczyk, J.; Cieślinska-Swider, J.; Plewa, M.; Zahorska-Markiewicz, B.; Markiewicz, A. Effects of excessive body weight on postural control. *J. Biomech.* **2009**, *42*, 1295–1300. [CrossRef]
15. Nashner, L.M. Computerized dynamic posturography. In *Handbook of Balance Function Testing*; Delmar: Clifton Park, NY, USA, 1993; pp. 280–334.
16. Trueblood, P.R.; Rivera, M.; Lopez, C.; Bentley, C.; Wubenhorst, N. Age-based normative data for a computerized dynamic posturography system that uses a virtual visual surround environment. *Acta Oto Laryngol.* **2018**, *138*, 597–602. [CrossRef]
17. Mohieldin, A.; Douaa, M.; Sherif, K.; Thabat, I.; Fawzy, H.; Walid, A.-B. Evaluation of dynamic posturography in anterior cruciate ligament injury patients. *Maced. J. Med. Sci.* **2011**, *4*, 167–173.
18. Dittmar, M. Functional and Postural Lateral Preferences in Humans: Interrelations and Life-Span Age Differences. *Hum. Biol.* **2002**, *74*, 569–585. [CrossRef]

19. Vanicek, N.; King, S.A.; Gohil, R.; Chetter, I.C.; Coughlin, P.A. Computerized dynamic posturography for postural control assessment in patients with intermittent claudication. *J. Vis. Exp.* **2013**, *82*, e51077. [CrossRef]
20. NeuroCom International Clinical Interpretation Guide. In *Balance Manager Systems*; NeuroCom International, Inc.: Clakamas, OR, USA, 2008.
21. Carey, D.P.; Smith, G.; Smith, D.T.; Shepherd, J.W.; Skriver, J.; Ord, L.; Rutland, A. Footedness in world soccer: An analysis of France '98. *J. Sports Sci.* **2001**, *19*, 855–864. [CrossRef]
22. Bergier, J. In the Search of the Tendency to Symmetrize the Shots in Female Soccer at Top Level Competitions. *Afr. J. Phys. Act. Health Sci.* **2015**, *21*, 1024–1029.
23. Barone, R.; Macaluso, F.; Traina, M.; Leonardi, V.; Farina, F.; Di Felice, V. Soccer players have a better standing balance in nondominant one-legged stance. *Open Access J. Sports Med.* **2010**, *2*, 1. [CrossRef]
24. Amiri-Khorasani, M.; Gulick, D.T. Acute effects of different stretching methods on static and dynamic balance in female football players. *Int. J. Ther. Rehabil.* **2015**, *22*, 68–73. [CrossRef]
25. Jakobsen, M.D.; Sundstrup, E.; Krustrup, P.; Aagaard, P. The effect of recreational soccer training and running on postural balance in untrained men. *Eur. J. Appl. Physiol.* **2011**, *111*, 521–530. [CrossRef]
26. Paillard, T. Effects of general and local fatigue on postural control: A review. *Neurosci. Biobehav. Rev.* **2012**, *36*, 162–176. [CrossRef]
27. Söderman, K.; Werner, S.; Pietilä, T.; Engström, B.; Alfredson, H. Balance board training: Prevention of traumatic injuries of the lower extremities in female soccer players? A prospective randomized intervention study. *Knee Surg. Sports Traumatol. Arthrosc.* **2000**, *8*, 356–363. [CrossRef]
28. Baghbaninaghadehi, F.; Ramezani, A.R.; Hatami, F. The effect of functional fatigue on static and dynamic balance in female athletes. *Int. Sportmed J.* **2013**, *14*, 77–85.
29. Brito, J.; Fontes, I.; Ribeiro, F.; Raposo, A.; Krustrup, P.; Rebelo, A. Postural stability decreases in elite young soccer players after a competitive soccer match. *Phys. Ther. Sport* **2012**, *13*, 175–179. [CrossRef]
30. Gioftsidou, A.; Malliou, P.; Pafis, G.; Beneka, A.; Godolias, G.; Maganaris, C.N. The effects of soccer training and timing of balance training on balance ability. *Eur. J. Appl. Physiol.* **2006**, *96*, 659–664. [CrossRef]
31. Mohammadi, V.; Alizadeh, M.; Gaieni, A. The Effects of six weeks strength exercises on static and dynamic balance of young male athletes. *Procedia Soc. Behav. Sci.* **2012**, *31*, 247–250. [CrossRef]
32. Pau, M.; Mereu, F.; Melis, M.; Leban, B.; Corona, F.; Ibba, G. Dynamic balance is impaired after a match in young elite soccer players. *Phys. Ther. Sport* **2016**, *22*, 11–15. [CrossRef]
33. Doettl Steven, M. Sports Concussions (TBI), Imbalance, and Dizziness. *Perspect. Neurophysiol. Neurogenic Speech Lang. Disord.* **2015**, *25*, 36–41. [CrossRef]
34. Iacono, A.D.; Martone, D.; Alfieri, A.; Ayalon, M.; Buono, P. Core Stability Training Program (CSTP) effects on static and dynamic balance abilities. *Gazz. Med. Ital. Arch. Per Le Sci. Med.* **2014**, *173*, 197–206.
35. Cankaya, S.; Gokmen, B.; Tasmektepligil, M.Y.; Con, M. Special Balance Developer Training Applications on Young Males' Static and Dynamic Balance Performance. *Anthropologist* **2015**, *19*, 31–39. [CrossRef]
36. Gribble, P.A.; Robinson, R.H.; Hertel, J.; Denegar, C.R. The Effects of Gender and Fatigue on Dynamic Postural Control. *J. Sport Rehabil.* **2009**, *18*, 240–257. [CrossRef] [PubMed]
37. Hrysomallis, C.; McLaughlin, P.; Goodman, C. Relationship between static and dynamic balance tests among elite Australian Footballers. *J. Sci. Med. Sport* **2006**, *9*, 288–291. [CrossRef]
38. Pau, M.; Arippa, F.; Leban, B.; Corona, F.; Ibba, G.; Todde, F.; Scorcu, M. Relationship between static and dynamic balance abilities in Italian professional and youth league soccer players. *Phys. Sport* **2015**, *16*, 236–241. [CrossRef]

9

Texture Analysis is a Useful Tool to Assess the Complexity Profile of Microcirculatory Blood Flow

Henrique Silva [1,2,*], Hugo A. Ferreira [3], Clemente Rocha [1] and Luís Monteiro Rodrigues [1,2]

1 CBIOS (Research Center for Biosciences and Health Technologies), School of Health Sciences and Technologies, Lusófona University, 1749-024 Lisboa, Portugal; c.rocha.dr@gmail.com (C.R.); monteiro.rodrigues@ulusofona.pt (L.M.R.)
2 Department of Pharmacological Sciences, Faculty of Pharmacy, University of Lisboa, 1649-003 Lisboa, Portugal
3 IBEB Institute of Biophysics and Biomedical Engineering, Faculty of Sciences, University of Lisboa, 1749-016 Lisboa, Portugal; hatdferreira@gmail.com
* Correspondence: henrique.silva@ulusofona.pt

Abstract: The quantitative assessment of cardiovascular functions is particularly complicated, especially during any physiological challenge (e.g., exercise), with physiological signals showing intricate oscillatory properties. Signal complexity is one of such properties, and reflects the adaptability of the physiological systems that generated them. However, it is still underexplored in vascular physiology. In the present study, we calculate the complexity of photoplethysmography (PPG) signals and their frequency components obtained with the wavelet transform (WT), with two analytical tools—(i) texture analysis (TA) of WT scalograms, and (ii) multiscale entropy (MSE) analysis. PPG signals were collected from twelve healthy young subjects (26.0 ± 5.0 y.o.) during a unilateral leg lowering maneuver to evoke the venoarteriolar reflex (VAR) while lying supine, with the contralateral leg remaining stationary. Results showed that TA was able to detect a decrease in complexity, viewed as an increase in texture entropy (TE), of the PPG scalograms during VAR, similarly to MSE, suggesting that a decrease in the competence of vascular regulation mechanisms might be present during VAR. Nonetheless, TA showed lower sensitivity than MSE for low frequency spectral regions. TA seems to be a promising and straightforward analytical tool for the assessment of the complexity of PPG perfusion signals.

Keywords: signal complexity; texture analysis; multiscale entropy analysis; wavelet transform; photoplethysmography

---

1. Introduction

The regulation of the cardiovascular system results from the adjustment of several biophysical phenomena, both electrical and mechanical. Their coordination is highly complex, depending on the continuous feedback and cross-talk between effector organs and controlling systems [1]. The heart pump and respiration are the most notorious "central" processes governing the performance of the cardiovascular system, while on a more "peripheral" level, the phenomena that control vascular tone, such as the myogenic activity of the vessel wall, the sympathetic activity and the endothelial release of vasoactive substances, play crucial roles [2–4]. Microcirculation signals are composed of both these central and peripheral components and therefore provide an "integrated" view of cardiovascular function [4,5]. The contributions from these multiple regulation systems and their intricate interplay explain the oscillatory properties of microcirculation signals. From an analytical standpoint, these oscillatory properties are increasingly considered as a means to extract more sensible information not apparent from the general analysis of the raw signals, in particular their spectral origin and the significance of their fractal and chaotic profiles [5–7]. In recent years, much attention has been given to the study of the complexity of physiological signals, a property that reflects the adaptability of the systems that generated them. Intuitively, the term complexity is often associated with "structural richness" [8], which can be applied to the study of biological signals and images. Complexity is typically assessed as "entropy," a general measure of "disorganization" in physical, chemical and biological phenomena [9]. In biomedical research, entropy is used as a quantitative parameter, and is typically assessed in continuous, but temporally unpredictable, physiological signals, such as electrocardiography [10], electroencephalography [11], blood pressure [12], laser Doppler flowmetry (LDF) [13], and photoplethysmography (PPG) [14]. Physiological signals may be regular (e.g., more periodic) or irregular. The higher entropy measured in irregular signals reflects the adaptation capability to changing internal and external conditions of the biological system that generated them [15]. Overall, the entropy of physiological signals tends to decrease whenever the systems that generated them lose adaptability, which can result in a compromise of their function or even in disease. Therefore, a suitable metric of complexity should assign higher values to the output signal of a "healthier" system with a rich and meaningful structure and lower values to either random dynamics or predictable systems, which are often associated with disease [8,16,17]. This has been observed in the aging process [18,19] and in cardiovascular, metabolic and neurological diseases [18], among several others. In addition to pathological states, some experimental procedures are sufficiently "challenging" to temporarily provoke tissue dysfunction, especially those that reduce perfusion [6]. For continuous signals, the multiscale entropy analysis (MSE) is considered a robust analytical tool, having shown superiority over other measures for its ability to assess entropy over different time scales [19]. Entropy can also be assessed in texturally rich biological images, reflecting their textural "disorganization." Texturally rich images can be assessed with texture analysis (TA), an analytical tool allowing the detection of various features on a gray-level image to discriminate textural differences, such as texture entropy (TE), contrast, correlation, homogeneity, and energy. Entropy calculated from TA of images may reflect different information than that conveyed by the entropy assessment of continuous numerical series. When applied to a grayscale image, high entropy means that the pixels can adopt a high number of gray levels, expressing richer information [20]. TA has been used in medical imaging with the purpose of improving diagnostic capacity, given that human visual inspection constitutes a process that is expensive, time-consuming and prone to interpretation errors [21]. Thus far, TA in medical imaging has been more frequently applied to mammography [22], ultrasonography, computerized tomography (CT) [23], and magnetic resonance imaging (MRI) [24] techniques [25], as well as to dermatoscopy [26] and microscopy images [27]. In particular, TE has been used to explore immune competence of lymphoid tissue in microscopic images [28], to assess the onset organ (liver) disease and tumor (colorectal cancer) evolution in CT scans [29–31], and to assess bone regeneration in fractures [32] and osteoarthritis [33], among others. In medical imaging, TE does not necessarily decrease when images display abnormal features. In fact, since abnormal or dysmorphic features often increase the coarseness of smooth or uniform images from healthy subjects, increases in TE are often seen in pathological images, such as in the case of aged tissues and organs [34] as well as the case of neoplastic formations [30,31]. In these situations, a richer texture and therefore, higher entropy, is associated with dysfunction. Although currently underexplored in vascular physiology, the complexity assessment of microcirculation signals, both raw and decomposed, may deepen our knowledge of the mechanisms underlying perfusion regulation. Microcirculation signals are easily decomposed into their frequency components by the wavelet transform (WT) [4]. One of the WT main outputs is a scalogram, i.e., a multi-patterned image representation of the time evolution of all components of the decomposed signal. Given their textural richness, WT scalograms seem suitable candidates for TE analysis, however, to our knowledge this analysis has not been previously attempted. Since WT scalograms are not medical images, the interpretation of TE in this context must be necessarily different from the one performed in medical diagnosis. Given the fact that a WT scalogram is a 2D projection of a 3D frequency spectrum, (i.e., the 3D spectrum seen from above), it is only logical to assume that a change in the entropy of the numerical series that constitute the 3D spectrum would also be observed in corresponding WT scalograms. Therefore, the assumption that similar trends in complexity would be observed with MSE and TA seems legitimate. Our objective was to compare the complexity of microcirculation PPG signals calculated with TE against MSE during a typical venoarteriolar reflex (VAR).

2. Materials and Methods

2.1. Experimental

Twelve healthy young adult subjects (26.0 ± 5.0 y.o., seven females, five males) participated in this study after giving informed written consent. All subjects were healthy, with no cardiovascular diseases, were non-smokers, and abstained from consuming alcohol and caffeine-containing beverages 24 hours prior to the experimental procedure. The protocol was approved by the School of Health Sciences and Technologies' Ethical Commission. All subjects gave written informed consent, and the study was conducted in accordance with the Declaration of Helsinki and subsequent amendments [35]. After 20 minute acclimatization to room conditions (temperature: 22 ± 1 °C, humidity: 40–60%), a postural challenge to elicit the VAR was applied, as previously described [4]—10 minutes lying supine with both legs extended (baseline, Phase I); 10 minutes with one foot lowered 50 cm from heart level (challenge, Phase II); and 10 minutes resuming the initial posture (recovery, Phase III). The contralateral foot remained stationary and served as control. Blood flow signals, expressed in arbitrary units (AU), were acquired from the first toe of both feet at a 100 Hz sampling rate with a reflection photoplethysmography Blood Pulse Volume sensor (Biosignals Plux, Lisboa, Portugal) connected to a BITalino Plugged microprocessor board (Biosignals Plux).

2.2. Numerical

The raw PPG signals were imported to Matlab (Mathworks R2012, Natick, MA, USA) and smoothed with a moving average filter.

The WT (http://noc.ac.uk/using-science/crosswavelet-wavelet-coherence) was then applied to the smoothed signals, which allowed the decomposition into their main frequency components. Wavelets are a family of functions constructed from translations and dilations of a single function called the "mother wavelet" $\psi(t)$, collectively defined by:

$$\psi_{a,b}(t) = \frac{1}{\sqrt{|a|}}\psi\left(\frac{t-b}{a}\right),\ a, b \in R,\ a \neq 0 \tag{1}$$

The parameter a is the scaling parameter or scale, measuring the degree of compression, while parameter b is the translation parameter, determining the time location of the wavelet. If $|a| < 1$, then the wavelet in the above equation is the compressed version of the mother wavelet and corresponds mainly to higher frequencies. If $|a| > 1$, then $\psi_{a,b}(t)$ has a larger time-width than $\psi(t)$ and corresponds to lower frequencies. Thus, wavelets have time-widths adapted to their frequencies.

In this case, the central frequency of the wavelet was 6 Hz, with a discretization factor of 10 scales per octave. The detected components of the PPG signals occurred at the following frequency ranges: cardiac [1.6–0.7 Hz], respiratory [0.7–0.26 Hz], myogenic [0.26–0.1 Hz], neurogenic/sympathetic [0.1–0.045 Hz], endothelial NO-dependent (NOd) [0.045–0.015 Hz] and NO-independent (NOi) [0.015–0.007 Hz], which were in line with the ranges previously described for LDF [36]. From the WT, two main outputs were generated for each subject: (1) a scalogram and (2) a 3D periodogram. The WT scalogram (Figure 1) shows the time (here converted to sample number) evolution of the amplitude with a factor of 2^n (here in color scale) for each signal scale. The approximate frequency of a component is obtained by dividing the central wavelet frequency by the scale of the component. From a visual inspection, the WT scalogram also presents an oscillatory pattern in pixel distribution on different scales, making it a suitable candidate for TA. The scalogram was then used as a grayscale image, where several regions of interest (ROI) were marked, each per component per phase of the protocol. Each ROI was then converted to a gray-level co-occurrence matrix (GLCM), a matrix where the number of rows and columns is equal to the number of gray levels (G) in the image, from which the TE was calculated as follows [37]:

$$\text{Entropy} = -\sum_{i=0}^{G-1}\sum_{j=0}^{G-1} P(i,j).\log[P(i,j)] \tag{2}$$

where $P(i, j)$ denotes the probability of occurrence of a given element in the matrix.

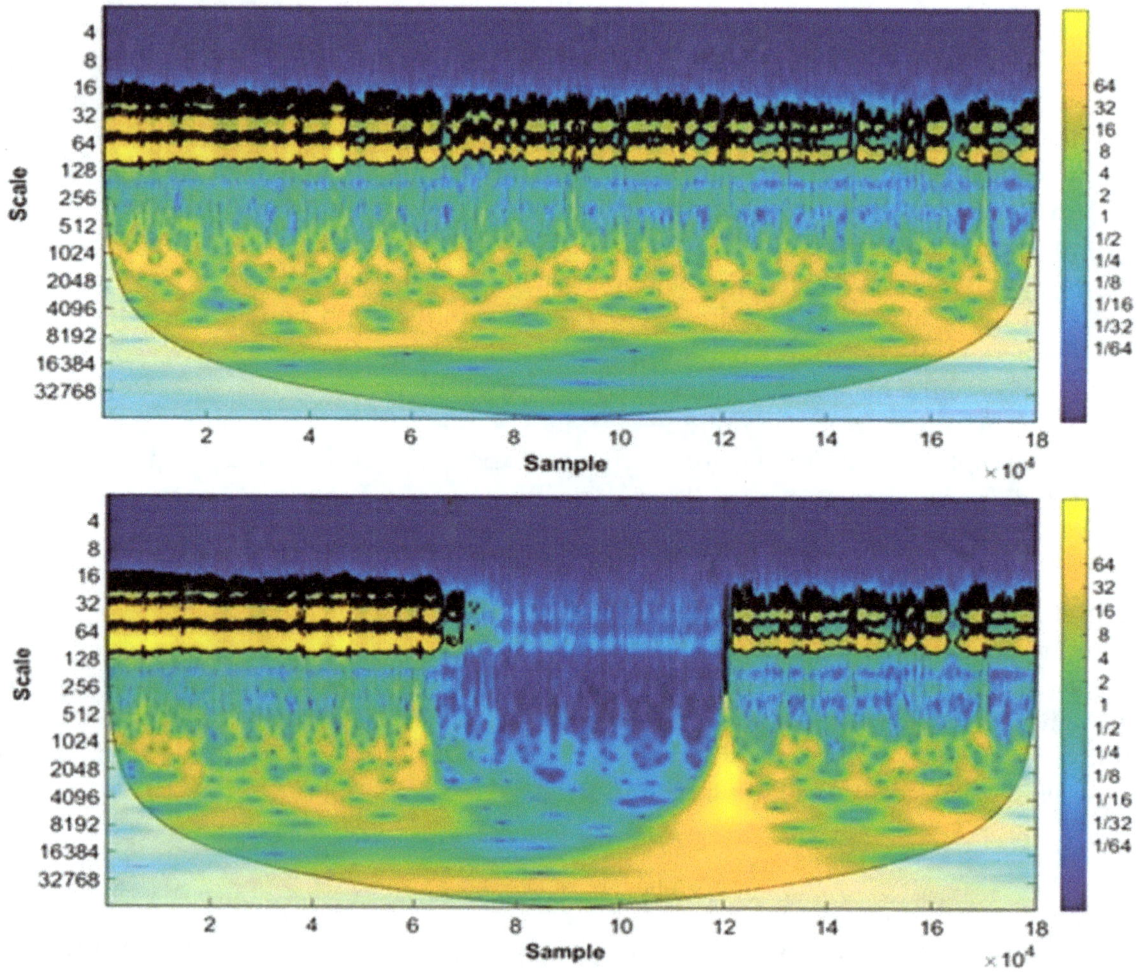

Figure 1. WT scalogram of the PPG signal from the control (top) and test (bottom) feet from a representative subject (20 y.o.).

To correctly select each ROI, a control sine wave signal was generated with multiple components occurring at known frequencies (f_1 = 3.2 Hz; f_2 = 1.6 Hz; f_3 = 0.7 Hz, f_4 = 0.26 Hz; f_5 = 0.1 Hz; f_6 = 0.045 Hz; f_7 = 0.015 Hz; f_8 = 0.007 Hz), where each frequency is close to the ones that define the borders of the PPG components' detected frequency ranges. The sine wave signal was then deconstructed with the WT, and a reference scalogram was generated (Figure 2).

From the 3D periodogram (Figure 3), a 2D time evolution of the amplitude of each component was constructed by averaging the amplitude at each time point for each spectral interval (Figure 4). Signals were acquired at a 100 Hz sampling rate, which translates to a total number of 180,000 samples for the entire 30 minute protocol. The wavelet period is a natural logarithmic representation of the wavelet scale, with the frequency in Hz exponentially related to this period. The time evolution was analyzed for both the raw PPG signal and its components with MSE, an algorithm that quantifies the randomness/unpredictability of a signal over different time scales as follows [19]:

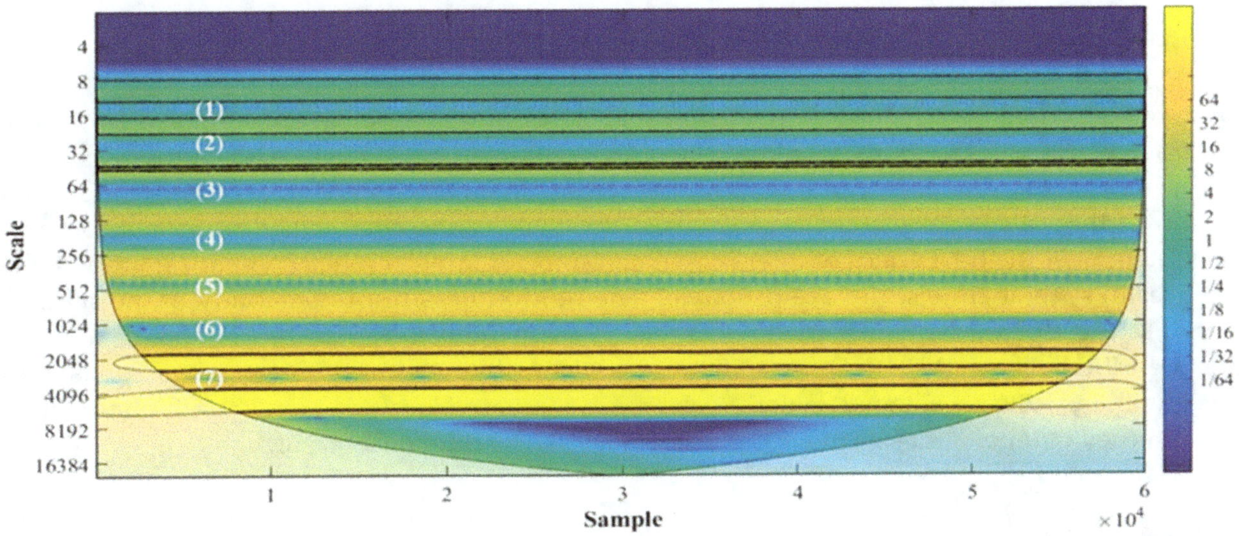

Figure 2. WT scalogram of the reference sine wave signal. The region corresponding to each component frequency interval is shown (1—first harmonic of the cardiac component; 2—cardiac; 3—respiratory; 4—myogenic; 5—sympathetic; 6—endothelial NO-dependent; 7—endothelial NO-independent).

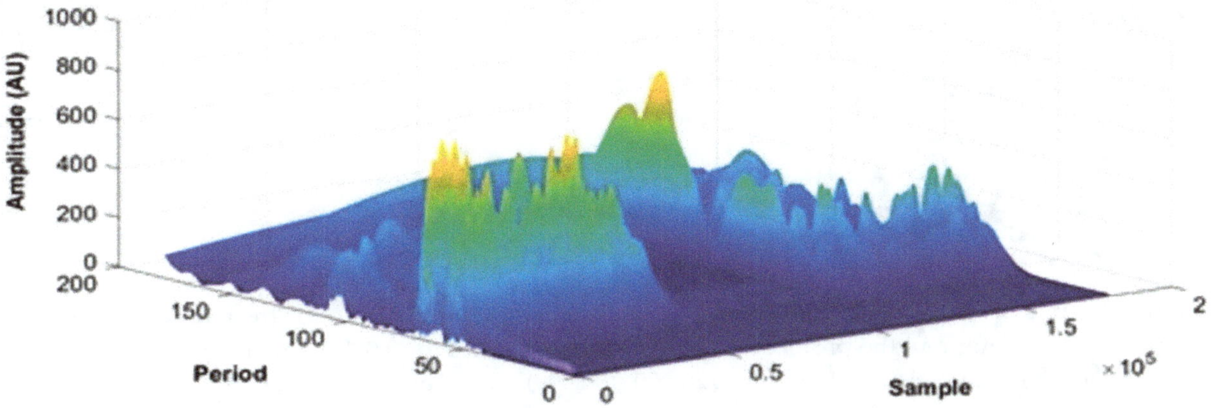

Figure 3. PPG 3D frequency spectrum (period vs. sample vs. amplitude) for the test foot of a representative subject (20 y.o.). Signals were acquired at a 100 Hz sampling rate, which translates to a total of 180,000 signal samples for a 30 minute acquisition period. Period is a natural logarithmic representation of the wavelet scale.

Given a time series $x_i = 1,\ldots, N$, a consecutive coarse-grained time series $y(\tau)$ is constructed:

$$y_j^{(\tau)} = \frac{1}{\tau} \sum_{i=(j-1)\tau+1}^{j\tau} x_i \tag{3}$$

where τ represents the scale factor and $1 \leq j \leq N/\tau$. The sample entropy (*SampEn*) of each coarse-grained time series is then computed. *SampEn(m, r, N)* is the negative natural logarithm of the conditional probability that a dataset of length N, having repeated itself with a tolerance of r points, will also repeat itself for $m+1$ points, without allowing self matches:

$$\mathrm{SampEn(m,r,N)} = -\ln \frac{\mathrm{A^m(r)}}{\mathrm{B^m(r)}} \tag{4}$$

where $A^m(r)$ is the probability that two sequences will match for $m+1$ points and $B^m(r)$ is the probability that two sequences will match for m points. The more regular and predictable a time series is, the lower the value of *SampEn*. The more random a time series is, the higher the value of *SampEn*. Plotting the *SampEn* over the scale factor yields the MSE curve, which gives insight into the integrated complexity of the system over the time scales of interest, which can be of interest when comparing groups where differences in specific time scales are probable. The randomness/unpredictability of the signal can finally be straightforwardly summarized as the complexity index (CI), which corresponds to the area under the MSE curve [38]. The CI and TE were statistically compared between each phase of the protocol with the Wilcoxon signed-rank test, and were compared between feet for each phase with the Mann-Whitney independent sample test, adopting a 95% confidence interval.

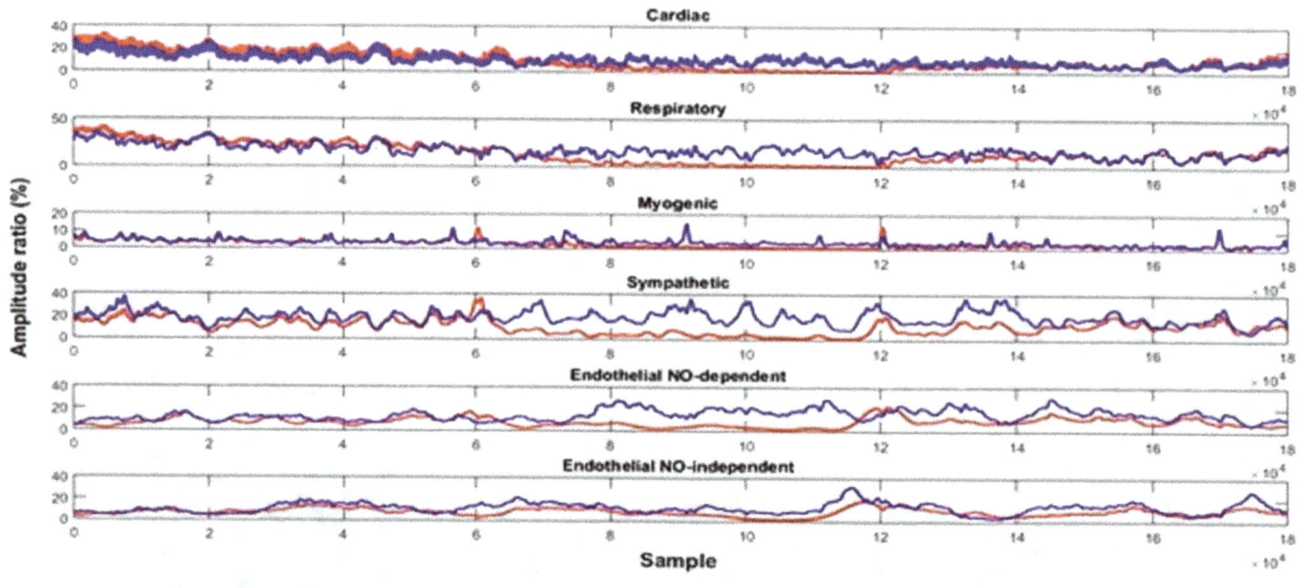

Figure 4. Time evolution of the PPG signal components' amplitude ratio for the control (blue) and test (red) feet throughout the protocol (baseline: signal samples 0–60,000; challenge: signal samples 60,000–120,000; recovery: signal samples 120,000–180,000) for a representative subject (20 y.o.).

3. Results

As previously published, during the postural challenge, perfusion decreased significantly on both the test and control feet [4]. The mean and standard deviation (SD) of the entropy parameter (CI) calculated with MSE is presented in Table 1. For the test foot, the CI of the raw PPG signal and all its components decreased significantly during the challenge (Phase II, raw signal: $p = 0.005$; cardiac: $p = 0.012$; respiratory: $p = 0.002$; myogenic: $p = 0.003$; sympathetic: $p = 0.002$; NOd: $p = 0.002$; NOi: $p = 0.002$). For the control foot, the CI of the raw PPG signal showed an increase without statistical significance. All the components' CI decreased, with the exception of the cardiac, although not so pronounced as in the test foot (respiratory: $p = 0.002$; myogenic: $p = 0.003$; sympathetic: $p = 0.002$; NOd: $p = 0.002$; NOi: $p = 0.002$). During recovery (Phase III), significant differences were still detected on both feet regarding baseline for the respiratory (test: $p = 0.002$; control: $p = 0.002$), myogenic (test: $p = 0.008$; control: $p = 0.008$), sympathetic (test: $p = 0.002$; control: $p = 0.002$), NOd (test: $p = 0.002$; control: $p = 0.002$) and NOi (test: $p = 0.002$; control: $p = 0.003$). The mean and SD of the entropy parameter (TE) calculated for the sine wave and PPG signals with TA is shown in Table 2. For the sine wave signal scalogram, TE decreased from the cardiac component towards the low frequency components, where it increased again for the NOi. For the test foot PPG scalogram, TE decreased significantly in the cardiac ($p = 0.004$), respiratory ($p = 0.013$), and myogenic ($p = 0.008$) components, increased significantly in the NOd ($p = 0.012$) and NOi ($p = 0.010$), and showed no change in the sympathetic component. During recovery, all components' TE returned except for the NOd, which showed a significant difference regarding baseline ($p = 0.007$). For the control foot PPG scalogram, changes in TE were not so pronounced as in the test foot, with only the cardiac component showing a significant difference regarding baseline ($p = 0.001$). During recovery, only the cardiac component showed a significant difference ($p = 0.022$) regarding baseline. No significant differences in entropy were found between feet at baseline (Tables 1 and 2) either with CI or TE. During the challenge phase, significant differences were found for the raw signal ($p < 0.001$) and all components (p=0.001 for the respiratory; $p < 0.001$ for the remaining) with CI. Similarly, TE showed significant differences in all components (cardiac: $p = 0.001$; respiratory: $p = 0.045$; myogenic: $p = 0.028$; NOd: $p = 0.001$; NOi: $p = 0.001$), except the sympathetic. During recovery, the CI of the sympathetic ($p = 0.012$), NOd ($p = 0.002$) and NOi ($p < 0.001$) were significantly different, while with TE no statistical differences were found.

Table 1. Mean and standard deviation (SD) of the MSE complexity index for each foot on each phase of the protocol (card—cardiac, resp—respiratory, myo—myogenic, sym—sympathetic, NOd—endothelial NO-dependent, NOi—endothelial NO-independent). Statistical comparison to Phase I is shown (*—$p < 0.05$).

Complexity Index		Test Foot		Control Foot		*p*-Value (T vs. C)
		Mean ± SD	*p*-Value	Mean ± SD	*p*-Value	
raw signal	Phase I	34.8 ± 6.1	-	34.2 ± 8.2	-	0.843
	Phase II	15.0 ± 11.5	0.005 *	35.9 ± 8.7	0.182	<0.001 *
	Phase III	31.4 ± 7.3	0.182	37.0 ± 6.7	0.239	0.089
card	Phase I	25.9 ± 6.1	-	29.3 ± 7.2	-	0.347
	Phase II	15.6 ± 9.0	0.012 *	28.7 ± 6.5	0.754	<0.001 *
	Phase III	23.8 ± 7.3	0.224	29.7 ± 7.8	0.875	0.089
resp	Phase I	25.9 ± 6.1	-	29.3 ± 7.2	-	0.347
	Phase II	6.7 ± 4.2	0.002 *	14.3 ± 4.8	0.002 *	0.001 *
	Phase III	10.1 ± 5.5	0.002 *	13.7 ± 4.9	0.002 *	0.160
myo	Phase I	23.2 ± 8.7	-	25.9 ± 7.5	-	0.378
	Phase II	3.9 ± 3.1	0.003 *	12.0 ± 2.8	0.003 *	<0.001 *
	Phase III	7.9 ± 5.4	0.008 *	10.9 ± 5.8	0.008 *	0.160
sym	Phase I	25.9 ± 6.1	-	29.3 ± 7.2	-	0.347
	Phase II	2.6 ± 2.4	0.002 *	10.5 ± 1.9	0.002 *	<0.001 *
	Phase III	6.8 ± 2.2	0.002 *	10.7 ± 4.0	0.002 *	0.012 *
NOd	Phase I	25.9 ± 6.1	-	29.3 ± 7.2	-	0.347
	Phase II	2.5 ± 3.5	0.002 *	11.5 ± 2.6	0.002 *	<0.001 *
	Phase III	5.5 ± 2.1	0.002 *	11.0 ± 4.8	0.002 *	0.002 *
NOi	Phase I	25.9 ± 6.1	-	29.3 ± 7.2	-	0.347
	Phase II	1.9 ± 0.9	0.002 *	10.2 ± 3.6	0.002 *	<0.001 *
	Phase III	6.2 ± 3.4	0.002 *	13.6 ± 5.0	0.003 *	<0.001 *

Table 2. Mean and standard deviation (SD) of the texture entropy for each foot on each phase of the protocol (card—cardiac, resp—respiratory, myo—myogenic, sym—sympathetic, NOd—endothelial NO-dependent, NOi—endothelial NO-independent). Statistical comparison to Phase I and between the test and control limbs are shown (*—$p < 0.05$).

Texture Entropy		Sine Wave Signal	Test Foot		Control Foot		p-Value (T vs. C)
			Mean ± SD	p-Value	Mean ± SD	p-Value	
card	Phase I	6.1	6.6 ± 0.5	-	6.8 ± 0.3	-	0.198
	Phase II		6.2 ± 0.7	0.004 *	6.9 ± 0.3	0.011 *	0.001 *
	Phase III		7.0 ± 0.2	0.563	7.0 ± 0.2	0.022 *	0.713
resp	Phase I	5.4	6.5 ± 0.2	-	6.5 ± 0.2	-	0.551
	Phase II		5.5 ± 1.3	0.013 *	6.3 ± 0.2	0.286	0.045 *
	Phase III		6.5 ± 0.2	0.638	6.4 ± 0.2	0.530	0.478
myo	Phase I	5.2	6.6 ± 0.3	-	6.7 ± 0.1	-	0.089
	Phase II		6.3 ± 0.4	0.008 *	6.6 ± 0.1	0.433	0.028 *
	Phase III		6.5 ± 0.2	0.289	6.7 ± 0.2	0.754	0.266
sym	Phase I	5.3	6.2 ± 0.3	-	6.2 ± 0.4	-	0.671
	Phase II		6.2 ± 0.2	0.147	6.2 ± 0.2	0.814	0.887
	Phase III		6.0 ± 0.2	0.594	6.1 ± 0.3	0.239	0.630
NOd	Phase I	5.3	5.8 ± 0.5	-	5.9 ± 0.4	-	0.630
	Phase II		6.4 ± 0.2	0.012 *	5.7 ± 0.5	0.272	0.001 *
	Phase III		6.1 ± 0.3	0.007 *	5.9 ± 0.3	0.307	0.060
NOi	Phase I	6.2	6.0 ± 0.4	-	5.9 ± 0.4	-	0.551
	Phase II		6.2 ± 0.3	0.010 *	5.5 ± 0.7	0.753	0.001 *
	Phase III		6.2 ± 0.3	0.594	5.8 ± 0.8	0.126	0.060

4. Discussion

In this study, the acquired PPG signals and an artificial sine wave signal were decomposed with the WT into their respective components so that TE and CI could be calculated. The relative contributions of each of the components to the overall signal, expressed as amplitude ratios, are typical WT outputs but were not considered for this study as these results were previously published [4]. During leg lowering, perfusion decrease in the test foot is explained by a constriction of arterioles secondary to the increased venous distension when the foot is in a pendent posture, which constitutes the VAR [39]. The fast perfusion decreases in the control foot (not so pronounced as in the test foot) is thought to be due to a centrally mediated neurogenic reflex initiated to maintain the vascular homeostasis in the lower limb [4]. The sine wave signal scalogram showed TE values generally invariant regarding the component, which reflects the regularity of these signals. The highest TE values were recorded for both the highest (cardiac) and lowest (NOi) frequency components, meaning a richer texture was found in the corresponding ROIs, likely explained by the particular overlap of the spectral waves that define them. Contrarily, the PPG signal scalogram showed that the higher frequency (HF) components (cardiac, respiratory, myogenic) displayed higher TE values in either foot, meaning the corresponding ROIs are more texturally rich, i.e., more complex in comparison to the lower frequency components. This suggests that TE assessment of PPG scalograms is sensitive to the underlying phenomena that explain the physiological complexity of these signals. In our data, both TE and MSE analyses showed an overall decrease in the PPG signal and in the respective components' entropies during leg lowering in both the test and control feet. This result seems to indicate a bilateral decrease in the vascular adaptation capacity to the lower perfusion levels observed during leg lowering. This apparent decrease in adaptation capacity is further reinforced by the observation that several PPG components' entropies show significant differences between the recovery and baseline phases, suggesting that full recovery was not attained at the end of the protocol. In our view, these results indicate that that VAR creates a state of reduced perfusion that, while not compromising tissue viability, destabilizes the evoked regulatory mechanisms. When considering the test foot, MSE detected a significant decrease in the entropy of all components during VAR. TE, however, detected an entropy decrease in the cardiac, respiratory, and myogenic components, an increase in both endothelial components and no change in the sympathetic. Regarding the control foot, an overall entropy decrease was observed with both tools. MSE recorded a decrease in the complexity of all components, although not so pronounced as in the test foot, which again is likely attributable to the magnitude of the perfusion decrease. Again, TE showed more subtle changes, only significant for the respiratory and NOi components. Overall, MSE and TE showed similar responses in the high frequency components (cardiac, respiratory, myogenic), and dissimilar responses in the low frequency components (sympathetic, NOd, NOi), suggesting that TE loses analytical sensitivity in the latter regions. This loss of sensitivity may be attributed to an incomplete visual resolution of the scalogram bands of the low frequency components, leading to a less precise identification of the respective ROIs. Nevertheless, TE was able to differentiate the entropies of most components during VAR between the test and control limbs. Overall, although both TE and MSE were able to detect differences in entropy, MSE was consistently more sensitive. One should keep in mind that MSE and TE ensure different scale evaluations—frequency for TE and time for MSE, which are two aspects of the same reality (i.e., perfusion signal). Thus, both analytical strategies provide different views into the same physiological event, which can also help to explain the differences in sensitivity found. MSE detected changes in entropy between limbs during both VAR and recovery phases, while TE was only able to detect the more pronounced changes that occurred during VAR. Furthermore, MSE was sensitive to changes in entropy for a greater number of components in comparison to TE. Although the performance of the reference MSE method was superior under the conditions studied, these results suggest that TE is an interesting and suitable tool for assessing the complexity of PPG microcirculation signals considered as WT scalograms, in particular for the analysis of high frequency components.

5. Conclusions

In this paper we present for the first time the use of texture entropy (TE) for the quantification of complexity in microcirculatory perfusion signals, using MSE as a reference analytical tool. Our results show that TE was able to detect a decrease in complexity of the PPG scalograms during VAR, similarly to MSE. This complexity decrease suggests that a decrease in the competence of vascular regulation mechanisms might be present during VAR and should be further investigated. Results from both tools were aligned for the high frequency components, but not for the low frequency components, suggesting a decrease in sensitivity of TE in the latter spectral regions. Recognizing the value of increasing the sample size (and heterogeneity) in future studies, our results have shown Texture Analysis (TA) to be a promising method to assess the complexity of PPG perfusion signals.

Author Contributions: Conceptualization, H.S.; Methodology, H.S., C.R. and H.A.F.; Software, H.S. and H.A.F.; Validation, H.A.F., and L.M.R.; Formal Analysis, H.S.; Investigation, H.S. and C.R.; Resources, H.A.F. and L.M.R.; Data Curation, H.S. and H.A.F.; Writing—Original Draft Preparation, H.S.; Writing—Review & Editing, H.A.F.; Visualization, H.A.F. and L.M.R.; Supervision, L.M.R.; Project Administration, L.M.R.; Funding Acquisition, L.M.R. All authors have read and agreed to the published version of the manuscript.

Acknowledgments: The authors would like to express their thanks to all the volunteers for their participation in this study.

References

1. Stefanovska, A. Coupled Oscillators: Complex but Not Complicated Cardiovascular and Brain Interactions. *IEEE Eng. Med. Biol.* **2007**, *26*, 25–29. [CrossRef] [PubMed]
2. Stefanovska, A.; Lotric, M.B.; Strle, S.; Haken, H. The cardiovascular system as coupled oscillators? *Physiol. Meas.* **2001**, *22*, 535–550. [CrossRef]

3. Bernjak, A.; Stefanovska, A. Importance of wavelet analysis in laser Doppler flowmetry time series. In Proceedings of the 29th Annual International Conference of the IEEE Engeniring in Medicine and Biology Society, Lyon, France, 22–26 August 2007; pp. 4064–4067.
4. Silva, H.; Ferreira, H.A.; Da Silva, H.P.; Rodrigues, L.M. The Venoarteriolar Reflex Significantly Reduces Contralateral Perfusion as Part of the Lower Limb Circulatory Homeostasis in vivo. *Front. Physiol.* **2018**, *9*, 1–9. [CrossRef] [PubMed]
5. Silva, H.; Bento, M.; Vieira, H.; Rodrigues, L.M. Comparing the spectral components of laser Doppler flowmetry and photoplethysmography signals for the assessment of the vascular response to hyperoxia. *J. Biomed. Biopharm. Res.* **2017**, *14*, 187–194. [CrossRef]
6. Silva, H.; Ferreira, H.; Rodrigues, L.M. Studying the Oscillatory Components of Human Skin Microcirculation. In *Measuring the Skin*; Springer Science and Business Media LLC: Berlin, Germany, 2015; pp. 1–15.
7. Mizeva, I.; Di Maria, C.; Frick, P.; Podtaev, S.; Allen, J. Quantifying the correlation between photoplethysmography and laser Doppler flowmetry microvascular low-frequency oscillations. *J. Biomed. Opt.* **2015**, *20*, 37007. [CrossRef] [PubMed]
8. Costa, M.; Goldberger, A.L.; Peng, C.-K. Multiscale entropy analysis of biological signals. *Phys. Rev. E* **2005**, *71*, 021906. [CrossRef]
9. Rangel, J.A.O. The Systemic Theory of Living Systems and Relevance to CAM Part I: The Theory. *Evid-Based Compl. Alt.* **2005**, *2*, 13–18. [CrossRef]
10. Zhang, Y.; Wei, S.; Long, Y.; Liu, C. Performance Analysis of Multiscale Entropy for the Assessment of ECG Signal Quality. *J. Electr. Comput. Eng.* **2015**, *2015*, 1–9. [CrossRef]
11. Chung, C.-C.; Kang, J.-H.; Yuan, R.-Y.; Wu, D.; Chen, C.-C.; Chi, N.-F.; Chen, P.-C.; Hu, C.-J. Multiscale Entropy Analysis of Electroencephalography During Sleep in Patients With Parkinson Disease. *Clin. EEG Neurosci.* **2013**, *44*, 221–226. [CrossRef]
12. Trunkvalterova, Z.; Javorka, M.; Tonhajzerova, I.; Javorkova, J.; Lazárová, Z.; Javorka, K.; Baumert, M. Reduced short-term complexity of heart rate and blood pressure dynamics in patients with diabetes mellitus type 1: multiscale entropy analysis. *Physiol. Meas.* **2008**, *29*, 817–828. [CrossRef]
13. Humeau, A.; Buard, B.; Mahé, G.; Rousseau, D.; Chapeau-Blondeau, F.; Abraham, P. Multiscale entropy of laser Doppler flowmetry signals in healthy human subjects. *Med. Phys.* **2010**, *37*, 6142. [CrossRef] [PubMed]
14. Schack, T.; Harb, Y.S.; Muma, M.; Zoubir, A.M. Computationally efficient algorithm for photoplethysmography-based atrial fibrillation detection using smartphones. In *2017 39th Annual International Conference of the IEEE Engineering in Medicine and Biology Society (EMBC)*; Institute of Electrical and Electronics Engineers (IEEE): Piscataway, NJ, USA, 2017; pp. 104–108.
15. Zhang, X.D.; Shen, B. Entropy for the Complexity of Physiological Signal Dynamics. *Adv. Exp. Med. Biol.* **2017**, *1028*, 39–53. [PubMed]
16. Yang, D.; Luo, Z.; Ma, S.; Wong, W.T.; Ma, L.; Zhong, J.; He, H.; Zhao, Z.; Cao, T.; Yan, Z.; et al. Activation of TRPV1 by dietary capsaicin improves endothelium-dependent vasorelaxation and prevents hypertension. *Cell Metab.* **2010**, *12*, 130–141. [CrossRef] [PubMed]
17. Liu, Y.; Lin, Y.; Wang, J.; Shang, P. Refined generalized multiscale entropy analysis for physiological signals. *Phys. A: Stat. Mech. its Appl.* **2018**, *490*, 975–985. [CrossRef]
18. Vargas, B.; Cuesta-Frau, D.; Ruiz-Esteban, R.; Cirugeda, E.; Varela, M. What Can Biosignal Entropy Tell Us About Health and Disease? Applications in Some Clinical Fields. *Nonlinear Dyn. Psychol. Life Sci.* **2015**, *19*, 419–436.
19. Costa, M.; Goldberger, A.L.; Peng, C.-K. Multiscale Entropy Analysis of Complex Physiologic Time Series. *Phys. Rev. Lett.* **2002**, *89*, 068102. [CrossRef]
20. Tsai, D.-Y.; Lee, Y.; Matsuyama, E. Information Entropy Measure for Evaluation of Image Quality. *J. Digit. Imaging.* **2008**, *21*, 338–347. [CrossRef]
21. Larroza, A.; Bodí, V.; Moratal, D. Texture Analysis in Magnetic Resonance Imaging: Review and Considerations for Future Applications. In *Assessment of Cellular and Organ Function and Dysfunction using Direct and Derived MRI Methodologies*; IntechOpen: London, UK, 2016; pp. 75–106.
22. Pharwaha, A.P.S.; Singh, B. Shannon and Non-Shannon Measures of Entropy for Statistical Texture Feature Extraction in Digitized Mammograms. In Proceedings of the World Congres on Engineering nd Computer Science, San Francisco, CA, USA, 20–22 October 2009.

23. Al-Kadi, O.; Watson, D. Texture Analysis of Aggressive and Nonaggressive Lung Tumor CE CT Images. *IEEE Trans. Biomed. Eng.* **2008**, *55*, 1822–1830. [CrossRef]
24. Gibbs, P.; Turnbull, L.W. Textural analysis of contrast-enhanced MR images of the breast. *Magn. Reson. Med.* **2003**, *50*, 92–98. [CrossRef]
25. Castellano, G.; Bonilha, L.; Li, L.; Cendes, F. Texture analysis of medical images. *Clin. Radiol.* **2004**, *59*, 1061–1069. [CrossRef]
26. Shrestha, B.; Bishop, J.; Kam, K.; Chen, X.; Moss, R.H.; Stoecker, W.V.; Umbaugh, S.; Stanley, R.J.; Celebi, M.E.; Marghoob, A.A.; et al. Detection of atypical texture features in early malignant melanoma. *Skin. Res. Technol.* **2010**, *16*, 60–65. [CrossRef] [PubMed]
27. Gao, Y.; Helgeson, M.E. Texture analysis microscopy: quantifying structure in low-fidelity images of dense fluids. *Opt. Express* **2014**, *22*, 10046–10063. [CrossRef] [PubMed]
28. Pantic, I.; Pantic, S. Germinal Center Texture Entropy as Possible Indicator of Humoral Immune Response: Immunophysiology Viewpoint. *Mol. Imaging. Biol.* **2012**, *14*, 534–540. [CrossRef] [PubMed]
29. Mir, A.; Hanmandlu, M.; Tandon, S. Texture Analysis of CT. *IEEE Eng. Med. Biol.* **1995**, *14*, 781–786. [CrossRef]
30. Ng, F.; Ganeshan, B.; Kozarski, R.; Miles, K.A.; Goh, V. Assessment of Primary Colorectal Cancer Heterogeneity by Using Whole-Tumor Texture Analysis: Contrast-enhanced CT Texture as a Biomarker of 5-year Survival. *Radiology* **2013**, *266*, 177–184. [CrossRef] [PubMed]
31. Ng, F.; Kozarski, R.; Ganeshan, B.; Goh, V. Assessment of tumor heterogeneity by CT texture analysis: Can the largest cross-sectional area be used as an alternative to whole tumor analysis? *Eur. J. Radiol.* **2013**, *82*, 342–348. [CrossRef]
32. El Hassani, A.; El Hassouni, M.; Jennane, R.; Rziza, M.; Lespessailles, E. Texture Analysis for Trabecular Bone X-Ray Images Using Anisotropic Morlet Wavelet and Rényi Entropy. In *Image and Signal Processing, Proceedings of the 5th International Conference on Image and Signal Processing, Agadir, Morocco, 28–30 June 2012*; Elmoataz, A., Mammass, D., Lezoray, O., Nouboud, F., Aboutajdine, D., Eds.; Springer: Berlin, Germany, 2012; pp. 290–297.
33. Kołaciński, M.; Kozakiewicz, M.; Materka, A. Textural entropy as a potential feature for quantitative assessment of jaw bone healing process. *Arch. Med. Sci.* **2015**, *11*, 78–84. [CrossRef]
34. Shamir, L.; Wolkow, C.A.; Goldberg, I.G. Quantitative measurement of aging using image texture entropy. *Bioinformatics* **2009**, *25*, 3060–3063. [CrossRef]
35. WMA. World Medical Association Declaration of Helsinki: Ethical principles for medical research involving human subjects. *J. Am. Med. Assoc.* **2013**, *310*, 2191–2194. [CrossRef]
36. Kvandal, P.; Landsverk, S.A.; Bernjak, A.; Stefanovska, A.; Kvernmo, H.D.; Kirkebøen, K.A. Low-frequency oscillations of the laser Doppler perfusion signal in human skin. *Microvasc. Res.* **2006**, *72*, 120–127. [CrossRef]
37. Gonzalez, R.; Woods, R.E.; Eddins, S.L. *Digital Image Processing Using MATLAB*, 2nd ed.; Gatesmark Publishing: USA, 2009.
38. Ferreira, H.; Rodrigues, F.; Meyer, M.; Santos-Ribeiro, A.; Gonçalves-Pereira, P.; Manaças, R.; Andrade, A. Complexity analysis of resting-state networks. *MAGMA* **2013**, *26*, 2013.
39. Gabrielsen, A.; Norsk, P. Effect of spaceflight on the subcutaneous venoarteriolar reflex in the human lower leg. *J. Appl. Physiol.* **2007**, *103*, 959–962. [CrossRef] [PubMed]

10

Relationships between Body Build and Knee Joint Flexor and Extensor Torque of Polish First-Division Soccer Players

Jadwiga Pietraszewska [1], Artur Struzik [2,*], Anna Burdukiewicz [1], Aleksandra Stachoń [1] and Bogdan Pietraszewski [3]

1. Department of Physical Anthropology, University School of Physical Education, Paderewskiego 35 Avenue, 51-612 Wrocław, Poland; jadwiga.pietraszewska@awf.wroc.pl (J.P.); anna.burdukiewicz@awf.wroc.pl (A.B.); aleksandra.stachon@awf.wroc.pl (A.S.)
2. Department of Team Sport Games, University School of Physical Education, Mickiewicza 58 Street, 51-684 Wrocław, Poland
3. Department of Biomechanics, University School of Physical Education, Mickiewicza 58 Street, 51-684 Wrocław, Poland; bogdan.pietraszewski@awf.wroc.pl

* Correspondence: artur.struzik@awf.wroc.pl;

Featured Application: Body height, body mass and thigh and calf girths are the anthropometric variables that best describe the values of the torque of the knee flexors and extensors that can be achieved by soccer players. Based on these anthropometric variables, the coach can initially assess players' strength abilities, which can help plan individual training programmes.

Abstract: The aim of the study is to identify the relationships between anthropometric variables and knee joint extensor peak torque, knee joint flexor peak torque, and conventional hamstring-to-quadriceps ratio in Polish first-division soccer players. The study examined 37 soccer players aged 19 to 30 years (body mass: 76.8 ± 7.2 kg, body height 1.82 ± 0.06 m). Muscle torques of the knee joint were measured under isometric conditions using a Biodex 4 Pro dynamometer. The anthropometric variables such as body part lengths, breadths, and girths and skinfold thickness were measured. The strongest relationships of knee joint extensors were observed with body mass and variables describing skeleton size and lower-limb muscles. Regarding knee flexor torque, a significant relationship was found only with body mass. However, no significant relationships were observed between the conventional hamstring-to-quadriceps ratio and the anthropometric variables studied. The regression analysis results identified body height, body mass, and thigh and calf girth as the features most associated with knee joint torque. However, anthropometric measurements do not provide full information about the torque proportions of antagonist muscle groups, which is very important for injury prevention. Therefore, measurements using special biomechanical equipment are also necessary for the comprehensive analyses and control of the effects of sports training.

Keywords: anthropometric variables; hamstring-to-quadriceps ratio; H/Q ratio; injury prevention; isometric; lower limb; measurement acquisitions and techniques; strength and conditioning; sports training; strength abilities

---

1. Introduction

Measurements of muscle torque taken in isometric and isokinetic conditions have often been used for sports training [1–5]. Coaches use biomechanical measurement tools to analyse the sports skill level of athletes, improve movement techniques, or adjust tactics against the opponent [6,7].

Biomechanical analysis provides a fast and reliable evaluation of torque values, helps detect muscle strength imbalance, and screens for lower extremity injury [8,9]. Numerous studies have focused on the evaluation of the value of muscle torque in relation to lower limbs, which are particularly involved during sports movements. Appropriate force and proportion between antagonistic muscle groups are essential for optimal or maximum performance of various movements, which is also true in team sport games [10–14]. The dependence of force on the transverse cross-sectional area of muscles is known, but it should be noted that force is also affected by other factors related to the efficiency of the nervous system (that controls muscle function) and the properties of the muscles themselves [15].

Soccer is a sport in which the requirements for effective play are multi-factorial. The intervals and repetitive nature of the efforts during the match mean that the competitors should demonstrate adequate speed, endurance, strength, and coordination levels. In general, the players do not reach the highest levels of all these motor abilities. However, they must demonstrate a sufficiently high level of preparation in all aspects of motor abilities, with the dominance of some of them (depending on their playing position). Interindividual differences can also be observed in the anthropometric characteristics of soccer players [16]. In soccer, the lower limbs are particularly involved when kicking the ball, striking at a goal, and running at different velocities and with directional changes [17–20]. Soccer training is aimed, among other things, at increasing muscle mass and, consequently, muscle force. The adequate level of force of the knee extensors and flexors allows the player to achieve stronger strikes, jump higher, and sprint faster over short distances [21–23].

In addition to the absolute values of the generated torque, the correct ratio of the torque of extensors to that of flexors is also important. The commonly used conventional hamstring-to-quadriceps ratio (H/Q ratio) represents the ratio of concentric hamstring peak torque during lower limb flexion to concentric quadriceps peak torque during lower limb extension [24]. The functional hamstring-to-quadriceps ratio, in contrast, is a measure of the isokinetic eccentric peak torque of the hamstrings relative to the isokinetic concentric peak torque of the quadriceps during lower limb extension at equivalent angular velocities [25]. An adequately high value of these indexes is likely to effectively prevent injuries of the lower limbs (including those that occur without contact) due to effective eccentric activity to slow down or stop the movement [26].

Measurements of muscle torque under isometric conditions allow for the determination of the maximum values of force generated by a given muscle group to evaluate the potential of the player, the training programme, and muscle imbalance. It should also be noted that the amount of force generated depends on many factors, including physiological and biochemical factors. The aspect of morphological determinants is also important. Previous studies have investigated the relationships of muscle torque with body mass, body mass composition, and somatotype [27–31]. However, the results of such studies have been inconclusive. Norsuriani and Ooi [31] demonstrated positive relationships between muscle torque in the knee joint and body mass, fat-free mass, and body fat. Similar results were presented by Pietraszewski et al. [27]. Lewandowska et al. [28] emphasized positive relationships of muscle torque in the lower limb joints with characteristics of muscularity and skeletal mass (mesomorphy), negative relationships with body slenderness (ectomorphy) and lack of relationships with the fat component (endomorphy). Kim et al. [29] found that men with higher skeletal muscle mass are characterized by higher isokinetic muscle torque values in the lower limb joints. Furthermore, to our knowledge, no previous studies have examined the relationships between the conventional H/Q ratio and anthropometric variables. It should be pointed out that anthropometric measurements are the basic method used to assess the level of development of many morphological features. They can be performed anytime and anywhere, using mobile equipment. Measurements of body girths and skinfolds provide additional indirect information about changes in tissue components, which are very important in the context of functional capabilities of a player. Understanding the relationships between muscle torque and the anthropometric variables would allow coaches to easily make an initial assessment of the players' strength abilities and, at the same time, control the training effects.

Muscle torque is the product of the force *F* and the length of the lever arm *r*. The lever arm *r* is understood as the distance from the axis of rotation of the lever (joint) along a line perpendicular to the direction of the force *F*. Therefore, it can be expected that the torque of the flexors and extensors of the knee joint are related to the characteristics of muscle development (girths of the body parts) and the length of the individual lower limb parts. These features are related to the overall body size but may also show interpersonal differentiation due to the modifying effect of various environmental factors, including sports training. Due to the specificity of the training, the knowledge gained from the research of players practising various sports cannot be used uncritically. Substantial values of anthropometric variables (e.g., girths of body parts) may result from both muscularity and body fat. However, due to the characteristics of the research group (soccer players) resulting from the specificity of the motor activities performed by such athletes and the usually low body fat content in lower limbs, the relationships should be expected between muscle torque and variables indirectly describing muscularity of the lower limbs. It is important to examine morphofunctional relations in a specific sport.

The aim of the study is to identify the relationships between anthropometric variables and the values of knee joint extensor peak torque, knee joint flexor peak torque, and conventional hamstring-to-quadriceps ratio in a group of Polish first-division soccer players. Furthermore, the authors intended to identify the anthropometric variables that allow for the best possible estimation of the abovementioned biomechanical variables, which would allow coaches to monitor more frequently the effect of training loads used at different stages of the annual training cycle. Knowledge of the abovementioned biomechanical variables is also important during the choice of training loads to reduce the injury risk of athletes.

2. Materials and Methods

The study examined 37 soccer players aged 19 to 30 years. They were players playing in the Polish Ekstraklasa league. The study included only the players who had actively participated in training and league matches since the beginning of the season and had not been injured. They were previously qualified for the examinations by a sports physician. Their mean training experience was 14 years (8 to 20 years). The mean body mass (±SD) of the subjects was 76.8 ± 7.2 kg, and the body height was 1.82 ± 0.06 m. The tests were conducted in the morning, before the training sessions. On the day before the tests, the players did not play any league matches.

The study was carried out in the Biomechanical Analysis Laboratory and Scientific Research Laboratory of the Faculty of Sport (both with PN-EN ISO 9001:2009 certification) at the University School of Physical Education in Wrocław, Poland. All subjects gave their informed consent for inclusion before they participated in the study. The study was conducted in accordance with the Declaration of Helsinki, and the protocol was approved by the Senate's Research Bioethics Commission of the University School of Physical Education in Wrocław, Poland. Measurements were performed according to International Standards for Anthropometric Assessment (ISAK) [32].

The following anthropometric variables were measured: sitting height (B-vs), lower extremity length (B-tro), shank length (B-ti), biacromial diameter (a-a), biiliocristal diameter (ic-ic), humerus breadth (cl-cm), femur breath (epl-epm), chest girth, waist girth, hip girth, relaxed and flexed biceps girth, thigh girth, and calf girth. Skinfold thickness was measured at the subscapular, abdominal, suprailiac, triceps, and calf locations to assess body fat. Body height, lengths, and breadths were measured to the nearest 0.1 cm with the use of the GPM Anthropological Instruments (Siber Hegner Machinery Ltd., Zürich, Switzerland). Skinfold thickness was measured with a Tanner/Whitehouse skinfold calliper (Holtain LTD, Crosswell, Crymych, Pembs, UK) with a 0.2 mm graduation. Body mass was measured with an electronic weighing scale with an accuracy of 0.1 kg. Body mass index (BMI) was also calculated.

The peak muscle torque under isometric conditions was measured to assess the strength of the lower limbs. Peak muscle torque for extensors and flexors of the knee joint was measured at 75° and

30°, respectively; 0° at the knee joint was considered to be a full extension. The measurements were performed separately for the right and left lower limbs. The results of measurements of the dominant limb were used for analyses. Biodex System 4 Pro (Biodex Medical Systems, Inc., Shirley, NY, USA) was used for the torque measurements. The conventional hamstring-to-quadriceps ratio (H/Q ratio) was calculated using the following equation:

$$\text{H/Q ratio} = (T_f \,/\, T_e) \cdot 100\%, \tag{1}$$

where T_f denotes the concentric peak torque value of knee joint flexors of the dominant lower limb and T_e is the concentric peak torque value of extensors of the same joint and limb. The conventional H/Q ratio is possible to calculate during the measurement of peak torque only under isometric conditions [33]. Furthermore, the muscle torques of extensors and flexors were added together, and the muscle torque for the knee joint relative to body mass was calculated:

$$(T_e + T_f) \,/\, \text{BM}. \tag{2}$$

To supplement the information about the general strength abilities of the soccer players studied, back and handgrip strengths were measured using TAKEI dynamometers (Takei Scientific Instruments Co., Ltd., Niigata City, Japan).

Cluster analysis (k-means) was used in the statistical analysis to distinguish two groups significantly differing in the magnitude of muscle torque. The intergroup differentiation of anthropometric variables in these clusters was evaluated by means of Student's t-test for independent samples. Pearson's r correlation coefficient was used to evaluate the relationships of anthropometric variables with muscle torque.

3. Results

The soccer players studied were characterized by small and moderate intragroup variability in the anthropometric variables (Table 1). The mass-to-height ratios were correct and were confirmed by the BMI values in the entire group (23.3 ± 1.5 kg/m^2).

The obtained values of muscle torque showed a clear interindividual differentiation. To create relatively homogeneous groups in terms of the values of muscle torque generated in the knee extensors and flexors, the k-mean cluster analysis was used to identify two subgroups significantly differing in the magnitude of these variables: Group 1—weaker group and Group 2—stronger group. With the adopted criterion of division, the groups differed significantly in terms of the generated muscle torque and in terms of the sum of muscle torque relative to body mass (Table 2). All of the above values were significantly higher in Group 2 (stronger). Higher values were also found in most of the anthropometric variables in this group of players. However, significant intergroup differences were recorded only for body mass, BMI; chest, thigh and calf girths; and humerus and femur breadths, which are a measure of skeleton size. The soccer players from Group 2 also showed significantly higher values in the remaining strength tests, although these variables were not included in the grouping variables. Both back strength and handgrip strength were greater in the athletes from the second cluster. The mean conventional H/Q ratios were 47.0% (Group 1) and 45.6% (Group 2).

The values of correlation coefficients between muscle torque of the knee extensors and flexors and anthropometric variables were quite low, yet statistically significant in some cases (Table 3). The strongest relationships were observed for knee joint extensors with body mass, BMI, and variables describing skeleton size and lower limb muscles. In the case of the torque of knee flexors, a significant relationship was found only with body mass and BMI. However, no significant relationships were observed between the conventional H/Q ratio and the anthropometric variables studied.

Table 1. Statistical characterization of the variables analysed for the entire group of soccer players studied (n = 37).

Variables	Mean	Minimum	Maximum	SD
Body height (cm)	181.6	170.0	192.5	5.5
Body mass (kg)	76.8	65.0	94.5	7.2
BMI (kg/m^2)	23.3	18.6	26.0	1.5
b-vs (cm)	95.2	89.5	104.3	3.3
b-tro (cm)	95.6	88.0	105.2	4.0
b-ti (cm)	48.5	38.5	54.0	2.7
a-a (cm)	41.8	38.0	46.5	1.8
ic-ic (cm)	28.6	25.4	32.5	1.8
cl-cm (cm)	7.1	6.4	7.8	0.3
epl-epm (cm)	10.1	9.2	11.1	0.5
Chest girth (cm)	88.4	80.0	100.0	4.9
Waist girth (cm)	79.5	70.0	89.0	4.6
Relaxed biceps girth (cm)	30.3	26.0	35.0	2.4
Flexed biceps girth (cm)	33.4	29.5	37.5	2.3
Hip girth (cm)	98.5	90.0	106.0	3.5
Thigh girth (cm)	58.5	50.4	65.0	3.0
Calf girth (cm)	37.9	33.2	41.0	1.8
Subscapular skinfold (mm)	8.2	5.8	12.0	1.4
Triceps skinfold (mm)	4.3	2.8	7.0	1.0
Suprailiac skinfold (mm)	6.8	4.6	12.0	1.7
Abdominal skinfold (mm)	7.0	4.0	12.0	2.2
Calf skinfold (mm)	3.7	2.8	5.4	0.7
Right hand grip strength (kG)	47.5	36.0	62.0	6.3
Left hand grip strength (kG)	46.2	38.0	58.0	5.2
Back strength (kG)	127.0	91.5	169.5	18.7
T_e (Nm)	416.8	252.7	596.7	86.4
T_f (Nm)	191.7	106.0	294.4	46.3
H/Q ratio (%)	46.1	32.1	61.0	6.5
$(T_e + T_f)$ / BM (Nm/kg)	7.9	5.5	12.1	1.5

SD—standard deviation; BMI—body mass index; b-vs—sitting height; b-tro—lower extremity length; b-ti—shank length; a-a—biacromial diameter; ic-ic—biiliocristal diameter; cl-cm—humerus breadth; epl-epm—femur breath; T_e—peak torque value of knee joint extensors; T_f—peak torque value of knee joint flexors; H/Q ratio—conventional hamstrings-to-quadriceps ratio; $(T_e + T_f)$ / BM—sum of knee muscle torque relative to body mass.

Table 2. Statistical characteristics of the variables studied in separate clusters.

Variables	Group 1 (weaker) n = 14	Group 2 (stronger) n = 23	t	p
Body height (cm)	180.5 ± 5.0	182.2 ± 5.8	−0.95	0.349
Body mass (kg)	72.8 ± 5.1	79.2 ± 7.3	−2.91	0.006 *
BMI (kg/m^2)	22.4 ± 1.5	23.8 ± 1.3	−3.13	0.004 *
b-vs (cm)	94.7 ± 2.8	95.6 ± 3.5	−0.86	0.395
b-tro (cm)	95.6 ± 4.0	95.7 ± 4.0	−0.06	0.951
b-ti (cm)	48.4 ± 2.1	48.5 ± 3.1	−0.07	0.945
a-a (cm)	41.3 ± 1.8	42.1 ± 1.9	−1.33	0.191
ic-ic (cm)	28.4 ± 1.5	28.8 ± 2.0	−0.77	0.447
cl-cm (cm)	7.0 ± 0.3	7.2 ± 0.3	−2.60	0.014 *
epl-epm (cm)	9.9 ± 0.3	10.2 ± 0.5	−1.52	0.037 *
Chest girth (cm)	86.6 ± 5.2	89.6 ± 4.4	−1.83	0.076
Waist girth (cm)	78.0 ± 4.0	80.4 ± 4.9	−1.55	0.131
Relaxed biceps girth (cm)	29.8 ± 1.6	30.7 ± 2.7	−1.15	0.260
Flexed biceps girth (cm)	33.1 ± 1.8	33.6 ± 2.6	−0.67	0.505
Hip girth (cm)	97.3 ± 2.7	99.3 ± 3.8	−1.74	0.091
Thigh girth (cm)	57.1 ± 2.8	59.3 ± 2.8	−2.29	0.028 *
Calf girth (cm)	36.9 ± 2.0	38.5 ± 1.4	−2.83	0.008 *
Subscapular skinfold (mm)	7.5 ± 1.1	8.5 ± 1.5	−2.15	0.039 *
Triceps skinfold (mm)	4.4 ± 1.3	4.2 ± 0.9	0.36	0.719
Suprailiac skinfold (mm)	6.1 ± 1.1	7.2 ± 1.9	−1.97	0.057
Abdominal skinfold (mm)	6.4 ± 1.8	7.4 ± 2.3	−1.29	0.206
Calf skinfold (mm)	3.5 ± 0.5	3.9 ± 0.7	−1.95	0.060
Right hand grip strength (kG)	44.4 ± 5.5	49.4 ± 6.1	−2.53	0.016 *
Left hand grip strength (kG)	43.6 ± 4.6	47.8 ± 4.9	−2.56	0.015 *
Back strength (kG)	112.4 ± 11.9	135.9 ± 16.5	−4.62	0.000 *
T_e (Nm)	325.6 ± 37.2	472.2 ± 53.9	−8.93	0.000 *
T_f (Nm)	152.3 ± 26.1	215.6 ± 39.0	−5.37	0.000 *
H/Q ratio	47.0 ± 7.4	45.6 ± 6.0	0.61	0.546
$(T_e + T_f)$ / BM (Nm/kg)	6.6 ± 1.3	8.7 ± 0.8	−5.60	0.000 *

*—significant differences between Groups I and II group at the level of $p < 0.05$; p—probability of type I error; t—t-test value; BMI—body mass index; b-vs—sitting height; b-tro—lower extremity length; b-ti—shank length; a-a—biacromial diameter; ic-ic—biiliocristal diameter; cl-cm—humerus breadth; epl-epm—femur breath; T_e—peak torque value of knee joint extensors; T_f—peak torque value of knee joint flexors; H/Q ratio—conventional hamstrings-to-quadriceps ratio; $(T_e + T_f)$ / BM—sum of knee muscle torques relative to body mass.

Table 3. The correlation coefficients between the muscle torque of extensors (T_e) and flexors (T_f) of the knee joint and anthropometric variables for the entire group of soccer players ($n = 37$).

Anthropometric Variables	T_e	T_f	Anthropometric Variables	T_e	T_f
Body height	0.21	0.12	Flexed biceps girth	0.10	0.06
Body mass	0.46 *	0.34 *	Hip girth	0.26	0.13
BMI	0.45 *	0.37 *	Thigh girth	0.26	0.20
b-vs	0.21	0.18	Calf girth	0.40 *	0.31
b-tro	0.14	−0.01	Subscapular skinfold	0.34 *	0.14
b-ti	0.07	−0.09	Triceps skinfold	0.12	0.12
a-a	0.16	−0.02	Suprailiac skinfold	0.36 *	0.23
ic-ic	0.16	0.05	Abdominal skinfold	0.19	0.14
cl-cm	0.34 *	0.21	Calf skinfold	0.38 *	0.29
epl-epm	0.43 *	0.22	Right handgrip strength	0.33 *	0.27
Chest girth	0.31	0.13	Left handgrip strength	0.35 *	0.26
Waist girth	0.27	0.08	Back strength	0.56 *	0.25
Relaxed biceps girth	0.27	0.17			

*—statistically significant at $p < 0.05$; BMI—body mass index; b-vs—sitting height; b-tro—lower extremity length; b-ti—shank length; a-a—biacromial diameter; ic-ic—biiliocristal diameter; cl-cm—humerus breadth; epl-epm—femur breath.

Multiple regression analysis was performed, taking into account body height and anthropometric variables that were most significantly correlated with the examined muscle torque. A significant effect of anthropometric variables on the muscle torque measured in the knee joint was demonstrated. A regression model with four anthropometric variables estimating the biomechanical values was statistically significant, and all predictors explained 38% of the torque variation in the knee extensors and 25% of the torque variation in the knee flexors. Three of the four predictors in the model had a significant effect on the torque of the knee extensors and flexors. The results of the regression analysis are presented in Tables 4 and 5. The estimation error for the extensor Equation (3) was 72.3, whereas for the flexor Equation (4), this value was 42.5.

$$T_e = 1943.845 - (10.052 \cdot \text{body height}) - (25.424 \cdot \text{thigh girth}) + (13.383 \cdot \text{calf girth}) + (16.652 \cdot \text{body mass}). \quad (3)$$

$$T_f = 1019.404 - (5204 \cdot \text{body height}) - (11{,}878 \cdot \text{thigh girth}) + (5715 \cdot \text{calf girth}) + (7756 \cdot \text{body mass}). \quad (4)$$

Table 4. Results of regression analysis for knee joint extensor torque.

Independent Variables	Dependent Variable: Peak Torque Value of Knee Joint Extensors $R = 0.62$, $R^2 = 0.38$, Adj. $R^2 = 0.30$ F (4.32) = 4.86, $p < 0.01$ Standard Error of the Estimate: 72.3			
	b	Standard Error of b	t	p
Intercept coefficient *	1943.9	880.1	2.2	0.035
Body height *	−10.1	4.3	−2.4	0.025
Thigh girth *	−25.4	9.4	−2.7	0.011
Calf girth	13.4	9.8	1.4	0.180
Body mass *	16.7	5.1	3.3	0.003

*—statistically significant at $p < 0.05$.

Table 5. Results of regression analysis for knee joint flexor torque.

Independent Variables	Dependent Variable: Peak Torque Value of Knee Joint Flexors $R = 0.50$, $R^2 = 0.25$, Adj. $R^2 = 0.16$, F (4.32) = 2.71, $p < 0.05$ Standard Error of the Estimate: 42.5			
	b	Standard Error of b	t	p
Intercept coefficient	1019.4	516.7	2.0	0.057
Body height *	−5.2	2.5	−2.1	0.047
Thigh girth *	−11.9	5.5	−2.2	0.038
Calf girth	5.7	5.7	1.0	0.326
Body mass *	7.8	3.0	2.6	0.015

*—statistically significant at $p < 0.05$.

4. Discussion

The body build of the soccer players studied showed a typical profile of basic anthropometric variables typical for athletes participating in this sport. Interpersonal differences resulted from the different playing positions [34,35]. The mean body height of the soccer players studied (1.82 ± 0.06 m) was similar to the mean body height of the players of most of the best teams in the world and slightly exceeds the mean body height of young men in Poland (1.79 ± 0.07 m) [36]. Therefore, the results obtained in the study are consistent with the information provided in the literature on the body morphology of athletes. Norton and Olds [32] indicated that the mean body height of soccer players (1.79 ± 0.06 m) and its variations are very close to those of the general population. This finding was also confirmed by the research presented by Reilly and Doran [17]. However, these authors pointed to differences depending on sports skill level and nationality. The extreme values in their ranking were obtained from the players from Hong Kong (1.73 ± 0.06 m) and Norway (1.81 ± 0.05 m). The BMI of soccer players in the present study also showed values typical of soccer players [17]. The athletes tested were characterized by good musculature of all body parts, as evidenced by the values of chest and lower and upper limb girths. These features are similar to those of players on other soccer teams [34,35]. The results of our research indicated particularly muscular thighs, which enable players to generate high muscle torque. This ability is also very important when jumping, kicking, rotating, and changing the velocity of movement [14,17,19]. The harmonious development of limb and torso muscles contributes to maintaining player balance on a slippery field and allows for easier control of the ball [17]. Particularly valuable research, whose results can help athletes achieve top-level performance, was carried out among the players of the top teams. Therefore, it seems very valuable that we had an opportunity to conduct research on the Polish first-division soccer players.

Analysis of the muscle torque of knee extensors and flexors shows that human muscles are shaped to a large extent by the gravitational field. This finding is reflected in the significant muscle torque of the knee joint extensors (416.8 ± 86.4 Nm), which act against the gravitational force. The torque values of the knee flexors are approximately two times lower (191.7 ± 46.3 Nm). The mean values of isometric muscle torque in the knee joint obtained for the players in our study are much higher than the mean values obtained in Polish striker soccer players (315.3 ± 53.3 Nm for extensors and 167.7 ± 26.0 Nm for flexors) [37] and higher than those in lower-league soccer players (328.0 ± 69.7 Nm for extensors) [38]. The recorded large values of isometric muscle torque measured in our study may result from substantial training loads to which players were exposed. They trained four times a week in two sessions. In the morning, the athletes had a soccer training session (about 2.5 hours). In the afternoon, they exercised in the gym for about 1.5 hours. The exercises were selected individually. The high sports skill level of the players studied is also of great importance to the results obtained. Previous studies [1,39] indicated differences in the magnitude of muscle torque depending on the sports skill level. Measurements of muscle torque under isokinetic conditions are now also popular. However, these measurements have limitations [33,40]. Furthermore, the aim of the study was to determine the maximum strength abilities of the players, rather than the strength at a certain angular velocity of movement in the knee joint.

The relationship between the muscle torque of extensors and flexors of the knee joint is important from the standpoint of maintaining knee stability during some movement activities. For example, damage to the hamstrings can occur during the kicking of the ball with the lower limb. This damage may occur when, during knee extension, a group of antagonistic muscles does not ensure the effective eccentric deceleration of the movement [8,41,42]. It is assumed that conventional H/Q ratio values exceeding 60% can effectively prevent injuries and damage to the anterior cruciate ligament (ACL) and hamstring strains [43–48]. According to Kim and Hong [44], soccer players with a conventional H/Q ratio of more than 60% are less likely to suffer non-contact injuries to their lower limbs. In this study, the conventional H/Q ratio was 46.1% for all the soccer players studied, which is lower than the desired value and indicates unfavourable proportions of muscle torque in these muscle groups. This result suggests that coaches should pay more attention to the improvement of the strength level of the knee flexors during training. No injuries were reported the last time among the players studied. However, it can be presumed that this was influenced by motor control, which means mutual adjustment of the musculoskeletal and nervous systems [49]. In order to control movement, the central nervous system must integrate multiple sensory information (both external and proprioceptive) and trigger the signals necessary for muscle recruitment to achieve the intended goal. The performance of the movement consists in the planning of the motor strategy and its economic and flawless execution. Disturbed motor control has a negative effect on the quality of movement and increases the risk of injury. It should be expected that in elite players, sport training had led to the improved motor control. Disproportionate torque of agonist and antagonist muscle groups has been observed in male soccer players [27,37,48]. However, there are groups of soccer players for which the value of the conventional H/Q ratio remains within the recommended standard [45]. Cometti et al. [39] demonstrated that sports skill level in soccer players increases with higher H/Q ratios.

The lack of significant relationships between the conventional H/Q ratio and anthropometric variables indicates that low values of the conventional H/Q ratio in the group of soccer players (i.e., not entirely correct proportion of torque of antagonistic muscle groups) cannot be observed based on the variables describing body structure. Therefore, muscle imbalance cannot be diagnosed without special biomechanical measurements because the body build will not suggest such an abnormality. It should also be noted that high H/Q ratios may exist in the presence of relative weakness in both the hamstring and quadriceps muscle groups [50], which can also explain the lack of the above relationships. Another limitation may be that the peak values of extensors and flexors occur at different knee flexion angles [26,33].

Dividing the soccer players studied into two clusters allowed for the assessment of body build differences between the players, who significantly differed in terms of muscle torque generated within the knee joint. The athletes from both clusters did not show any differences in body height or its components, which is attributable to the genetic determinants of this feature [51]. Furthermore, the differences observed in body mass and girths that describe the size of the skeleton and muscles indicate relationships between these features and strength abilities. This is also confirmed by significant correlation coefficients for some anthropometric features (body mass, humerus breadth, femur breadth, calf girth, subscapular skinfold, suprailiac skinfold, and calf skinfold) and isometric muscle torque of the knee joint extensors and flexors. As in other studies, positive relationships were obtained between muscle torque and body mass, breadths and girths that describe the size of the skeleton and muscles [27–31]. However, contrary to previous reports, positive relationships between muscle torque and skinfolds were also found [28].

The regression analysis was used to identify the variables that can be indirectly used to estimate torque values for knee joint extensors and flexors generated by the player. The results of this analysis identify the body height, body mass, and thigh and calf girth as the features that best describe these variables. Therefore, based on these anthropometric variables, the coach may initially assess the strength abilities of soccer players, and these assessments can lead to the adjustment of training programmes to the individual predispositions of the players.

The limitations of our study are incomplete information about the applied training loads (resulting, e.g., from club changes of the players studied), the sex of the players (slightly different results can be expected in female groups, which are characterized by higher body fat), and the type of sport being practised (it is not advisable to directly refer to the results of people practising other sports, e.g., individual sports). On the other hand, all of the players studied belonged to the national soccer elite, which allows for the assumption that their training was carried out professionally, translating into a high sports skill level.

5. Conclusions

The results allow for the conclusion that the muscle torque of the knee joint extensors and flexors in soccer players is significantly related to some anthropometric variables. Due to the less complicated nature of anthropometric apparatuses and the high mobility of this type of equipment, the prediction of muscle torque in the knee joint based on anthropometry seems to be useful for screening soccer players for preliminary estimation of the abovementioned biomechanical variables. However, anthropometric methods do not provide full information about the mutual relationships between the muscle torque of the knee joint extensors and flexors, which is very important from the standpoint of injury prevention. For this reason, measurements using special biomechanical equipment are also necessary for the comprehensive analyses and control of the effects of sports training.

Author Contributions: Conceptualization, J.P. and B.P.; methodology, J.P. and B.P.; software, J.P. and B.P.; validation, J.P., A.S. (Artur Struzik), A.B., A.S (Aleksandra Stachoń). and B.P.; formal analysis, J.P., A.S. (Artur Struzik) and B.P.; investigation, J.P., A.B., A.S. (Aleksandra Stachoń) and B.P.; resources, J.P., A.B., A.S. (Aleksandra Stachoń) and B.P.; data curation, J.P. and A.S. (Artur Struzik); writing—original draft preparation, J.P., A.S. (Artur Struzik) and B.P.; writing—review and editing, J.P., A.S. (Artur Struzik) and B.P.; visualization, J.P. and A.S. (Artur Struzik); supervision, J.P.; project administration, J.P.; and funding acquisition, B.P. All authors have read and agreed to the published version of the manuscript.

Acknowledgments: The authors thank the study participants for their effort, time devotion, and collaboration during the study.

References

1. Wit, A.; Eliasz, J.; Gajewski, J.; Janiak, J.; Jaszczuk, J.; Trzaskoma, Z. Maximal isometric muscle torque assessment in elite athletes. *Acta Bioeng. Biomech.* **2002**, *4*, 591–592.
2. Ergün, M.; Işlegen, C.; Taşkiran, E. A cross-sectional analysis of sagittal knee laxity and isokinetic muscle strength in soccer players. *Int. J. Sports Med.* **2004**, *25*, 594–598. [CrossRef] [PubMed]
3. Zakas, A. Bilateral isokinetic peak torque of quadriceps and hamstring muscles in professional soccer players with dominance on one or both two sides. *J. Sports Med. Phys. Fitness* **2006**, *46*, 28–35. [PubMed]
4. Ellenbecker, T.S.; Roetert, E.P.; Sueyoshi, T.; Riewald, S. A descriptive profile of age-specific knee extension flexion strength in elite junior tennis players. *Br. J. Sports Med.* **2007**, *41*, 728–732. [CrossRef]
5. Ruas, C.V.; Minozzo, F.; Pinto, M.D.; Brown, L.E.; Pinto, R.S. Lower-extremity strength ratios of professional soccer players according to field position. *J. Strength Cond. Res.* **2015**, *29*, 1220–1226. [CrossRef]
6. Lech, G.; Chwała, W.; Ambroży, T.; Sterkowicz, S. Muscle torque and its relation to technique, tactics, sports level and age group in judo contestants. *J. Hum. Kinet.* **2015**, *45*, 167–175. [CrossRef]
7. Sterkowicz, S.; Lech, G.; Sterkowicz-Przybycień, K.; Chwała, W.; Ambroży, T.; Pałka, T. Relationship of maximal isometric torque produced in flexors and extensors rate to technique by judo athletes. *Acta Bioeng. Biomech.* **2018**, *20*, 65–71.
8. Croisier, J.L.; Ganteaume, S.; Binet, J.; Genty, M.; Ferret, J.M. Strength imbalances and prevention of hamstring injury in professional soccer players: A prospective study. *Am. J. Sports Med.* **2008**, *36*, 1469–1475. [CrossRef]
9. Ruas, V.C.; McManus, T.R.; Bentes, M.C.; Costa, B.P. Acute effects of proprioceptive neuromuscular facilitation on peak torque and muscle imbalance. *J. Funct. Morphol. Kinesiol.* **2018**, *3*, 63. [CrossRef]
10. Bamaç, B.; Çolak, T.; Özbek, A.; Çolak, S.; Cinel, Y.; Yenigün, Ö. Isokinetic performance in elite volleyball and basketball players. *Kinesiology* **2008**, *40*, 183–189.
11. Hadzic, V.; Sattler, T.; Markovic, G.; Veselko, M.; Dervisevic, E. The isokinetic strength profile of quadriceps and hamstrings in elite volleyball players. *Isokinet. Exerc. Sci.* **2010**, *18*, 31–37. [CrossRef]
12. Teixeira, J.; Carvalho, P.; Moreira, C.; Carneiro, A.; Santos, R. Muscle strength assessment of knee flexors and extensors. Comparative study between basketball, football, handball and volleyball athletes. *Int. J. Sports Sci.* **2015**, *5*, 192–200.
13. Jones, P.A.; Thomas, C.; Dos'Santos, T.; McMahon, J.J.; Graham-Smith, P. The role of eccentric strength in 180° turns in female soccer players. *Sports* **2017**, *5*, 42. [CrossRef] [PubMed]
14. Struzik, A.; Pietraszewski, B. Relationships between hamstrings-to-quadriceps ratio and variables describing countermovement and drop jumps. *Appl. Bionics Biomech.* **2019**, *2019*, 4505481. [CrossRef] [PubMed]

15. Zatsiorsky, V.M.; Kraemer, W.J. *Science and Practice of Strength Training*, 2nd ed.; Human Kinetics: Champaign, IL, USA, 2006; pp. 17–46.
16. Reilly, T.; Bangsbo, J.; Franks, A. Anthropometric and physiological predispositions for elite soccer. *J. Sports Sci.* **2000**, *18*, 669–683. [CrossRef] [PubMed]
17. Reilly, T.; Doran, D. Fitness assessment. In *Science and Soccer*; Reilly, T., Williams, A.M., Eds.; Routledge: London, UK; New York, NY, USA, 2003; pp. 21–46.
18. Pietraszewski, B.; Siemieński, A.; Bober, T.; Struzik, A.; Rutkowska-Kucharska, A.; Nosal, J.; Rokita, A. Lower extremity power in female soccer athletes: A pre-season and in-season comparison. *Acta Bioeng. Biomech.* **2015**, *17*, 129–135.
19. Bona, C.C.; Filho, H.T.; Izquierdo, M.; Ferraz, R.M.P.; Marques, M.C. Peak torque and muscle balance in the knees of young U-15 and U-17 soccer athletes playing various tactical positions. *J. Sports Med. Phys. Fitness* **2017**, *57*, 923–929.
20. Zago, M.; Sforza, C.; Dolci, C.; Tarabini, M.; Galli, M. Use of machine learning and wearable sensors to predict energetics and kinematics of cutting maneuvers. *Sensors* **2019**, *19*, 3094. [CrossRef]
21. Newman, M.A.; Tarpenning, K.M.; Marino, F.E. Relationships between isokinetic knee strength, single-sprint performance, and repeated-sprint ability in football players. *J. Strength Cond. Res.* **2004**, *18*, 867–872.
22. Stølen, T.; Chamari, K.; Castagna, C.; Wisløff, U. Physiology of soccer: An update. *Sports Med.* **2005**, *35*, 501–536. [CrossRef]
23. Cerrah, A.O.; Gungor, E.O.; Soylu, A.R.; Ertan, H.; Lees, A.; Bayrak, C. Muscular activation patterns during the soccer in-step kick. *Isokinet. Exerc. Sci.* **2011**, *19*, 181–190. [CrossRef]
24. Dvir, Z.; Eger, G.; Halperin, N.; Shklar, A. Thigh muscle activity and anterior cruciate ligament insufficiency. *Clin. Biomech.* **1989**, *4*, 87–91. [CrossRef]
25. Aagaard, P.; Simonsen, E.B.; Magnusson, S.P.; Larsson, B.; Dyhre-Poulsen, P. A new concept for isokinetic hamstring: Quadriceps muscle strength ratio. *Am. J. Sports Med.* **1998**, *26*, 231–237. [CrossRef] [PubMed]
26. Struzik, A.; Siemieński, A.; Bober, T.; Pietraszewski, B. Ratios of torques of antagonist muscle groups in female soccer players. *Acta Bioeng. Biomech.* **2018**, *20*, 153–158.
27. Pietraszewski, B.; Zawadzki, J.; Pietraszewska, J.; Burdukiewicz, A. Body composition and muscle torques of lower limbs. *Biol. Sport* **1997**, *14*, 104–107.
28. Lewandowska, J.; Buśko, K.; Pastuszak, A.; Boguszewska, K. Somatotype variables related to muscle torque and power in judoists. *J. Hum. Kinet.* **2011**, *30*, 21–28. [CrossRef]
29. Kim, S.E.; Hong, J.; Cha, J.Y.; Park, J.M.; Eun, D.; Yoo, J.; Jee, Y.S. Relative appendicular skeletal muscle mass is associated with isokinetic muscle strength and balance in healthy collegiate men. *J. Sports Sci.* **2016**, *34*, 2114–2120. [CrossRef]
30. Camic, C.L.; Housh, T.J.; Mielke, M.; Zuniga, J.; Hendrix, C.; Johnson, G.O.; Housh, D.J.; Schmidt, R.J. Validity of fat-free weight equations for predicting isokinetic peak torque in young wrestlers. *Int. J. Sport Sci. Health* **2018**, *5*, 69–78.
31. Norsuriani, S.; Ooi, F. Bone health status, isokinetic muscular strength and power, and body composition of Malay adolescent female silat and taekwondo practitioners. *Int. J. Public Health Clin. Sci.* **2018**, *5*, 244–262.
32. Norton, K.; Olds, T. *Anthropometrica: A Textbook of Body Measurement for Sports and Health Courses*; UNSW Press: Sydney, Australia, 2002.
33. Cozette, M.; Leprêtre, P.-M.; Doyle, C.; Weissland, T. Isokinetic strength ratios: Conventional methods, current limits and perspectives. *Front. Physiol.* **2019**, *10*, 567. [CrossRef]
34. Matković, B.R.; Mišigoj-Duraković, M.; Matković, B.; Janković, S.; Ružić, L.; Leko, G.; Kondrič, M. Morphological differences of elite Croatian soccer players according to the team position. *Coll. Antropol.* **2003**, *27*, 167–174. [PubMed]
35. Hazir, T. Physical characteristics and somatotype of soccer players according to playing level and position. *J. Hum. Kinet.* **2010**, *26*, 83–95. [CrossRef]
36. Kulaga, Z.; Litwin, M.; Tkaczyk, M.; Różdżyńska, A.; Barwicka, K.; Grajda, A.; Świąder, A.; Gurzkowska, B.; Napieralska, E.; Pan, H. The height-, weight-, and BMI-for-age of Polish school-aged children and adolescents relative to international and local growth references. *BMC Public Health* **2010**, *10*, 109. [CrossRef] [PubMed]
37. Buśko, K.; Górski, M.; Nikolaidis, P.T.; Mazur-Różycka, J.; Łach, P.; Staniak, Z.; Gajewski, J. Leg strength and power in Polish striker soccer players. *Acta Bioeng. Biomech.* **2018**, *20*, 109–116.

38. Váczi, M.; Tollár, J.; Meszler, B.; Juhász, I.; Karsai, I. Short-term high intensity plyometric training program improves strength, power and agility in male soccer players. *J. Hum. Kinet.* **2013**, *36*, 17–26. [CrossRef]
39. Cometti, G.; Maffiuletti, N.A.; Pousson, M.; Chatard, J.C.; Maffulli, N. Isokinetic strength and anaerobic power of elite, subelite and amateur French soccer players. *Int. J. Sports Med.* **2001**, *22*, 45–51. [CrossRef]
40. Zawadzki, J.; Bober, T.; Siemieński, A. Validity analysis of the biodex system 3 dynamometer under static and isokinetic conditions. *Acta Bioeng. Biomech.* **2010**, *12*, 25–32.
41. Struzik, A.; Pietraszewski, B.; Bober, T. The biodex system used in the evaluation of the proportion of muscle torque and hamstring muscle injury risk. *Pol. J. Sports Med.* **2015**, *1*, 11–17.
42. Chen, Y.; Li, J.X.; Hong, Y.; Wang, L. Plantar stress-related injuries in male basketball players: Variations on plantar loads during different maximum-effort maneuvers. *Biomed. Res. Int.* **2018**, *2018*, 4523849. [CrossRef]
43. Hewett, T.E.; Myer, G.D.; Zazulak, B.T. Hamstrings to quadriceps peak torque ratios diverge between sexes with increasing isokinetic angular velocity. *J. Sci. Med. Sport* **2008**, *11*, 452–459. [CrossRef]
44. Kim, D.; Hong, J. Hamstring to quadriceps strength ratio and noncontact leg injuries: A prospective study during one season. *Isokinet. Exerc. Sci.* **2011**, *19*, 1–6. [CrossRef]
45. Cheung, R.T.; Smith, A.W.; Wong del, P. H:Q ratios and bilateral leg strength in college field and court sports players. *J. Hum. Kinet.* **2012**, *33*, 63–71. [CrossRef] [PubMed]
46. Dervišević, E.; Hadžić, V. Quadriceps and hamstrings strength in team sports: Basketball, football and volleyball. *Isokinet. Exerc. Sci.* **2012**, *20*, 293–300. [CrossRef]
47. Orchard, J.W.; Driscoll, T.; Seward, H.; Orchard, J.J. Relationship between interchange usage and risk of hamstring injuries in the Australian Football League. *J. Sci. Med. Sport* **2012**, *15*, 201–206. [CrossRef] [PubMed]
48. Daneshjoo, A.; Rahnama, N.; Mokhtar, A.H.; Yusof, A. Bilateral and unilateral asymmetries of isokinetic strength and flexibility in male young professional soccer players. *J. Hum. Kinet.* **2013**, *36*, 45–53. [CrossRef]
49. Latash, M. *Fundamentals of Motor Control*; Academic Press: Amsterdam, The Netherlands, 2012.
50. Wilkerson, G.B.; Colston, M.A.; Short, N.I.; Neal, K.L.; Hoewischer, P.E.; Pixley, J.J. Neuromuscular changes in female collegiate athletes resulting from a plyometric jump-training program. *J. Athl. Train.* **2004**, *39*, 17–23.
51. Silventoinen, K.; Kaprio, J.; Lahelma, E.; Koskenvuo, M. Relative effect of genetic and environmental factors on body height: Differences across birth cohorts among Finnish men and women. *Am. J. Public Health* **2000**, *90*, 627–630.

11

Electromyographic Evaluation of Specific Elastic Band Exercises Targeting Neck and Shoulder Muscle Activation

Ying Gao [1,2], Lars A. Kristensen [3], Thomas S. Grøndberg [3], Mike Murray [3], Gisela Sjøgaard [3] and Karen Søgaard [3,4,*]

1 Department of Sports Science, College of Education, Zhejiang University, Hangzhou 310028, China; yigao@zju.edu.cn
2 Faculty of Sport and Health Sciences, University of Jyväskylä, 40700 Jyväskylä, Finland
3 Department of Sports Science and Clinical Biomechanics, University of Southern Denmark, DK-5230 Odense, Denmark; larsakristensen1@gmail.com (L.A.K.); thomas-stig@hotmail.com (T.S.G.); mike_ster@hotmail.com (M.M.); gsjogaard@health.sdu.dk (G.S.)
4 Department of Clinical Research, University of Southern Denmark, DK-5230 Odense, Denmark
* Correspondence: ksogaard@health.sdu.dk;

Featured Application: This electromyographic evaluation of elastic band exercises documents that the type and intensity of exercise played a role in the activity in three muscle groups of the neck and shoulder. However, importantly, shrugs and reverse flyes are simple to perform and also highly effective training exercises as they induced high muscle activity of both shoulder and neck muscles at 12RM. The practical implications of these findings are that these simple exercises can be preferred for training programs targeting neck and shoulder muscle either for increased general strength or as prevention for work related pain and disorders.

Abstract: Background: Specific strength training at a high intensity is effective in reducing work related neck/shoulder pain. However, it remains to be documented as to which exercises most specifically target neck and shoulder muscles at high activation level while using simple equipment as e.g., elastic bands. We hypothezised that selected exercises would specifically target the respective muscles, as follows: (1) shrugs and reverse flyes: the upper trapezius muscle, (2) cervical extension and lateral flexion: the upper neck extensor muscle, and (3) cervical flexion and rotation: the sternocleidomastoideus muscle. Methods: Eleven healthy males (25.9 ± 1.4 years, BMI 24.3 ± 1.4) with no neck/shoulder pain (VAS = 0) performed the six exercises with elastic bands at 12RM (repetition maximum) and 20RM in a randomized order. Electromyography was bilaterally recorded from the three muscles and it was normalized to maximal voluntary activation (%MVE). Exercises that evoke more than 60%MVE were considered as high intensity activation. Results: High muscle activation level was attained during 12RM in the upper trapezius muscle during shrugs (100.3 ± 29.8%MVE) and reverse flyes (91.6 ± 32.8%MVE) and in the upper neck extensor muscle during cervical extension (67.6 ± 29.8%MVE) and shrugs (61.9 ± 16.8%MVE). In the sternocleidomastoideus muscle, the highest activity was recorded during cervical flexion (51.7 ± 16.4%MVE) but it did not exceed 60%MVE. The overall activity was ~10% higher during 12RM when compared to 20RM. Conclusion: The simple exercises shrugs and reverse flyes resulted in high intensity activation of both the upper trapezius and neck extensors, while no exercises activated sternocleidomastoideus at high intensity.

Keywords: physical training intensity; therapeutic exercises; work related neck pain; musculoskeletal pain

1. Introduction

Neck and shoulder pain are frequent in the general population and within several occupational groups that are characterized by monotonous work tasks that require the stability of the head and neck in constrained postures [1–6]. In often male dominated jobs, helmets add to the weight of the head increasing the demands on the neck muscles and a high prevalence of neck pain is reported among e.g., construction workers, helicopter, and fighter pilots [7–9]. Physical exercise—in particular specific high intensity strength training at the job—has been shown to effectively reduce musculoskeletal pain in the neck and shoulders [10–13].

In clinical practice, at work sites, and in home-based rehabilitation the use of conventional resistance training equipment, such as mascines or free weight, may not be a possibility, as it requires high financial cost and advanced facilities. Thus, it is important to identify more feasible alternatives that are easy to perform at the workplace and still effectively target muscles in the neck and shoulder regions. One alternative is the use of elastic resistance bands that has recently gained interest, because they are simple to handle, low in cost, and easy to transport. However, with elastic bands, it might specifically for the neck extensor muscles be difficult to add enough external load as resistance to achieve the requested high activity level. To attain this, a special headband has been invented for more specific, but also more complex, elastic band neck exercises. These complex exercises have been applied in training interventions of helicopter pilots [8]. However, the attendance rate was low, which was possibly due to the more complex head band exercises; and, in that study, it was not investigated whether the more complex exercises actually resulted in a higher activation for the specific muscles when compared to the more simple neck exercises, like shrugs and reverse flyes [8,14]. The aim of the present study was to assess whether simple exercises as compared to the more complex exercises may suffice for sufficient activation of the neck and shoulder muscles.

Regarding the level of sufficient exercise intensity in strength training programs, this is often defined as the percentage of maximal voluntary force exerted [15]. In practice, one repetition maximum (RM) weight is often used as reference for the maximal weight that can be lifted in an exercise for a given number of repetitions. Activation levels of >60% of maximal voluntary contraction force (MVC) are generally recommended to attain a physiological effect of resistance training [15]. A higher force per contraction can be performed the lower the number of repetitions per set, e.g., at 1RM the performed force is close to 100% MVC, decreasing to around 60% MVC when performing 12RM—depending highly on training status. In well trained persons 60% MVC might be repeated more times, e.g., corresponding to 20RM.

To access the activation level, electromyography (EMG) is commonly used to measure the activity of the specific muscles that are involved in an exercise [16,17]; the bilateral upper trapezius muscle (mUTR), upper neck extensor muscles (mUNE), and sternocleidomastoideus muscle (mSCM) were the muscle groups included here. In the prevention and treatment of neck and shoulder pain such EMG measurements can ensure that a given mode and intensity of training will activate the target muscles to the sufficient level [18]. In addition, EMG measures allow for exploratory analysis, such as the development of muscle fatigue during multiple repetitions that might be an indicator of the long-term effect on hypertrophy, as well as the reduced perception of pain. The myoelectrical manifestations used as an indication of muscle fatigue is an increase in the amplitude and a shift in the power spectrum towards lower frequencies [19–21]. Previous studies with advanced exercises have presented important knowledge for selecting the most adequate exercises to target specific health effects [16,17]. However, studies using simple exercises have similarly shown an effect on both pain relieve and increase in strength [2,22]. The present study will expand on this by using simple (shrugs, SH, and reverse flyes, RF), as well as more advanced (cervical extension, CE and cervical flexion, CF), and quite difficult (cervical lateral flexion, CL and cervical rotation, CR) neck/shoulder exercises and compare the activation in the muscles specifically targeted with each exercise at 20RM and 12RM.

The main hypothesis was that specific training exercises were requested to maximize the activation of the individual neck and shoulder muscles: with mUTR activation being the highest during SH and

RF, mUNE during CE and CL, and mSCM during CF and CR. Further, it was hypothesized that the intensity of the exercises significantly affected muscle activity: 12RM, resulting in higher activity than 20RM during the specific training exercises. Finally, we hypothesized that the muscle activity in the concentric phase was higher than in the eccentric phase and fatigue development was present in each set of an exercise being shown as an increase in EMG amplitude and a decrease in EMG frequency in the targeted muscle groups.

2. Materials and Methods

2.1. Study Design and Subjects

This study was conducted over three separate days that were interspaced with at least three days with no exercises. On the first day participants were familiarized with the elastic band training exercises and practiced the proper technique under supervision. On the second day, individual loadings were determined for each training exercise during low intensity, high repetition sets (20RM), and during high intensity, moderate repetition sets (12RM). All of the exercises were performed while using concentric and eeccentric muscle contractions in a controlled manner, with slow to moderate lifting velocity corresponding to the execution in earlier intervention studies [16]. Subsequently, the actual duration of concentric and eccentric phases were measured and shown to have an equal duaration each of minimum three seconds. The length and color code of elastic bands were adjusted to reduce or increase the resistance to match 12RM and 20RM for each participant. The task was repeated until the participant was exhausted and/or not able to continue the exercise according to the basics of procedures in the literature to define the individual 12RM and 20RM loads for each exercise [15]. The participant was deemed not able to continue the exercise if making compensating adjustment in body posture or not obeying contraction time and range of movement. The exercise was repeated until the loading corresponding to 20RM and 12RM was determined. On the third day, the determined loadings for each participant were applied and all EMG measurements were performed, while the participant performed all exercises at the intensity of 20RM sets, followed by 12RM sets. The order of exercises was randomized and each exercise was separated by 3-minutes rest intervals to avoid a gradient of fatigue through the test protocol. At the end, isometric maximal voluntary contractions (MVC) were performed for the normalization of the EMG data. For each targeted muscle, three MVCs with a duration of 5 s and 1 minute rest between consecutive trials were performed to induce the maximal muscle activity in a seated position and according to standardized procedures described in details in a recent study [23]. In short, maximal activity in mUTR was obtained during resisted bilateral shoulder elevation, with resistance being placed above the acromions. Maximal activity for mUNE was obtained during a resisted cervical extension and for mSCM during a resisted cervical flexion with resistance being placed on the external occipital protuberance and above the eyebrows, respectively.

The subjects participating were a group of 11 healthy males (age 25.9 ± 1.4 years, height 183.6 ± 5.0 cm, body mass 82.1 ± 6.0 kg, BMI 24.3 ± 1.4), with no pain in neck or shoulders (VAS = 0). The inclusion of only males was justified by the aviation personell—who used these exercises in a previous RCT study—all being males [8]. All of the subjects were informed regarding the benefits and risks of the investigation prior to signing the institutionally approved informed consent document to participate in the study. The local Ethics Committee of Southern Denmark (S-20120121) approved the procedures in the study.

2.2. Procedures

2.2.1. Electromyography (EMG)

The activity of the neck and shoulder muscles was measured through a bipolar surface EMG configuration (Neuroline 720-01-K, Medicotest A/S, Ølstykke, Denmark). The electrodes (Ag/AgC1, Ambu Blue Sensor, N-00-S/25, Denmark) were positioned bilaterally, in accordance with the SENIAM recommendations and earlier studies [24–27]) with an inter-electrode distance of 20 mm. The electrodes were placed (1) above the upper trapezius muscle (mUTR), 20% medially from the centerpoint between the lateral edge of the acromion and seventh cervical vertebra, (2) above the upper neck extensor (mUNE) muscle, on the most prominent part of the muscle at the level of the fourth cervical vertebra, and (3) above the sternocleidomastoideus muscle (mSCM), over the main muscle belly at the 1/3 distance from the sternal notch to the mastoid process (Figure 1). Before affixing the electrodes, skin was shaved and cleaned with scrubbing gel (Acqua gel, Meditec, Parma, Italy) and 70% alcohol, to effectively lower the impedance to less than 10 kΩ.

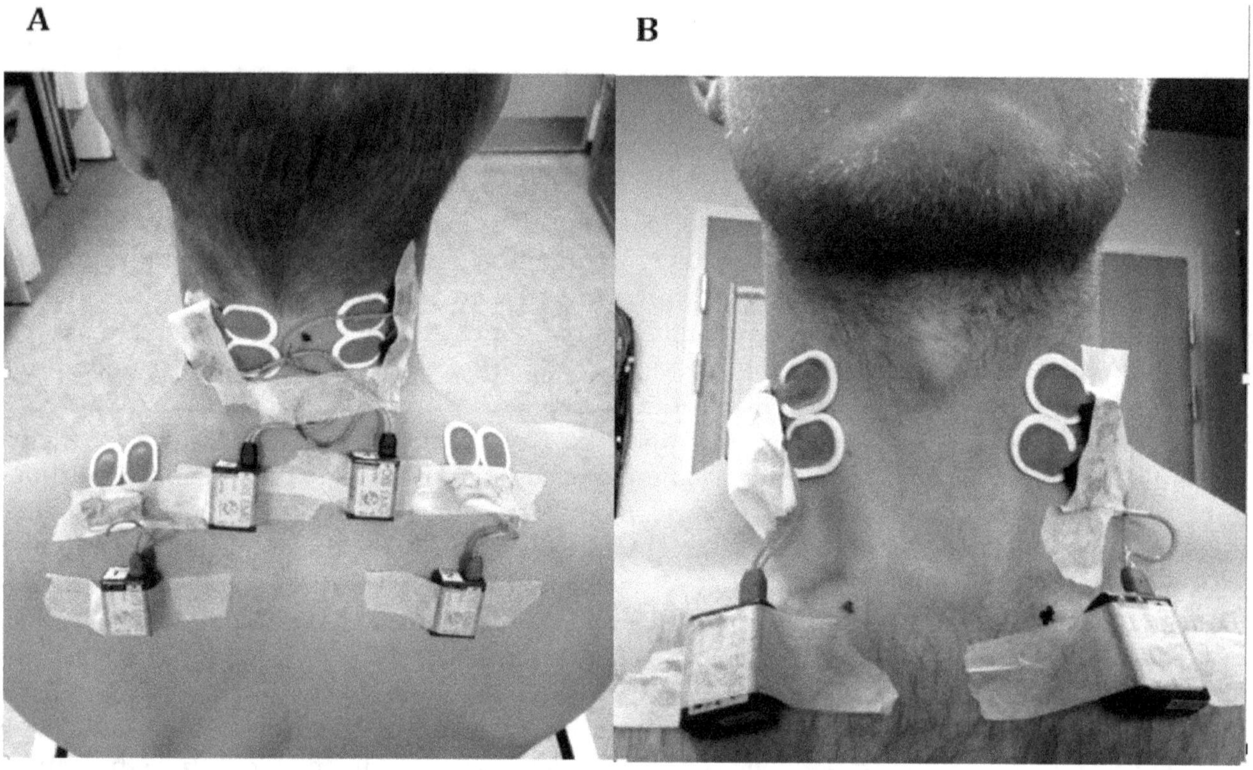

Figure 1. Bilateral electrode placement above the upper trapezius muscle (mUTR) and upper neck extensors muscles (mUNE) (**A**) and sternocleidomastoideus muscles (mSCM) (**B**).

The EMG signal was pre-amplified with a gain of 400 and then transferred through an EMG probe (Direct Transmission System (DTS), Noraxon Inc, Scottsdale, AZ, USA) to a belt-receiver (TELEMyo ™ 2400T, DTS, Noraxon Inc, Scottsdale, AZ, USA) with a bandwidth of 10–500 Hz and a common mode rejection ratio better than 100 dB. The signal was sampled at 1000 Hz while using a 16-bit A/D converter (DAQCard Al 16XE 50, National Instruments, Austin, TX, USA) and stored on a computer via the laboratory interface (CED 1401, Spike2 software, Cambridge Electronic Devices, Cambridge, UK).

2.2.2. Elastic Band Training Exercises

Six specifically tailored elastic band training exercises were performed targeting the neck and shoulder muscles. The choice of exercises was evidence-based and designed by an interdisciplinary team, including sports exercise training specialists, physical therapists, medical doctors, and chiropractors. The exercises were performed with a head harness (Neck Flex ®, Leesburg, VA, USA) while using different color-coded elastic resistance bands (Thera-Band®, The Hygenic Corporation, Akron, OH, USA). The individual exercises are briefly presented below, as a detailed description can be found in an earlier publication [14] and video material is available online: Neck exercises.

In short the exercises are the following:

(1) Shrugs (SH) were performed in standing position with the elastic band fixated under the feet and arms placed along the side of the body and shoulders relaxed. The head was held in an anatomically neutral position with eyes looking straight forward. During the exercise, shoulders were elevated as high as possible toward the ears against resistance and lowered again.
(2) Reverse Flyes (RF) were performed seated with the elastic band fixated under the feet and with a straight back. Participants were instructed to position their head in an anatomically neutral position, lean the trunk forward (~20–30°), and place both arms pointing towards the floor. Elbows were kept in a static and slightly flexed position (~5°). During the exercise, both of the arms were raised toward a horizontal level against resistance and lowered again.
(3) Cervical Extension (CE) was performed seated. The participants were instructed to keep a straight back, position their head in an anatomically neutral position, and lean the trunk forward (~20–30°). Arms were held strait with the hands placed underneath the knees. An elastic band was stretched between the hands and front of the head harness. The exercise was performed with a low cervical spine flexion, followed by a low cervical spine extension (against resistance).
(4) Cervical Flexion (CF) was performed in the same way as during cervical extension, but the elastic band was stretched between a door anchor and the back of the head harness. During the exercise, the participants performed a low cervical spine flexion (against resistance), followed by a low cervical spine extension.
(5) Cervical Lateral flexion (CL) was performed standing erect with the head in an anatomically neutral position. One hand was placed horizontally against a wall and an elastic band was stretched between the hand and side of the head harness. The exercise was performed with a low lateral spine flexion against resistance, followed by a low lateral spine extension. The exercise was performed for the right and left side, respectively.
(6) Cervical rotation (CR) was performed seated with a straight back and trunk leaned forward (~20°). The head was held in an anatomically neutral position and rotated approximately 45° to either the right or left side. An elastic band was stretched between the head harness and a door anchor. Keeping a static upper body, the hips were flexed and the body flexed (against resistance), followed by an extension. The exercise was performed to the right and left side.

2.3. Outcomes

Analyses of the EMG signals were the outcome data. All data analysis was performed while using a custom-made script in Matlab (MathWorks Inc. USA) and Hedera 2.0 (University of Southern Denmark, Denmark). The peak EMG amplitude was calculated by root mean square (RMS) in a 500 ms moving window. For each repetition during exercises, the peak RMS was normalized to the peak RMS that was obtained during the MVC of each muscle as percentage of maximal voluntary EMG signal (%MVE) in standardized postures [23]. The 3rd, 4th, and 5th repetition of each exercise were averaged and used as the muscle activation for the exercises. The EMG activity in the concentric and eccentric phases of the muscle contraction was analyzed for each muscle during the exercise, resulting in the highest activation. The concentric and eccentric phases of each exercise were marked as an event in a separate channel in the Spike2 software, during each recording, As each repetition was performed with a 3 s concentric and 3 s eccentric phase, the midpoint was used to divide these phases. Additionally, the mean power frequency (MPF) was calculated in the last 1000 ms of the concentric phase of each contraction for the muscle groups during the exercise that represents the highest activation during the contraction.

2.4. Statistical Analysis

All of the data are presented as mean ± SD. The Q-Q plot and the Shapiro-Wilk test with skewness were used to test for normal distribution of data. Differences between left and right muscles during the symmetrical exercises SH, RF, CE, and CF, or between ipsilateral and contralateral muscles during CL and CR performed towards left and right side were examined while using paired-t test. In the case of no difference, the mean value of the two sides was used. If significant differences were found, the side specific values are reported and the highest used to represent the muscle activation level for that exercise. Regarding the main hypotheses of the muscle activity (%MVE) for each muscle group, one way repeated measures ANOVA was used to compare the different exercises (SH, RF, CE, CF, CL, and CR). If the assumption of Sphericity was violated, the Greenhouse-Geisser correction was used. Planned contrasts were used to localize the differences between the exercise, resulting in the highest activation of specific muscle group and the other exercises. Paired t-test was used for testing possible differences between the two exercise intensities. Furthermore, paired t-test was used to compare muscle activity in the concentric phase and eccentric phase of each muscle group. The fatigue development was tested by paired t-test to compare the third repetition and the last one repetition in normalized EMG amplitude (%MVE) and EMG frequency (MPF). A substantial addition in muscle activation level of at least 20% was requested in order to recommend an advanced, instead of a simple, exercise. This level is well above the SD of approx. 10% in mean level of trapezius activation both found within groups and variability of repeated EMG recordings during high intensity contractions, see, for instance, mean activation levels for trapezius in [17]. A power analysis showed that eight subjects would be sufficient to reveal a difference in muscle activation level of 20%. Within the recruiting period, we managed to recruit 11, who all conducted the full protocol. All of the results were analyzed using SPSS 16.0 statistical software (SPSS Inc, Chicago, IL, USA). A probability level of $p < 0.05$ (two-tailed) was considered to be statistically significant.

3. Results

Table 1 presents the muscle activation levels for the six exercises at two intensities. There were no differences between left and right side of muscles during the symmetrical exercises and no difference between ipsilateral and contralateral when the exercises CL and CR were performed to right versus left side. Therefore, the data were averaged over left and right muscles or ipsilateral and contralateral muscles, except during CL for mUNE and mSCM. This is due to the higher muscle activity during CL in ipsilateral than contralateral for mUNE (30.2% ± 13.6% vs. 12.8% ± 6.8%, $p < 0.001$, for 20RM, and 45.5% ± 14.6% vs. 17.2% ± 7.1%, $p < 0.001$, for 12RM) and for mSCM (25.6% ± 7.7% vs. 11.6% ± 6.3%, $p = 0.001$, for 20RM, and 41.5% ± 14.6% vs. 15.3% ± 8.4%, $p = 0.001$, for 12RM). Therefore, for CL the higher value of %MVE in ipsilateral of mUNE and mSCM were used as the results (Table 1).

Table 1. Mean muscle activity (%MVE) for representative muscle groups shown for each exercise at 12RM and 20RM intensities. Values are presented as mean ± SD. Values > 60% MVE are marked in bold. Italic values are unilateral data, see text.

Muscle	Intensity	Exercise					
		SH	RF	CE	CF	CL	CR
mUTR	20RM	**78.8 ± 24.0**	**75.9 ± 30.7**	3.4 ± 1.8	1.9 ± 1.3	8.1 ± 4.6	3.7 ± 2.3
	12RM	**100.3 ± 29.8**	**91.6 ± 32.8**	4.8 ± 2.5	2.4 ± 2.0	9.1 ± 4.1	4.3 ± 2.8
mUNE	20RM	45.7 ± 16.7	39.1 ± 22.3	50.9 ± 25.8	7.6 ± 3.2	*30.2 ± 13.6*	10.4 ± 4.6
	12RM	**61.9 ± 16.8**	55.4 ± 16.3	**67.6 ± 29.8**	8.5 ± 3.8	*45.5 ± 14.6*	12.0 ± 4.7
mSCM	20RM	16.7 ± 13.5	14.2 ± 8.9	15.1 ± 11.3	44.8 ± 16.6	*25.6 ± 7.7*	28.8 ± 9.9
	12RM	26.2 ± 16.5	22.9 ± 14.8	10.1 ± 6.3	51.7 ± 16.4	*41.5 ± 14.6*	42.5 ± 11.6

The repeated measures ANOVAs revealed significantly different muscle activation between the types of exercise for: mUTR ($F(1.099, 10.987) = 97.622$, $p < 0.001$), mUNE ($F(2.359, 23.59) = 29.038$, $p < 0.001$), and mSCM ($F(5, 50) = 18.045$, $p < 0.001$), respectively. Figure 2 presents the contrast of muscle activity during the exercise, which induced the highest activation with other exercises. For mUTR, SH induced highest activity, and this was significantly higher than all of the remaining exercises, except RF. For mUNE, CE induced the highest activity and this was higher than during CF, CL and CR, but not significantly different from SH, and RF. For mSCM, CF induced the highest activity and this was higher than in all the remaining exercises. Furthermore, when compared with 20RM, the mean muscle activity of all exercises was significantly higher (relative increase 34%) during 12RM. For the specific muscle groups the relative increase were 26% in mUTR ($p < 0.001$), 41% in mUNE ($p < 0.001$), and 35% in mSCM ($p < 0.001$). (Figure 3).

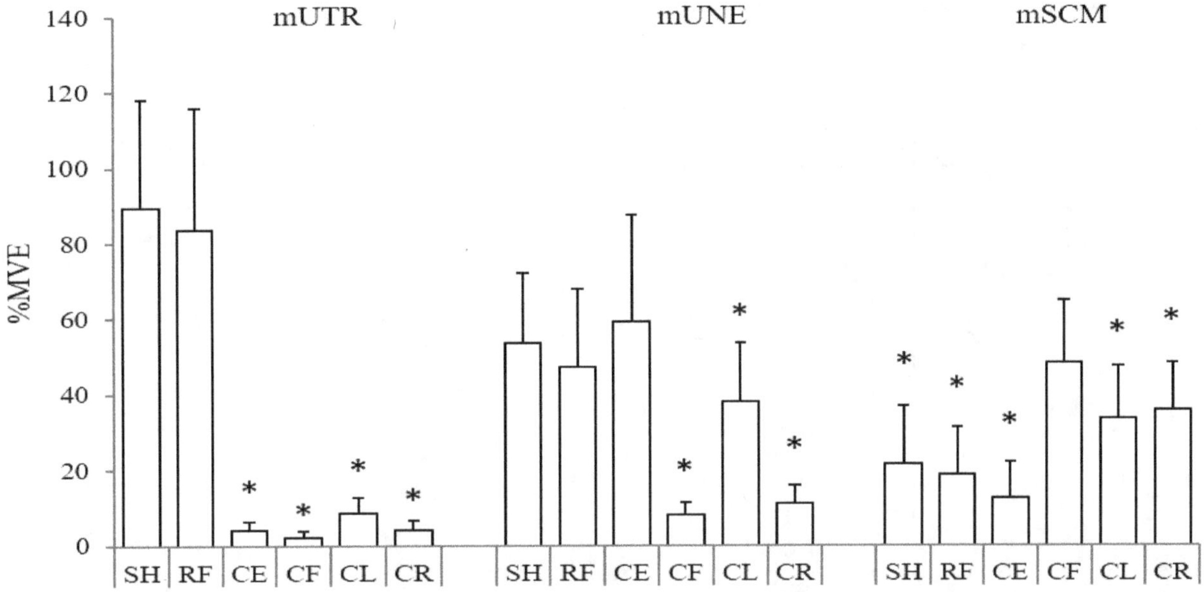

Figure 2. The muscle activity of the upper trapezius muscle (mUTR), upper neck extensors muscles (mUNE) and sternocleidomastoideus muscles (mSCM) were compared in six different types of exercises. The highest muscle activation (%MVE) was found during SH for mUTR, during CE for mUNE and during CF for mSCM. * marks exercises with significantly lower activation than the exercise inducing the highest muscle activation.

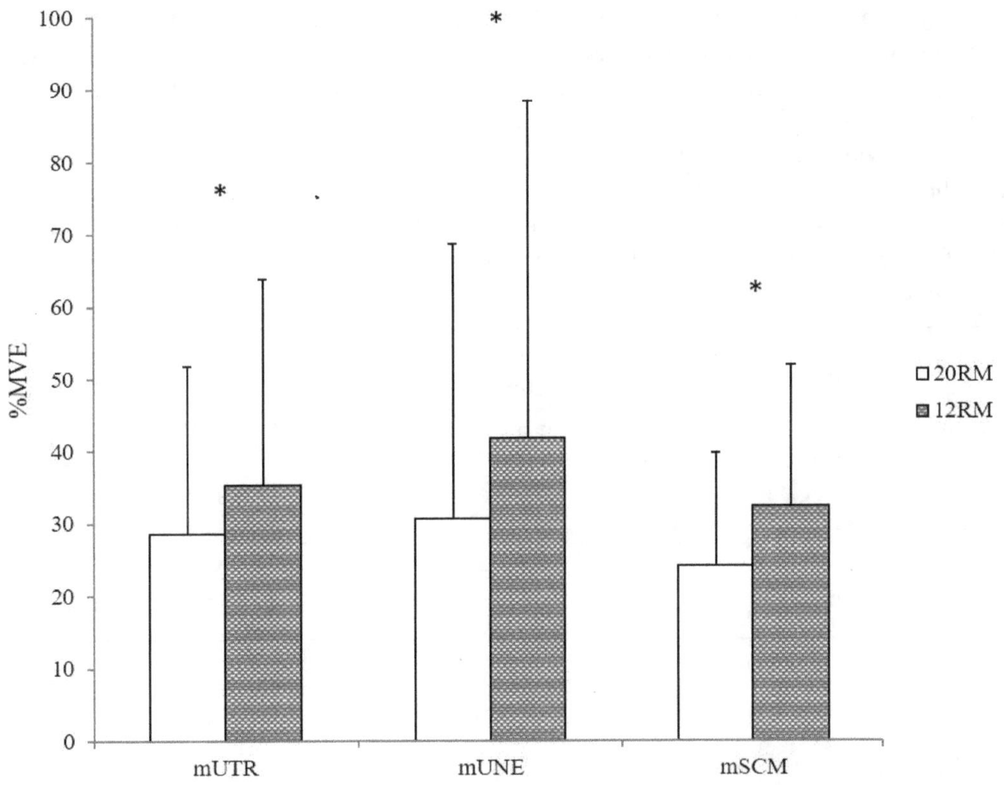

Figure 3. Mean muscle activity (%MVE) for all exercises in the upper trapezius muscle (mUTR), upper neck extensors muscles (mUNE), and sternocleidomastoideus muscles mSCM during intensities of 12RM and 20RM. * indicates significant difference between training intensities.

Analysis while considering activity separately in the concentric and eccentric contraction modes showed that the muscle activity of mUTR, mUNE, and mSCM in the concentric phase when compared to the eccentric phase was significantly increased by relative 75% for SH ($p < 0.001$), 32% for CE ($p = 0.009$), and 22% for CF ($p = 0.002$) (Figure 4).

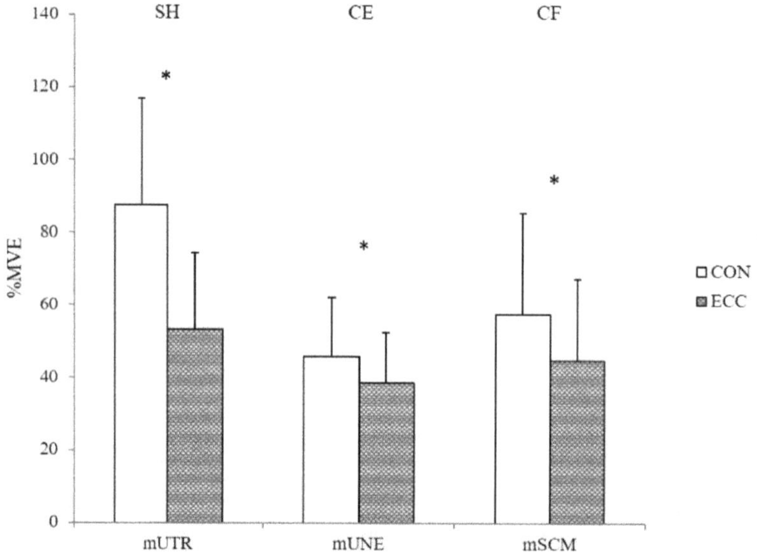

Figure 4. The muscle activity (%MVE) of the upper trapezius muscle (mUTR), upper neck extensors muscles (mUNE), and sternocleidomastoideus muscles (mSCM) in the concentric phase (CON) and eccentric phase (ECC) during shugs (SH), cervical extension (CE), and cervical flexion (CF), respectively. * Indicates significant difference between CON and ECC within exercise.

Analysis of fatigue development showed that, in each set of an exercise, a significant increase occurred in %MVE and a significant decrease occurred in EMG frequency (MPF) during SH, CE, and CF for each muscle groups of mUTR, mUNE, and mSCM, respectively (Table 2).

Table 2. The fatigue development of mean muscle activity (%MVE) and mean power frequency (MPF) for the upper trapezius muscle (mUTR), upper neck extensors muscles (mUNE), and sternocleidomastoideus muscles mSCM at intensities of 12 and 20RM. #Values are presented as mean ± SD for the exercises shrugs (SH), cervical extension (CE), and cervical extension (CF) that resulted in the highest activation of each muscle.

Muscle	Exercise	Fatigue Development	20RM			12RM		
			Rep 3.	Rep 19.	p-Values	Rep 3.	Rep 11.	p-Values
mUTR	SH	%MVC	81.2 ± 27.1	95.6 ± 25.6	0.001	94.3 ± 31.4	114.1 ± 30.2	<0.001
		MPF	78.5 ± 5.9	69.8 ± 8.2	<0.001	80.3 ± 12.0	71.6 ± 10.2	<0.001
mUNE	CE	%MVC	50.7 ± 26.2	67.5 ± 33.7	0.006	64.5 ± 28.7	82.4 ± 33.7	0.010
		MPF	66.0 ± 7.6	57.2 ± 8.9	0.004	63.6 ± 9.4	57.6 ± 10.6	0.005
mSCM	CF	%MVC	43.9 ± 17.4	53.5 ± 20.7	0.016	51.4 ± 17.1	65.0 ± 21.5	0.027
		MPF	104 ± 14.4	95.2 ± 14.4	0.005	104.0 ± 13.4	99.1 ± 12.7	0.012

4. Discussion

4.1. Main Finding

Specific activation patterns were identified in the three neck/shoulder muscles that were studied, in accordance with the hypothesis exercise type. Interestingly, the simple exercises, SH and RF, elicited muscle activities of >60% MVE in mUNE as well as in mUTR. The more advanced exercise, CE, showed numerically slightly higher—but not significantly—activation of mUNE, and CF produced the highest activity in mSCM, but this did not attain >60% MVE neither during 20RM nor 12RM and can therefore, not be recommend in case of mSCM insufficiencies. The two muscle groups most often attracting work related pain are mUTR and mUNE [1,3–5]. It is therefore interesting that both muscles can be intensively activated by two simple exercises (SH and RF), as this might potentially counteract the work related pain. The CL and CR, which are the most difficult exercises to perform correctly, did not elicit significantly higher percentages of muscle activation than any of the other exercises and can therefore be disregarded, unless for extra training variation. Thereby, our main hypothesis was rejected.

Earlier studies have reported significantly higher activation levels of mUTR during SH than RF [17,28], but this was not the case in the present study. The similar activation levels of mUTR during SH and RF may have great clinical importance due to the difference in force resistance that is required for performing the exercises. When performing the SH exercise for all subjects, a combination of three high resistance elastic bands were needed, whereas only one low resistance elastic band was used during RF. Thus, the SH exercise requires significant grip strength and core stability, which might be challenging for some populations. The mUTRs role as a scapula up- and outward rotator in combination with the significant external moment arm during the RF exercise may explain the high muscle activation in spite of low external resistance. Therefore, the RF exercise might, for some populations, be a more appropriate choice of exercise as compared to the SH.

The activity of mUNE was not significantly higher in CE compared to SH and RF. To our knowledge this is the first study to demonstrate high activity of neck muscles during SH and RF. This observation implies that the use of sophisticated exercises might not be needed as simple exercises effectively can activate both neck and shoulder muscles. This finding is supported by an earlier finding on high (>60% MVE) muscle activity of m. splenius capitis during lateral raise, which is similar to the RF that was used in the present study [29]. As splenius capitis is a part of the upper neck extensor muscle group, it will contribute to the gross activity measured as mUNE in the present study. Based on functional anatomy, the cervical spine will be forced in a protracted position during SH and RF, when performed with an external loading [30–32]. The neck muscles must be activated in order to stabilize and keep a neutral positio. This essential role of neck stability during SH, RF, and lateral raise may thus be a possible explanation for the high muscle activity in neck extensor muscle group. In this regard, it must be noted that the stabilizing effect arrives from static muscle contractions and the subsequent physiological effect might not be the same as from dynamic muscle contractions during the CE exercise [33–35]. Studies using wire electrodes to separate activity in the deep and superficial neck extensor muscles have pointed out the importance of activity specifically in the deep extensor muscles for patients with chronic neck pain [36]. Since surface EMG records from all of the underlying muscles, we cannot rule out that the same activity in SH and CE represent different contribution from the neck extensor muscles that may be of importance for specific patient groups. However, this distinction might not be equally important for the purpose of general strengthening of the neck extensors to relieve work related pain.

4.2. *Contraction Intensities*

In general, it is assumed that muscle activation increases with increased external load. Our hypothesis regarding a higher intensity during 12RM as compared 20RM was confirmed. We found that the EMG activity increased by 9% MVE from an overall mean of 28% MVE at 20RM to 37% MVE at 12RM. This corresponds to the estimated increase from 60% of 1RM at 20RM to the 70% of 1RM at 12RM. However, this general increase consisted of largely different increases for each of the targeted muscles. The muscles have a rather different function in each exercise and a high degree of co-contraction occurring in the neck region. Only for the mUTR would the 20RM evoke intensities >60% MVE that is normally considered to be most efficient for a training effect. From a pain reduction perspective, the high intensive exercises have been shown to be most effective and, therefore, the 12RM might be the best gain for the work time invested into exercises at the workplace [11,18].

4.3. Muscle Activation Patterns

The exercises included a concentric and an eccentric phase and EMG recordings clearly demonstrated that the highest activation occurred in the concentric phase, which is in concert with general physiological findings of the recruitment pattern explained by the force-velocity relationship [37,38]. Elastic band training exercises has been shown to compare well to activation patterns seen during traditional dumbbell exercises [29] and this underpins that elastic band exercise training might well substitute training with more advanced equipment. EMG recording also demonstrated that, during each set of contractions, significant muscle fatigue developed in all recorded muscle groups. In spite of the difference in activation level between the 12RM and 20RM in the first contraction of the sets then at the last contraction of the 12RM and 20RM both attained levels >60%MVE, which may potentially evoke an increase in muscle capacity [15]. Hereby, the present hypotheses regarding the contraction mode and fatigue EMG patterns were confirmed.

4.4. Study Strenghts and Limitations

We consider this study as a first step in the investigation of recommendable training and rehabilitation exercises for the neck/shoulder muscle based on elastic bands. The strengths of the study is the direct measures using EMG to assess the activation of representative neck muscle groups and instead of subjective assessment. Additionally, the design of the study using randomization of the exercises is a strength, since this ensures that the fatigue development within each type of exercise is not biased by its timewise performance.

The limitations of present study relate to the population only including a small group of males similar to majority of employees in the job groups specifically challenged with high exposures of the neck muscles due to helmet wearing or high accelerations (fighter pilots, helicopter pilots, construction workers, etc.). Additionally, the population consist of healthy subjects without serious neck/shoulder disorders. Therefore, extrapolation of our results to patients with neck/shoulder injury should be undertaken with caution. We cannot conclude that patients suffering from neck/shoulder pain will show similar muscle activation patterns when performing the exercises that are studied here.

Furthermore, EMG activity during the dynamic exercises was normalized to measurements of EMG activity during static MVCs to quantify the level of muscle activation. Given the inherent methodological limitations that are associated with surface EMG, only a rough estimate of the absolute level of muscle activation can be inferred while using this method. Fine wire electrodes for some of the deeper layers of neck extensor muscles could have further detailed the contribution of activity from each of the neck extensors. Finally, more muscles and contraction intensities could be studied to give an even more complete activation pattern for optimal recommendations of training exercises.

4.5. Future Perspectives

While considering the limitations above, future studies should include participants with work-related neck pain in a randomized controlled trial preferably designed with three groups: (A) training only using the simple exercises, (B) training with a variety of exercises, including the advanced and difficult exercises, and (C) a control group. Importantly the training volume, progression, undulation, and duration should be similar for groups A and B, as we have exemplified in previous studies [9–11,13]. The primary outcome should be neck pain testing the hypothesis that groups A and B would have equally positive effects. Additionally, secondary outcomes should be included, like muscle strength and adherence to the exercises; the latter in particular to test the hypothesis implied in the present study that adherence for group A would be larger that for group B.

5. Conclusions

The simple exercises (SH and RF) were highly effective, as they induced high muscle activation level of both shoulder and neck muscles and induced fatigue within the set of exercises. The more advanced neck exercises (CE and CF) and quite difficult exercises (CL and CR) did not, in general, add significantly higher muscle activation levels. The practical implications of these findings are that these simple exercises can be preferred for self-administered training programs—e.g., at the worksite—targeting neck and shoulder muscle either for increased general strength or as prevention for work related pain and disorders.

Author Contributions: Responsible for the conceptualization of the study were, M.M., G.S. and K.S.; the methodology, software, and validation was taken care of by M.M., L.A.K. and T.S.G.; formal analysis, M.M., L.A.K. and T.S.G.; investigation and experimental work, M.M., L.A.K. and T.S.G.; resources, G.S., K.S. and Y.G.; data curation and statistics, Y.G.; writing—original draft preparation, Y.G.; writing—review and editing, all authors.; visualization, Y.G., L.A.K. and T.S.G.; supervision, G.S. and K.S.; project administration, K.S. All authors have read and agreed to the published version of the manuscript.

References

1. Sjøgaard, G.; Lundberg, U.; Kadefors, R. The role of muscle activity and mental load in the development of pain and degenerative processes at the muscle cell level during computer work. *Eur. J. Appl. Physiol.* **2000**, *83*, 99–105. [CrossRef]
2. Hagberg, M.; Harms-Ringdahl, K.; Nisell, R.; Hjelm, E.W. Rehabilitation of neck-shoulder pain in women industrial workers: A randomized trial comparing isometric shoulder endurance training with isometric shoulder strength training. *Arch. Phys. Med. Rehabil.* **2000**, *81*, 1051–1058. [CrossRef]
3. Unge, J.; Ohlsson, K.; Nordander, C.; Hansson, G.A.; Skerfving, S.; Balogh, I. Differences in physical workload, psychosocial factors and musculoskeletal disorders between two groups of female hospital cleaners with two diverse organizational models. *Int. Arch. Occup. Environ. Health* **2007**, *81*, 209–220. [CrossRef]
4. Van den Heuvel, S.G.; van der Beek, A.J.; Blatter, B.M.; Bongers, P.M. Do work-related physical factors predict neck and upper limb symptoms in office workers? *Int. Arch. Occup. Environ. Health* **2006**, *79*, 585–592. [CrossRef]
5. Van den Oord, M.H.; De Loose, V.; Meeuwsen, T.; Sluiter, J.K.; Frings-Dresen, M.H. Neck pain in military helicopter pilots: Prevalence and associated factors. *Mil. Med.* **2010**, *175*, 55–60. [CrossRef]
6. Adam, J. *Results of NVG-Induced Neck Strain Questionnaire Study in CH-146 Griffon Aircrew*; DRDC Toronto, Defence R&D Canada: Toronto, ON, Canada, 2004.
7. Lange, B.; Toft, P.; Myburgh, C.; Sjøgaard, G. Effect of targeted strength, endurance, and coordination exercise on neck and shoulder pain among fighter pilots: A randomized-controlled trial. *Clin. J. Pain* **2013**, *29*, 50–59. [CrossRef]
8. Murray, M.; Lange, B.; Nornberg, B.R.; Sogaard, K.; Sjogaard, G. Self-administered physical exercise training as treatment of neck and shoulder pain among military helicopter pilots and crew: A randomized controlled trial. *BMC Musculoskelet. Disord.* **2017**, *18*, 147. [CrossRef]
9. Gram, B.; Andersen, C.; Zebis, M.K.; Bredahl, T.; Pedersen, M.T.; Mortensen, O.S.; Jensen, R.H.; Andersen, L.L.; Sjøgaard, G. Effect of training supervision on effectiveness of strength training for reducing neck/shoulder pain and headache in office workers: Cluster randomized controlled trial. *BioMed Res. Int.* **2014**, *2014*, 693013. [CrossRef]
10. Blangsted, A.K.; Sogaard, K.; Hansen, E.A.; Hannerz, H.; Sjogaard, G. One-year randomized controlled trial with different physical-activity programs to reduce musculoskeletal symptoms in the neck and shoulders among office workers. *Scand. J. Work. Environ. Health* **2008**, *34*, 55–65. [CrossRef]
11. Andersen, L.L.; Kjaer, M.; Sogaard, K.; Hansen, L.; Kryger, A.I.; Sjogaard, G. Effect of two contrasting types of physical exercise on chronic neck muscle pain. *Arthritis Rheum.* **2008**, *59*, 84–91. [CrossRef]
12. Zebis, M.K.; Andersen, L.L.; Pedersen, M.T.; Mortensen, P.; Andersen, C.H.; Pedersen, M.M.; Boysen, M.; Roessler, K.K.; Hannerz, H.; Mortensen, O.S.; et al. Implementation of neck/shoulder exercises for pain relief among industrial workers: A randomized controlled trial. *BMC Musculoskelet. Disord.* **2011**, *12*, 205. [CrossRef]
13. Dalager, T.; Bredahl, T.G.; Pedersen, M.T.; Boyle, E.; Andersen, L.L.; Sjøgaard, G. Does training frequency and supervision affect compliance, performance and muscular health? A cluster randomized controlled trial. *Man. Ther.* **2015**, *20*, 657–665. [CrossRef] [PubMed]

14. Murray, M.; Lange, B.; Nornberg, B.R.; Sogaard, K.; Sjogaard, G. Specific exercise training for reducing neck and shoulder pain among military helicopter pilots and crew members: A randomized controlled trial protocol. *BMC Musculoskelet. Disord.* **2015**, *16*, 198. [CrossRef] [PubMed]
15. Ratamess, N.A.; Alvar, B.A.; Evetoch, T.K.; Housh, T.J.; Kibler, W.B.; Kraemer, W.J.; Triplett, N.T. American College of Sports Medicine position stand. Progression models in resistance training for healthy adults. *Med. Sci. Sports Exerc.* **2009**, *41*, 687–708. [CrossRef]
16. Andersen, C.H.; Zebis, M.K.; Saervoll, C.; Sundstrup, E.; Jakobsen, M.D.; Sjogaard, G.; Andersen, L.L. Scapular muscle activity from selected strengthening exercises performed at low and high intensities. *J. Strength Cond. Res.* **2012**, *26*, 2408–2416. [CrossRef]
17. Andersen, L.L.; Kjaer, M.; Andersen, C.H.; Hansen, P.B.; Zebis, M.K.; Hansen, K.; Sjogaard, G. Muscle activation during selected strength exercises in women with chronic neck muscle pain. *Phys. Ther.* **2008**, *88*, 703–711. [CrossRef]
18. Chen, X.; Coombes, B.K.; Sjogaard, G.; Jun, D.; O'Leary, S.; Johnston, V. Workplace-Based Interventions for Neck Pain in Office Workers: Systematic Review and Meta-Analysis. *Phys. Ther.* **2018**, *98*, 40–62. [CrossRef]
19. Beck, T.W.; Stock, M.S.; Defreitas, J.M. Shifts in EMG spectral power during fatiguing dynamic contractions. *Muscle Nerve* **2014**, *50*, 95–102. [CrossRef]
20. Farina, D.; Merletti, R.; Enoka, R.M. The extraction of neural strategies from the surface EMG: An update. *J. Appl. Physiol.* **2014**, *117*, 1215–1230. [CrossRef]
21. Enoka, R.M.; Duchateau, J. Muscle fatigue: What, why and how it influences muscle function. *J. Physiol.* **2008**, *586*, 11–23. [CrossRef]
22. Ris, I.; Sogaard, K.; Gram, B.; Agerbo, K.; Boyle, E.; Juul-Kristensen, B. Does a combination of physical training, specific exercises and pain education improve health-related quality of life in patients with chronic neck pain? A randomised control trial with a 4-month follow up. *Man. Ther.* **2016**, *26*, 132–140. [CrossRef] [PubMed]
23. Murray, M.; Lange, B.; Chreiteh, S.S.; Olsen, H.B.; Nornberg, B.R.; Boyle, E.; Sogaard, K.; Sjogaard, G. Neck and shoulder muscle activity and posture among helicopter pilots and crew-members during military helicopter flight. *J. Electromyogr. Kinesiol.* **2016**, *27*, 10–17. [CrossRef] [PubMed]
24. Holtermann, A.; Roeleveld, K.; Mork, P.J.; Gronlund, C.; Karlsson, J.S.; Andersen, L.L.; Olsen, H.B.; Zebis, M.K.; Sjogaard, G.; Sogaard, K. Selective activation of neuromuscular compartments within the human trapezius muscle. *J. Electromyogr. Kinesiol.* **2009**, *19*, 896–902. [CrossRef] [PubMed]
25. Gosselin, G.; Rassoulian, H.; Brown, I. Effects of neck extensor muscles fatigue on balance. *Clin. Biomech.* **2004**, *19*, 473–479. [CrossRef] [PubMed]
26. Juul-Kristensen, B.; Kadefors, R.; Hansen, K.; Bystrom, P.; Sandsjo, L.; Sjogaard, G. Clinical signs and physical function in neck and upper extremities among elderly female computer users: The NEW study. *Eur. J. Appl. Physiol.* **2006**, *96*, 136–145. [CrossRef]
27. Falla, D.; Dall'Alba, P.; Rainoldi, A.; Merletti, R.; Jull, G. Location of innervation zones of sternocleidomastoid and scalene muscles-a basis for clinical and research electromyography applications. *Clin. Neurophysiol.* **2002**, *113*, 57–63. [CrossRef]
28. Jakobsen, M.D.; Sundstrup, E.; Andersen, C.H.; Zebis, M.K.; Mortensen, P.; Andersen, L.L. Evaluation of muscle activity during a standardized shoulder resistance training bout in novice individuals. *J. Strength Cond. Res.* **2012**, *26*, 2515–2522. [CrossRef]
29. Andersen, L.L.; Andersen, C.H.; Mortensen, O.S.; Poulsen, O.M.; Bjornlund, I.B.; Zebis, M.K. Muscle activation and perceived loading during rehabilitation exercises: Comparison of dumbbells and elastic resistance. *Phys. Ther.* **2010**, *90*, 538–549. [CrossRef]
30. Rivard, J.; Unsleber, C.; Schomacher, J.; Erlenwein, J.; Petzke, F.; Falla, D. Activation of the semispinalis cervicis and splenius capitis with cervical pulley exercises. *Musculoskelet. Sci. Pract.* **2017**, *30*, 56–63. [CrossRef]
31. Schomacher, J.; Erlenwein, J.; Dieterich, A.; Petzke, F.; Falla, D. Can neck exercises enhance the activation of the semispinalis cervicis relative to the splenius capitis at specific spinal levels? *Man. Ther.* **2015**, *20*, 694–702. [CrossRef]

32. Gabriel, D.A.; Matsumoto, J.Y.; Davis, D.H.; Currier, B.L.; An, K.N. Multidirectional neck strength and electromyographic activity for normal controls. *Clin. Biomech.* **2004**, *19*, 653–658. [CrossRef]
33. Folland, J.P.; Williams, A.G. The adaptations to strength training: Morphological and neurological contributions to increased strength. *Sports Med.* **2007**, *37*, 145–168. [CrossRef]
34. Higbie, E.J.; Cureton, K.J.; Warren, G.L., 3rd; Prior, B.M. Effects of concentric and eccentric training on muscle strength, cross-sectional area, and neural activation. *J. Appl. Physiol.* **1996**, *81*, 2173–2181. [CrossRef]
35. Vikne, H.; Refsnes, P.E.; Ekmark, M.; Medbo, J.I.; Gundersen, V.; Gundersen, K. Muscular performance after concentric and eccentric exercise in trained men. *Med. Sci. Sports Exerc.* **2006**, *38*, 1770–1781. [CrossRef]
36. Jull, G.; Falla, D. Does increased superficial neck flexor activity in the craniocervical flexion test reflect reduced deep flexor activity in people with neck pain? *Man. Ther.* **2016**, *25*, 43–47. [CrossRef]
37. Aura, O.; Komi, P.V. Mechanical efficiency of pure positive and pure negative work with special reference to the work intensity. *Int. J. Sports Med.* **1986**, *7*, 44–49. [CrossRef]
38. Komi, P.V.; Kaneko, M.; Aura, O. EMG activity of the leg extensor muscles with special reference to mechanical efficiency in concentric and eccentric exercise. *Int. J. Sports Med.* **1987**, *8* (Suppl. 1), 22–29. [CrossRef]

12

Immediate Effect of Whole-Body Vibration on Skin Temperature and Lower-Limb Blood Flow in Older Adults with Type 2 Diabetes

Kennedy Freitas Pereira Alves [1], Ana Paula de Lima Ferreira [1], Luana Caroline de Oliveira Parente [1], François Talles Medeiros Rodrigues [1], Thais Vitorino Marques [1], Gabriel Barreto Antonino [1], Luiz Carlos de Melo [1], Débora Wanderley Villela [1], Marcelo Renato Guerino [1], Wagner Souza Leite [1], Shirley Lima Campos [1], Larissa Coutinho de Lucena [2], Redha Taiar [3] and Maria das Graças Rodrigues de Araújo [1,*]

1 Department of Physical Therapy, Universidade Federal de Pernambuco (UFPE), Recife-PE 50670-901, Brazil; kennedyfpa@hotmail.com (K.F.P.A.); apllima@yahoo.com.br (A.P.d.L.F.); luanaparente00@gmail.com (L.C.d.O.P.); francoismedeirosfisiot@gmail.com (F.T.M.R.); thaisvmarques@hotmail.com (T.V.M.); gabrielbarreto@live.com (G.B.A.); luiz-carlos-melo@hotmail.com (L.C.d.M.); deborawanderley84@hotmail.com (D.W.V.); marceloguerino@hotmail.com (M.R.G.); wagnerszleite@gmail.com (W.S.L.); shirleylcampos@uol.com.br (S.L.C.)

2 Faculdade Nova Esperança (FACENE), João Pessoa-PB 58067-698, Brazil; larissacoutinho@gmail.com

3 GRESPI, Université de Reims Champagne-Ardenne, 51100 Reims, France; rtaiar@chu-reims.fr

* Correspondence: mgra@ufpe.br

Abstract: The purpose of this study was to evaluate the response of a single whole-body vibration (WBV) training session to peripheral skin temperature and peripheral blood flow of older adults with type 2 diabetes. A double-blind, controlled clinical trial was conducted following the Consolidated Standards of Reporting Trials (CONSORT) guidelines. A single session of WBV (24 Hz; amplitude 4 mm; vibration time 45 s, with a series of eight repetitions with recovery between repetitions of 30 s; total time of 10 min) or sham vibration on the Kikos P204 Vibrating Platform was employed. To assess skin temperature, the FLIR E40bxs thermographic camera and the ultrasonic vascular Doppler for flow velocity were used. Evaluation occurred before and after a WBV or sham intervention. The sample consisted of three men and 17 women. In the WBV group, there was a decrease in the temperature from 29.7 °C (±1.83) to 26.6 °C (±2.27), with $p = 0.01$. Temperature following sham decreased from 28.6 °C (±1.84) to 26.3 °C (±2.49), with $p = 0.01$. Regarding blood flow, there was a decrease in the analyzed arteries, especially the left posterior tibial artery, where there was a statistically significant flow reduction from 27.1 m/s (±25.36) to 20.5 m/s (±19.66), post WBV ($p = 0.01$). In the sham group, an increased flow velocity was observed for all the arteries analyzed, except for the left dorsal artery. Immediately following a full-body vibration session, peripheral skin temperature and lower-limb blood flow tend to decrease in diabetic patients. However, from the design of study developed, we cannot infer the maintenance of this effect in the medium and long term.

Keywords: type 2 diabetes mellitus; blood flow velocity; skin temperature; vibration

---

1. Introduction

Diabetes mellitus (DM) is one of the largest global health emergencies of the 21st century and, each year, more people develop and live with this condition. In addition to the 415 million adults diagnosed with diabetes, there are 318 million adults with glucose intolerance, resulting in a high risk of aggravating the condition and improving future disease development [1]. In Brazil, the number increased from 4.5 million in 2000 to 11.3 million in 2013, with an estimated range of 19.2 million by 2035 [2].

DM is a metabolic disorder of multiple etiologies characterized by hyperglycemia, which may be caused by defects in insulin secretion and/or action, involving specific pathological causes, such as the destruction of pancreatic β-cells responsible for the production of this hormone. This condition generates numerous side effects, such as the consequent disturbance mainly of carbohydrates, as well as proteins and fats, which leads to complications in various organs and may be accompanied by dyslipidemia, systemic arterial hypertension (SAH), endothelial dysfunction, obesity, smoking, and physical inactivity. Other macrovascular complications are either myocardial infarction and stroke, whereas microvascular complications include retinopathies and nephropathies [3–6].

The classification of the Brazilian Diabetes Society (BDS) includes four types defined according to specific disabilities or processes. Type 2 DM has an unknown etiology and is linked to relative insulin deficiency when it has a state of resistance combined with failure to secrete insulin, requiring the use of synthetic insulin to achieve glycemic control. It covers about 90% of diabetes cases in the population and usually manifests in adults aged over 45 with overweight or central fat deposition, physical inactivity, and family history of type 2DM [6,7].

Endothelial dysfunction is an important early factor in the development of macrovascular and microvascular complications of diabetes. Vascular endothelium is a dynamic tissue lining the blood vessels and the heart, and its performance is essential for homeostasis. The endothelium has several functions like maintenance of vascular tone, intravascular homeostasis, participation in the inflammatory process, and maintenance of blood flow. Reduction in peripheral blood flow and, consequently, local cooling of the skin are relevant markers of endothelial dysfunction that can be used as predecessors of cardiovascular disease. In older adults with type 2 diabetes, vascularization of the lower limbs is compromised [7–9]. The basal skin temperature in patients with type 2 diabetes is significantly lower than in patients without diabetes [10]. and this fact can be explained by the dilation of arteriovenous anastomoses and reduced blood supply in the capillaries due to autonomic neuropathy [11].

Many studies showed reduced blood glucose, insulin resistance, dyslipidemia, hypertension, and improved vascular function after regular physical activity, which are recognized as an important tool in diabetes control. Evidence of vasodilation after aerobic exercise and resistance training in diabetic individuals suggests increased vascular diameter and glucose uptake in the musculoskeletal system, which contributes to blood supply and lower-limb irrigation [12–15].

Reduced exercise tolerance is an important feature in patient with type 2 diabetes, who often have muscle weakness, making exercise more challenging. Whole-body vibration (WBV) is an alternative therapy which consists of a training program that exposes the whole body to mechanical vibrations. It was shown to be a safe alternative intervention to stimulate balance, and to improve muscle strength, body composition, and endurance in sedentary individuals who cannot perform conventional exercises such as walking and functional training. Protocols vary according to number of sessions per week, number of weeks, and frequency used in WBV in hertz (Hz) and amplitude (mm) [16–19].

However, there are few reports in the literature about the immediate effect of WBV on skin temperature and blood flow in the lower limbs of older adults with type 2 diabetes. Thus, the aim of this study was to evaluate the response of a single whole-body vibration training session to peripheral blood circulation and peripheral skin temperature in older adults with type 2 diabetes.

2. Methods

This is a pilot, randomized, double-blind, controlled clinical study that followed the guidelines set out in the Consolidated Standards of Reporting Trials (CONSORT) conducted with patients diagnosed with type 2 diabetes mellitus.

The research was carried out in the Laboratório de Cinesioterapia e Recursos Terapêuticos Manuais (LACIRTEM) of the Physiotherapy Department of the Universidade Federal de Pernambuco (UFPE). This study was approved by the Research Ethics Committee of the CCS/UFPE (No.3.219.332) and registered at www.clinicaltrials.gov (NCT04207853), respecting the ethical aspects of Resolution 466/12 of the National Health Council and the Declaration of Helsinki. All participants signed the free and informed consent form (FICF) after being informed of the objectives, risks, and benefits of the research.

The study was disseminated in various ways to attract volunteers (social networks, leaflets, lectures, scientific events, etc.). Volunteers were instructed to contact the research team to receive information and study guidance. When the volunteer met the research criteria, they were instructed to attend the day and time scheduled for exams to confirm the disease, while wearing appropriate clothes for the study.

The study included 20 clinically classified type 2 diabetic men (three) and women (17) who were aged 60 to 80 years, functionally independent, without severe foot deformities requiring the use of therapeutic footwear, without orthopedic deficiencies, without indication of deep vein thrombosis, without the use of walking aids, and with cognitive ability to respond and perform the exercises assessed by the Mini-Mental State Examination (MMSE), using 19 points as the cutoff point for illiteracy [20].

Volunteers who performed another physical activity and those who presented peaks of hypertension during treatment or who reported discomfort during the session that prevented the completion of training were discontinued.

Randomization was performed by a researcher not involved in any research stage, using the tool offered by www.randomization.com, and the order of participants was placed in numbered, sealed, and opaque envelopes, which were only opened at the time of the survey intervention. Thus, participants were randomly divided into two groups: whole-body vibration training (WBV), simulated vibration training (sham), and a single treatment session for WBV and sham. All participants underwent an initial and final evaluation.

Initially, anthropometric data were collected: gender, age, body mass index (BMI), vital signs (heart rate (HR), blood pressure (BP), and peripheral oxygen saturation (SpO_2), capillary glucose, and clinical history at the time of evaluation. Subsequently, the volunteers were assessed for peripheral circulation through blood flow and peripheral skin temperature on both limbs and then instructed to perform training on the vibrating platform. At the end of the intervention, blood flow, peripheral skin temperature, vital signs, and capillary blood glucose were re-evaluated.

2.1. *Vital Signs*

Heart rate (HR) measured in beats per minute (BPM) and peripheral oxygen saturation (SpO_2) expressed as a percentage (%) were evaluated using a Contec model CMS50M digital pulse oximeter (Contec Medical System Co., Ltd., Qinhuangdao, Hebei Province, China) placed on the second left toe with pressure. Blood pressure (BP) was measured in millimeters of mercury (mmHg) using a PREMIUM aneroid sphygmomanometer and a Rappaport Premium adult stethoscope (Accumed-Produtos Medico-Hospitalares Ltda, Rio de Janeiro-RJ, Brazil) using the left arm supported during measurement, with the patient sitting comfortably after 15 min of rest at baseline and immediately after the intervention.

2.2. *Capillary Blood Glucose*

Capillary blood glucose expressed in milligrams per deciliter (mg/dL) was verified by an Accu-Chek Active GU blood glucose monitor (Roche Diabetes Care Ltda, São Paulo-SP, Brazil), with the participant sitting comfortably with their arms resting on their legs before and at the end of each intervention to monitor and control the patient's glycemic index.

2.3. *Anthropometric Data*

Body composition was evaluated using a digital electronic anthropometric scale with a retractable ruler model MIC 200PPA (Micheletti Industria e Comercio de Equipamentos EIRELI, São Paulo-SP, Brazil). Body mass index (BMI) was defined as weight in kilograms divided by the square of height in meters (kg/m^2).

2.4. *Blood Flow Velocity*

The evaluation of blood flow velocity expressed in meters per second (m/s) was performed by ultrasonic vascular Doppler BV-620VP (Shenzhen Bestman Instarument Co., Ltd., Shenzhen, Guangdong, China), with sine wave emission. Prior to evaluation, a wide trichotomy of the examination site was performed, and then the area was coated with a water-soluble gel to promote better contact between the transducer and the skin. The transducer was positioned at a 45° angle to the blood vessels and was analyzed for flow. For the posterior tibial artery and the dorsal artery of the foot, recordings of the high-frequency transducer (8 Hz) were made, using the distal third of the calf and the instep as a reference. Confirmation of the most appropriate site for the evaluation of each blood vessel was performed through the acoustic signals generated by the equipment and, at this point, a marking was made to facilitate re-evaluation after the intervention. Three measurements were taken at 30-s intervals, and the final result was the average of the values obtained in the three collections. The exam was repeated after the intervention via which the patient was submitted, respecting the markings of the previous collection.

2.5. *Skin Temperature*

Skin temperature was evaluated using an FLIR E40bx thermographic camera (FLIR Systems Inc., Wilsonville, OR, USA) with a thermal sensitivity of 0.05 °C and a resolution of 160 × 120 pixels. The camera was positioned at a distance of 1 m from the assessed region, at an angle of 90° to the camera lens. Participants were instructed regardingthe preparatory measures for the thermographic exam, according to the recommendations of Priego Quesada (2017). Prior to the exam, the volunteers rested for 10 min in a room with a temperature between 18 and 23 °C and relative humidity between 40% and 70%, monitored with the help of athermo-hygrometer (KT-908). Reflected temperature was measured by the "reflective method" described in ISO 18434-1: 2008 for thermographic camera calibration [21]. We noted that the human body emissivity is assumed to be constant (about 0.98) [22] to ensure that the influence of the environment reflection is negligible.

Image analyses were performed according to the Glamorgan (2008) protocol for the anterior and posterior leg and dorsal region and sole of the feet, using the average temperature of a polygon, which followed the contour of the studied areas [23].

Images were collected before and after the intervention. Subsequently, the images obtained were organized, stored, and analyzed in the FLIR Tools software (FLIR Systems Inc., Wilsonville, OR, USA) provided by the camera manufacturer (Figure 1).

2.6. *Whole-Body Vibration*

The vibratory platform used was the Kikos P204–110v (Kikos Fitness, São Paulo-SP, Brazil), whose vibration direction is of the lateral oscillatory type. The vibrating plate features non-slip material on its surface for better foot attachment at the time of training. The established vibration frequency was 24 Hz. The 4-mm displacement peak was maintained throughout the program and was determined by the width of the volunteers' position on the platform. The intervention time was 45 s, with eight series being performed and, for each, the recovery time was maintained at 30 s for all intervals, totaling 600 s of intervention.

The subjects, barefoot, adopted a 40° squat position, verified with a universal goniometer. The calcans were supported on a silicone insole, consisting of a particular type of semi-rigid sole used to correct the distribution of body weight and biomechanical changes found in the foot. Only the forefoot and midfoot were in direct contact with the platform in order to reduce the transmission of vibrations to the head. This posture was used for the both groups.

The simulated vibration "sham" was performed with the platform disconnected. A sound device was connected producing a noise similar to the connected platform for a time equivalent to the treatment protocol because the vibratory stimulus could not be visibly distinguished. Participants who experienced false vibration had no contact with those who performed the protocol effectively.

On the day of intervention, participants were instructed not to do intense exercises, requiring at least one week apart from the last moderate/high-intensity physical activity. In addition, all participants were instructed to wear comfortable and appropriate exercise clothing.

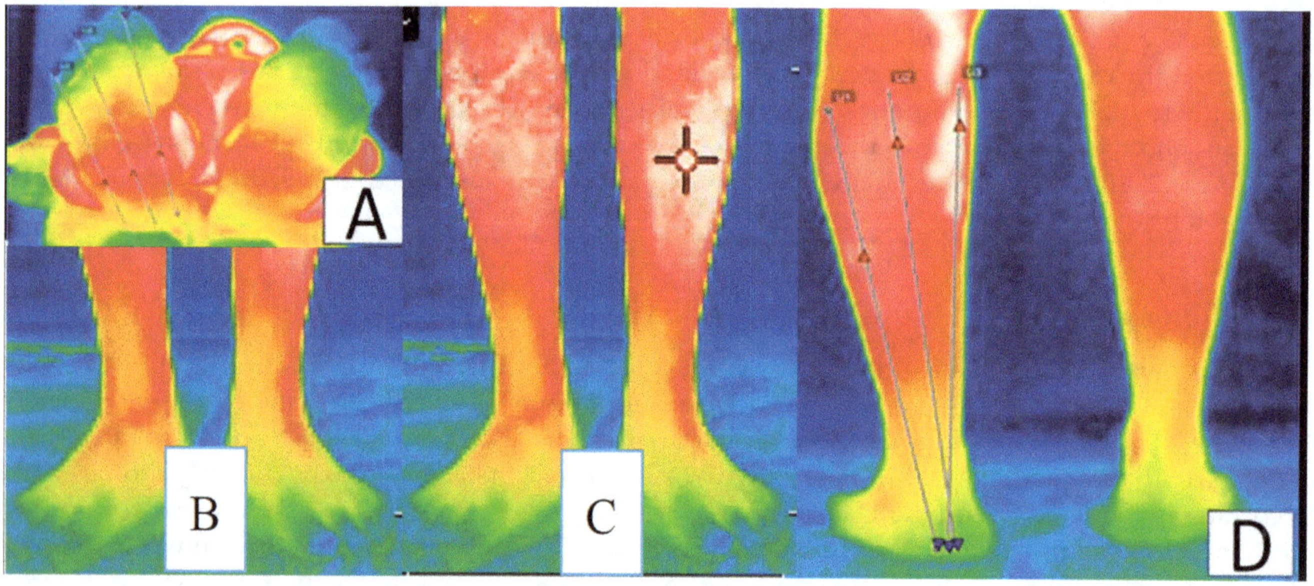

Figure 1. Regions of interest for infrared thermographic imaging: (**A**) sole of the feet; (**B**) back of the feet; (**C**) anterior leg; (**D**) back of the legs.

2.7. Data Analysis

Statistical analysis was performed using the statistical software SPSS version 23.0 (IMB Software Group, Chicago, IL, USA). To test the hypothesis of normality of each quantitative variable, the Shapiro–Wilk adherence test was used, and then the behavior of the quantitative variables was evaluated using the Mann–Whitney and Wilcoxon comparison test for the inter- and intragroup analysis, respectively.

The effect size was calculated by Cohen's d. An effect size of 0.2 was considered a small effect, an effect size of 0.5 was considered a moderate effect, and an effect size of 0.8 was considered a large effect. Descriptive statistical analysis was performed using the mean, standard deviation (SD), and percentage for qualitative variables. All tests were assigned a significance level of 95% ($p < 0.05$).

3. Results

Each group consisted of 10 participants, from WBV (two men and eight women) and sham (one man and nine women), as shown in Figure 2. For all variables, the groups were considered statistically comparable at baseline, as shown in Table 1).

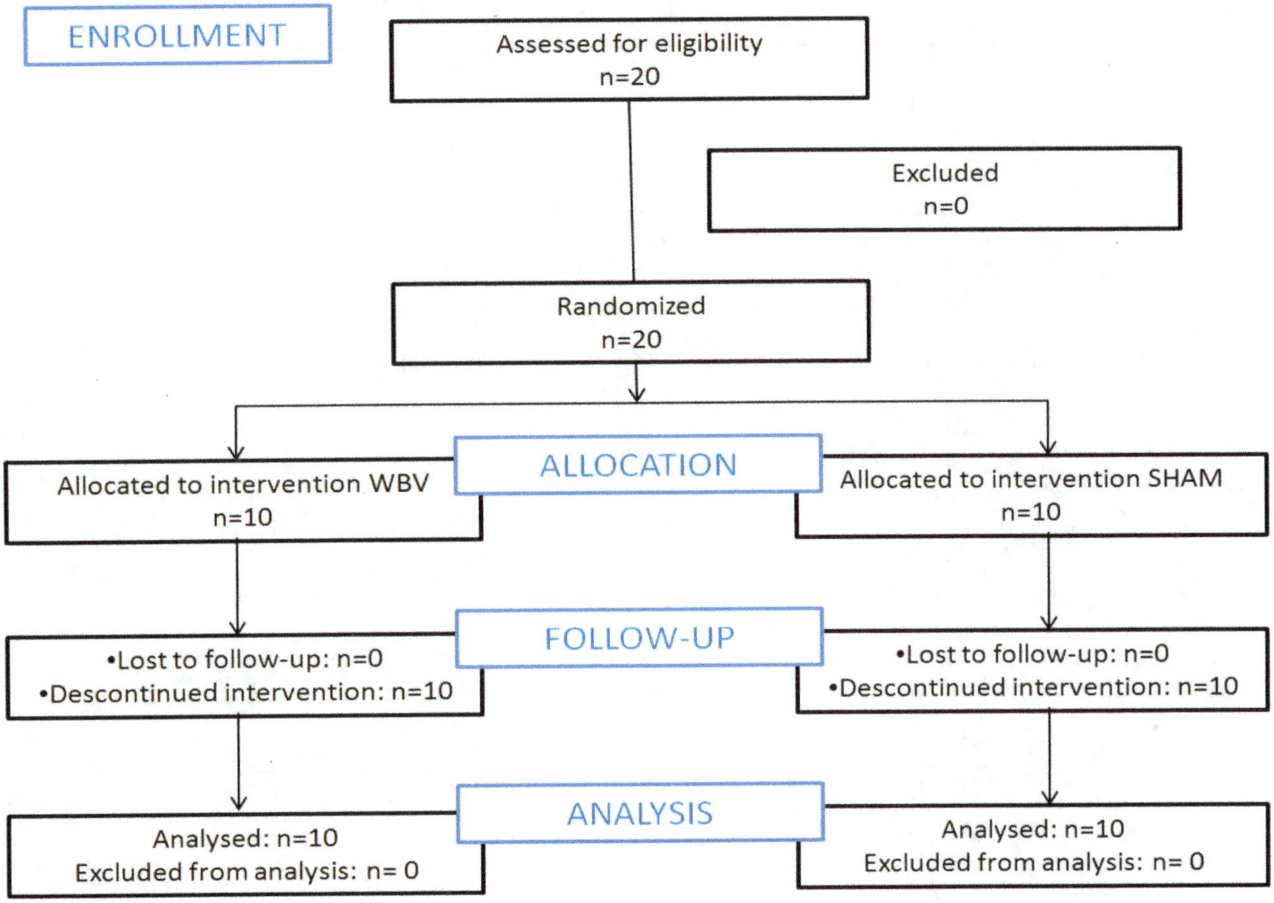

Figure 2. Flow chart which describes the recruitment, randomization, and allocation of patients.

Table 1. Baseline characteristics of patients in the whole-body vibration (WBV) and sham groups.

Variables	WBV G1 (n=10)	Sham G2 (n=10)	*p*-Value
Age (years)	64.4 (±3.99)	65.2 (±4.54)	0.83
Diagnostic Time (years)	7.29 (±4.53)	9.13 (±6.81)	0.55
Sex	10 (100%)	10 (100%)	
Male	2 (20%)	1 (10%)	0.54
Female	8 (80%)	9 (90%)	
Smoker			
Yes	3 (30%)	1 (10%)	
No	7 (70%)	9 (90%)	0.4
Former smoker	2 (28.6%)	3 (33.3%)	
Passive smoker	-	-	
Anthropometric data			
BMI	30.4 (±4)	27.9 (±3.9)	0.18

Table 1. *Cont.*

Variables	WBV G1 (n=10)	Sham G2 (n=10)	*p*-Value
Schooling			
Illiterate	-	-	
Incomplete elementary	1 (10%)	1 (10%)	
Complete elementary	2 (20%)	2 (20%)	
Incomplete medium	-	1 (10%)	0.42
Medium complete	2 (20%)	4 (40%)	
Incomplete higher	2 (20%)	1 (10%)	
Graduated	3 (30%)	-	
Postgraduate	-	1 (10%)	
Marital status			
Single	3 (30%)	-	
Married	4 (40%)	4 (40%)	0.24
Divorced	2 (20%)	3 (30%)	
Widowed	1 (10%)	3 (30%)	
Family income			
<1 MW	3 (30%)	3 (30%)	
1–3 MW	4 (40%)	4 (40%)	1
4–6 MW	2 (20%)	2 (20%)	
>7 MW	1 (10%)	1 (10%)	
HPAQ	8.49 (±1.19)	7.9 (±1.37)	0.32
Blood pressure			
SBP	120 (±9.43)	116 (±6.99)	0.3
DBP	77 (±8.23)	78 (±9.66)	0.81
Capillary blood glucose	133.6 (±36.75)	135.4 (±35.2)	0.91
SpO_2	98.3 (±0.82)	95.3 (4.8)	0.08
Diabetes knowledge	20.85 (±11.27)	21.42 (±9.54)	0.9

Data are expressed as mean (±standard deviation) or absolute frequency (relative frequency). Abbreviations: body mass index, BMI; minimum wage, MW; SpO_2, peripheral oxygen saturation; QAFH, usual physical activity questionnaire; BMI, body mass index; SBP, systolic blood pressure; DBP, diastolic blood pressure.

Only the plantar region of the right foot suffered a statistically significant reduction in skin temperature in both groups. In the WBV group, there was a reduction from 29.7 °C (±1.83) to 26.6 °C (±2.27), $p = 0.01$. In the sham group, the reduction was from 28.6 °C (±1.84) to 26.3 °C (±2.49), $p = 0.01$. There was no statistically significant difference between the groups. For all results, the effect size was considered low. Thermographic data are expressed in Table 2.

Table 2. Mean skin temperature analysis in °C (and standard deviation) before and after intervention (intra- and intergroup) and effect size.

Variables	WBV Before	WBV Post	p^+	Sham Before	Sham Post	p^+	Effect Size	*p*-Value
Plant right foot	29.7 (±1.83)	26.6 (±2.27)	0.01 *	28.6 (±1.84)	26.3 (±2.49)	0.01 *	0.12	0.78
Left foot plant	26.9 (±2.33)	26.7 (±1.89)	0.84	28.7 (±2)	26.3 (±2.21)	0.05	0.18	0.67
Back right foot	29.6 (±1.64)	29 (±1.7)	0.33	30.2 (±1.93)	29.2 (±1.23)	0.07	−0.16	0.77
Back left foot	27.9 (±1.85)	29.3 (±1.06)	0.06	30.2 (±1.93)	29.7 (±1.25)	0.30	−0.32	0.45
Anterior right leg	30.1 (±1.59)	30.1 (±1.59)	0.52	30.3 (±1.06)	30.3 (±1.06)	0.48	−0.19	0.74
Anterior left leg	30.1 (±1.52)	30.1 (±1.52)	0.21	30.4 (±1.26)	30.4 (±1.26)	0.36	−0.24	0.64
Posterior right leg	30.4 (±0.97)	30.3 (±1.06)	0.80	30.4 (±.97)	30.4 (±0.84)	1	0.12	0.82
Posterior left leg	30.6 (±0.97)	30.3 (±1.34)	0.54	30.5 (±1.08)	30.6 (±0.84)	0.76	−0.32	0.56

Data are expressed as mean (± standard deviation). Abbreviations: WBV, whole-body vibration; sham, dummy vibration. p^+, Wilcoxon; *p*-value, Mann–Whitney; * statistically significant result.

There was a reduction in blood flow in the WBV group after the intervention, but there was only a statistically significant reductionin the left tibial artery, from 27.1 m/s (±25.36) to 20.5 m/s (±19.66), $p = 0.01$. In the sham group, there was only a reduction in flow velocity in the left dorsal artery and an increase in all other evaluated arteries. However, none of them had a statistically significant difference, just as there was no statistically significant difference between the groups in this variable. Alow effect size was also observed for this variable. The complete analysis of blood flow velocity is detailed in Table 3.

Table 3. Analysis of mean blood flow velocity in m/s (and standard deviation) before and after intervention (intra and intergroup) and effect size.

Variables	WBV			Sham			Effect Size	p-Value
	Before	Post	p^+	Before	Post	p^+		
Right dorsal artery	29.3 (±25.79)	23.4 (±24.61)	0.31	27.9 (±29.14)	29.3 (±25.79)	0.81	−0.23	0.61
Left dorsal artery	24.6 (±21.65)	20.3 (±20.25)	0.37	26.8 (±23.58)	23.8 (±21.21)	0.13	−0.17	0.71
Right tibial artery	23.1 (±25.92)	21.4 (±23.68)	0.58	21.3 (±24.76)	23.2 (±26)	0.06	−0.07	0.87
Left tibial Artery	27.1 (±25.36)	20.5 (±19.66)	0.01 *	24 (±26.24)	27.2 (±25.42)	0.69	−0.26	0.52

Abbreviations: WBV, whole-body vibration; sham, dummy vibration. p^+ Wilcoxon; p-value, Mann–Whitney; * statistically significant result.

4. Discussion

In the present study, in both groups (WBV and sham), there was a reduction in skin temperature and blood flow velocity, corroborating previous studies. Fujiwara et al. (2000) evaluated 61 diabetic participants and 16 healthy subjects, and they reported that basal skin temperature in diabetic patients was significantly lower than in healthy patients, in addition to lower temperature variation and recovery after intervention. These findings agree with the present study, where there was little variation in some of the evaluated points and, in some of them, the temperature remained constant [10]. According to Uccioli et al. (1994), this fact can be explained by the dilation of arteriovenous anastomoses and reduced blood supply in the capillaries due to autonomic neuropathy [11].

The study by Kistler et al. (1998) inferred that capillary blood flow and blood pressure are lower in autonomic diabetic neuropathy because the anatomical walls are larger, directing flow and damaging peripheral sympathetic nerves. This promotes a slow recovery of skin temperature, justifying the smallest temperature variation in the present study [24].

Manimmanakorn et al. (2017) performed a study with a vibratory platform with 36 diabetic participants, of which 17 were trained on the platform for 12 weeks and 19 participants maintained their daily activities only. Reductions in peak systolic velocity and diastolic pressure were noticed in the WBV group, but without significant difference from the control group. In the present study, although no peak systolic velocity and diastolic pressure were evaluated, we observed a reduction in which there was a reduction in blood flow velocity in the evaluated arteries. This finding can be explained by the possible vibration-induced dilation of the smaller blood vessels present in the muscles, reducing peripheral vascular resistance by inhibiting endothelin, an important vasoconstrictor [25].

Saudoudo et al. (2013) evaluated 40 diabetics, 20 of whom underwent 12 weeks of whole-body vibration training, and reported increased blood flow velocity after 12 weeks of intervention, with a significant difference compared with the control group. This divergence in the results found in relation to the present study is possibly due to the accomplishment of a training program over a long period of time, enhancing the effects of vibration and promoting long-term results, which may not be the case in the first session of the study training [8].

Bagavathiappan et al. (2010) analyzed 112 patients diagnosed with type 2 diabetes through thermographic images of the plantar region, correlating the presence of diabetic neuropathy and the cutaneous temperature of these individuals. Higher values of mean and global foot temperature were found in patients with neuropathy, in addition to a positive correlation with temperature in the hallux regions, bilaterally. This finding may be justified by neuropathic feet being warm, with palpable pulses and distended veins, indicating increased blood flow, although slow, and possible congestion in this region [26].

Due to the neurovascular lesions triggered by hyperglycemia, as well as the response to lesions or infections, the vascular response of these individuals is slower, making them more susceptible to ulcer development and possible long-term necrosis and amputation. Thus, due to the increase in skin temperature after the use of WBV, it is plausible to think that the use of this equipment may be beneficial for the vascular maintenance of these individuals, and thermographic monitoring is an ally in the maintenance of these patients' lesions [26]. The findings cited are discordant with the present study.

However, Moreira-Marconi et al. (2019) evaluated 19 healthy subjects and reported a reduction in skin temperature in most participants, regardless of the frequency used in WBV (0 Hz, 30 Hz, and 50 Hz). This reduction can be explained by the fast and constant isometric muscle action that promotes work and increases the body's metabolic rate, increasing intramuscular temperature, modifying the thermal balance, activating the feedback-mediated heat loss mechanism. This change leads to redirection of blood flow from inactive to active areas. Then, during vibration, blood flow redistributes to the periphery, allowing heat exchange with the external environment, cooling the skin, and causing blood to flow to the lower-temperature muscle regions, thus preventing hyperthermia and maintaining homeostasis [27].

In addition, a larger blood supply is needed in the recruited musculature, requiring greater blood supply, initially diverting from adjacent peripheral areas. Under these conditions, a vasoconstrictor response induced by the mechanical action of vibration occurs, promoting a reduction in peripheral perfusion, and reducing the local skin temperature [26]. The above findings of the study corroborate the results found in the present study.

WBV training is an exercise program that does not increase excessive physical effort to the skeletal muscle system compared to conventional exercise. Mastering this training with WBV can help with choosing the most appropriate training program for older adults with type 2 diabetes.

5. Conclusions

Immediately following a full-body vibration session, peripheral skin temperature and lower-limb blood flow tend to be reduced in older adults with type 2 diabetes. However, from the design of study developed, we cannot infer the maintenance of this effect in the medium and long term.

6. Study Limitations

As this clinical trial was a pilot with a small number of participants, this study can serve as a basis for sample size estimation in future studies, taking into account the trends pointed out in the results presented. No condition in the metabolic control of diabetes was considered because it was a single-session study, given that glycated hemoglobin is the average glycaemia in the last 3–4 months. An increase in the sample size and a higher male presence (balanced gender repartition) in a future study should be considered to infer more robust results.

Author Contributions: Conceptualization, L.C.d.O.P., K.F.P.A. and M.d.G.R.d.A.; data curation, D.W.V. and A.P.d.L.F.; formal analysis, W.S.L. and S.L.C.; funding acquisition, M.d.G.R.d.A. and M.R.G.; Investigation, F.T.M.R., G.B.A., T.V.M. and L.C.d.O.P.; methodology, L.C.d.M., L.C.d.O.P., K.F.P.A., F.T.M.R., T.V.M., L.C.L, A.P.d.L.F., D.W.V., W.S.L. and M.d.G.R.d.A.; project administration, M.R.G., L.C.d.L. and M.d.G.R.d.A.; writing-original draft, L.C.d.O.P., K.F.P.A., G.B.A. and M.d.G.R.d.A.; writing-review and editing, K.F.P.A., S.L.C., R.T. and M.d.G.R.d.A. All authors have read and agreed to the published version of the manuscript.

References

1. International Diabetes Federation IDF. IDF Atlas, Seventhedition, Brussels, Belgium. 2015. Available online: www.diabetesatlas.org (accessed on 10 November 2019).
2. Cecilio, H.P.M.; Arruda, G.O.; Teston, E.F.; Santos, A.L.; Marcon, S.S. Comportamentos e comorbidades associados às complicações microvasculares do diabetes. *Acta Paul. Enferm.* **2015**, *28*. [CrossRef]
3. Brasil. Ministério da Saúde. Secretaria de Atenção à Saúde. Departamento de Atenção Básica. *Estratégias Para o Cuidado da Pessoa com Doença Crônica: Diabetes Mellitus;* Ministério da Saúde, Secretaria de Atenção à Saúde. Departamento de Atenção Básica: Brasília, Brazil, 2013.
4. Del Pozo-Cruz, J.; Alfonso-Rosa, R.M.; Ugia, J.L.; McVeigh, J.G.; Del Pozo-Cruz, B.; Sañudo, B. A Primary Care–Based Randomized Controlled Trial of 12-Week Whole-Body Vibration for Balance Improvement in Type 2 Diabetes Mellitus. *Arch. Phys. Med. Rehabil.* **2013**, *94*, 2112–2118. [CrossRef] [PubMed]
5. Irvine, C.; Taylor, N.F. Progressive resistance exercise improves glycaemic control in people with type 2 diabetes mellitus: A systematic review. *Aust. J. Physiother.* **2009**, *55*, 237–246. [CrossRef]
6. Sivanandam, S.; Anburajan, M.; Venkatraman, B.; Menaka, M.; Sharath, D. Medical thermography: A diagnostic approach for type 2 diabetes based on non-contact infrared thermal imaging. *Endocrine* **2012**, *42*, 343–351. [CrossRef]
7. Sociedade Brasileira de Diabetes. Diretrizes da Sociedade Brasileira de Diabetes (2017-2018). São Paulo: Editora Clannad. 2017. Available online: http://www.diabetes.org.br/profissionais/images/2017/diretrizes/diretrizes-sbd-2017-2018.pdf (accessed on 10 November 2019).
8. Sañudo, B.; Alfonso-Rosa, R.; De Pozo-Cruz, B.; De Pozo-Cruz, J.; Galiano, D.; E Figueroa, A. O treinamento de vibração do corpo inteiro melhora o fluxo sanguíneo das pernas e a adiposidade em pacientes com diabetes mellitus tipo 2. *Eur. J. Appl. Physiol.* **2013**, *113*, 2245–2252. [CrossRef]
9. Silber, H.A.; Lima, J.A.; Bluemke, D.A.; Astor, B.C.; Gupta, S.N.; Foo, T.K.; Ouyang, P. Arterial reactivity in lower extremities is progressively reduced as cardiovascular risk factors increase: Comparison with upper extremities using magnetic resonance imaging. *J. Am. Coll. Cardiol.* **2007**, *49*, 939–945. [CrossRef]
10. Fujiwara, Y.; Inukai, T.; Aso, Y.; Takemura, Y. Thermographic measurement of skin temperature recovery time of extremities in patients with type 2 diabetes mellitus. *Exp. Clin. Endocrinol. Diabetes* **2000**, *108*, 463–469. [CrossRef]
11. Uccioli, L.; Mormile, F.; Monticone, G.; Mennuni, G.; Durola, L.; Menzinger, G.; Russo, F. Autonomic neuropathy influences great toe blood pressure. *Diabetes Care* **1994**, *17*, 284–287. [CrossRef]
12. Sato, Y.; Nagasaki, M.; Kubota, M.; Uno, T.; Nakai, N. Clinical aspects of physical exercise for diabetes/metabolic syndrome. *Diabetes Res. Clin. Pract.* **2007**, *77* (Suppl. S1), S87–S91. [CrossRef]
13. Chudyk, A.; Petrella, R.J. Effects of exercise on cardiovascular risk factors in type 2 diabetes: A meta-analysis. *Diabetes Care* **2011**, *34*, 1228–1237. [CrossRef]
14. Okada, S.; Hiuge, A.; Makino, H.; Nagumo, A.; Takaki, H.; Konishi, H.; Goto, Y.; Yoshimasa, Y.; Miyamoto, Y. Effect of exercise intervention on endothelial function and incidence of cardiovascular disease in patients with type 2 diabetes. *J. Atheroscler. Thromb.* **2010**, *17*, 828–833. [CrossRef] [PubMed]
15. Bloor, C.M. Angiogenesis during exercise and training. *Angiogenesis* **2005**, *8*, 263–271. [CrossRef] [PubMed]
16. Behboudi, L.; Azarbayjani, M.A.; Aghaalinejad, H.; Salavati, M. Effects of aerobic exercise and whole body vibration onglycaemia control in type 2 diabetic males. *Asian J. Sports Med.* **2011**, *2*, 83–90. [CrossRef]
17. Regensteiner, J.G. Type 2 diabetes mellitus and cardiovascular exercise performance. *Rev. Endocr. Metab. Disord.* **2004**, *5*, 269–276. [CrossRef] [PubMed]
18. Egger, A.; Niederseer, D.; Diem, G.; Finkenzeller, T.; Ledl-Kurkowski, E.; Forstner, R.; Pirich, C.; Patsch, W.; Weitgasser, R.; Niebauer, J. Different types of resistance training in patients with type 2 diabetes mellitus: Effects on glycemic control, muscle mass and strength. *Eur. J. Prev. Cardiol.* **2013**. [CrossRef] [PubMed]
19. Machado, A.; Garcia Lupez, D.; Gonzalez Gallego, J.; Garstschea, N. Whole body vibration training increases muscle strength and mass in older women: A randomize controlled trial. *Scand. J. Med. Sci. Sports* **2010**, *20*, 200–207. [CrossRef] [PubMed]
20. Lourenço, R.A.; Veras, R.P. Mini-Exame do Estado Mental: Característicaspsicométricas em idosos ambulatoriais. *Revista de Saúde Pública* **2006**, *40*, 712–719. [CrossRef]

21. Quesada, J.I.P.; Kunzler, M.R.; Carpes, F.P. Methodological aspects of infrared thermography in human assessment. In *Application of Infrared Thermography in Sports Science. Biological and Medical Physics, Biomedical Engineering*; Priego Quesada, J.I., Ed.; Springer International Publishing: Cham, Switzerland, 2017; pp. 49–67. [CrossRef]
22. Polidori, G.; Renard, Y.; Lorimier, S.; Pron, H.; Derruau, S.; Taiar, R. Medical Infrared Thermography assistance in the surgical treatment of axillary Hidradenitis Suppurativa: A case report. *Int. J. Surg. Case Rep.* **2017**, *34*, 56–59. [CrossRef]
23. Ammer, K. The Glamorgan Protocol for recording and evaluation of thermal images of the human body. *Thermol. Int.* **2008**, *18*, 125–144.
24. Kistler, A.; Mariauzouls, C.; Von-Berlepsch, K. Fingertp temperature as an indicator for sympathetic responses. *Int. J. Psychophysiol.* **1998**, *29*, 35–41. [CrossRef]
25. Manimmanakorn, N.; Manimmanakorn, A.; Phuttharak, W.; Hamlin, M.J. Effects of whole body vibration on glycemic indices and peripheral blood flow in type II diabetic patients. *Malays. J. Med. Sci.* **2017**, *24*, 55–63. [CrossRef] [PubMed]
26. Bagavathiappan, S.; Philip, J.; Jayakumar, T.; Raj, B.; Rao, P.N.; Varalakshmi, M.; Mohan, V. Correlation between plantar foot temperature and diabetic neuropathy: A case study by using an infrared thermal imaging technique. *J. Diabetes Sci. Technol.* **2010**, *4*, 1386–1392. [CrossRef] [PubMed]
27. Moreira-Marconi, E.; Moura-Fernandes, M.C.; Lopes-Souza, P.; Teixeira-Silva, Y.; Reis-Silva, A.; Marchon, R.M. Evaluation of the temperature of posterior lower limbs skin during the whole body vibration measured by infrared thermography: Cross-sectional study analysis using linear mixed effect model. *PLoS ONE* **2019**, *14*, e0212512. [CrossRef] [PubMed]

13

Do Grade II Ankle Sprains Have Chronic Effects on the Functional Ability of Ballet Dancers Performing Single-Leg Flat-Foot Stance?

Bruno Dino Bodini [1], Giacomo Lucenteforte [2], Pietro Serafin [1], Lorenzo Barone [2], Jacopo A. Vitale [1,*], Antonio Serafin [1], Valerio Sansone [1,3] and Francesco Negrini [1]

1 IRCCS Istituto Ortopedico Galeazzi, Via Riccardo Galeazzi 4, 20161 Milan, Italy; bodinibruno@hotmail.com (B.D.B.); pietro.knw@gmail.com (P.S.); antonio.serafin@grupposandonato.it (A.S.); valerio.sansone@unimi.it (V.S.); francesco.negrini@gmail.com (F.N.)

2 Physical Medicine and Rehabilitation Residency Program, University of Catania, Piazza Università 2, 95124 Catania, Italy; giacomo.lucenteforte@outlook.com (G.L.); lorenzob100887@gmail.com (L.B.)

3 Department of Biomedical Sciences for Health, Università degli Studi di Milano, Via Mangiagalli 31, 20133 Milan, Italy

* Correspondence: jacopo.vitale@grupposandonato.it;

Abstract: Ballet dancers have a higher risk than the general population of ankle sprains. Ankle proprioception is of the utmost importance for executing static and dynamic positions typical of ballet dancing. Ankle sprains can create changes in functional ability that may affect ballet performance. The aim of this cross-sectional observational study is to evaluate if non-professional ballet dancers that were previously injured with a grade II ankle sprain carry a long-term stability deficit in ballet specific positions (passé, arabesque) and in single-leg flat-foot stance, thereby affecting ballet performance. We enrolled 22 amateur female ballet dancers, 11 who previously had a grade II ankle injury and 11 who had no history of ankle injury. Stabilometric data (Center of Pressure Speed and Elipse Area) were assessed with the postural electronic multisensory baropodometer in normal, arabesque, and passè positions with both open and closed eyes. Using an unpaired *t*-test, we compared healthy and pathological feet of the ankle injury group for a standard monopodalic position and two ballet-specific positions. No difference between pathological and healthy feet of non-professional ballet dancers who suffered grade II ankle injury was detected. According to the parameters considered in this study, grade II ankle sprains seem to have a favorable prognosis in the sample that we evaluated.

Keywords: stabilometry; ballet dancers; ankle injury; chronic ankle instability; balance

---

1. Introduction

During performance, ballet dancers have a great need for stability and balance control [1,2], along with a high level of general "flexibility", which are peculiar characteristics that improve with ballet training [1,3–5]. Ankle control is of the utmost importance for executing static and dynamic positions typical of ballet dancing [6,7]. In 2017, Vassallo et al. reported the epidemiology of dance-related injuries between 2000 and 2013, defining ankle sprains as the most common injury [8]. Later, Smith et al. and Smith et al. collected data about their incidence and prevalence [9,10]. Ankle sprains could cause chronic functional ability changes, as is common in groups of dancers and non-dancers alike [11,12], also increasing the risk of re-injury [13]. In addition, it was seen that people with functional ankle instability had a less refined kinesthesia, in particular for inversion movements [14]. However, a prospective study conducted in 1996 by Leanderson et al., based on stabilometry, demonstrated only short-term consequences after ankle sprain in ballet dancers [15]. Data about chronic ankle instability (CAI) in the general sporting population are, to date, not satisfactory to determine the presence of common aspects of CAI within individual sports [16]. However, an exploratory study conducted by Simon et al. revealed a condition of CAI in 75.9% of university dance majors [17]. Despite new wearable technologies, such as Inertial Measurament Unit IMU [18,19] and wireless electromyography (EMG) [20], having been proposed to investigate balance and postural control, stabilometry remains the most commonly used tool [21]. To date, there is a lack of studies about the chronic effects of an ankle injury in ballet dancers using stabilometry evaluation, but there is an increasing body of literature concerning this method [22,23], including not previously injured ballet dancers [24]. A study performed by Lin et al., using stabilometry to assess dancers with ankle injuries, found that non-acute ankle injuries could worsen postural stability of professional ballet-dancers during ballet-specific postures. However, they did not focus on a specific injury nor on a precise time-frame for the post-injury evaluation [25]. Another relevant aspect in the evaluation of balance control is represented by the visual system's role in proprioception, which has the potential to mask proprioceptive issues in athletes [26]. For this reason, it can be argued that in order to obtain reliable proprioceptive measures, visual occlusion is mandatory [27,28]. As ankle control is crucial for successfully executing ballet specific positions and it could be impaired in ankle sprains, a position specific testing with closed eyes is needed. Moreover, some studies showed that athletic and sport training is task specific and skills acquired in a specific task did not completely translate to the same skills in different tasks [29–31]. Recently, Thalassinos et al. discovered that there were many sport skill-specific bias about sensory inputs for spatial orientation and postural control between experienced soccer athletes, ballet dancers, and nonathletes [32]. Considering the high incidence and prevalence of ankle injuries in professional and non-professional ballet dancers (from 3% to 25.6% of all musculoskeletal ballet injuries [4,8,10,33]), and the primary role of ankle control to perform ballet-specific tasks, the aim of our study was to understand if non-professional ballet dancers, previously injured with a grade II ankle sprain, compared to dancers who did not suffer any ankle injury, carry a long-term stability deficit in ballet specific positions (passé, arabesque), thereby affecting ballet performance.

2. Materials and Methods

This was a cross-sectional observational multi-center study. We enrolled 22 subjects (N = 11 in the pathological group and N = 11 in the control group) from six different schools of classical ballet dance in Italy. The inclusion criteria were: age between 15 and 25 years old; classical ballet dancer; at least 10 years of training (average of 2–3 sessions of training a week); right footed in ballet practice; unilateral ankle injuries; clinical diagnosis of grade II inversion right ankle sprain that occurred at least 6 months before our evaluations made by an orthopedic surgeon [34]; and informed consent signed (parents' consent was collected if subjects were under 18 years old). The exclusion criteria were: professional dancer; another lower extremity injury; history of neurological or motor deficits; and any visual impairment. The control group had the same inclusion and exclusion criteria, except for the history of ankle injury. For grading the severity of the ankle injury, we used the classification proposed by Malliaropoulos et al. [34], and classified grade II ankle injury patients positive to anterior drawer test but negative to talar tilt test. We defined grade II ankle injury as a partial tear of the lateral ligament complex of the ankle without decreased motion and loss of function. All pathological subjects were treated conservatively with soft bandages applied for 2 weeks. No patient underwent a specific rehabilitation protocol. At the moment of inclusion in the study, all patients were symptom free and fully participating in dance at their pre-injury level. Before entering the study, the participants were fully informed about the study's aims and procedures, and written informed consent was obtained before testing. The study protcol was approved by the Ethics Committee of the University of Milan (approved on 12/10/15, Prot. N. 54/15) in accordance with current national and international laws and regulations governing the use of human subjects (Declaration of Helsinki II).

3. Sample Size Calculation

In order to determine the sample size of the study, we carried out an a-priori power analysis on the basis of the scientific literature. Since our main outcome was to determine if there was a difference in monopodalic stance ellipse area between healthy and previously pathological ballet dancers, we used data from the 2017 paper by de Mello et al. [24]. With a reported monopodalic ellipse area in ballet dancers of 155 ± 64 mm^2 and an expected difference of 70 mm^2 (effect size = 1.1), we calculated that we would need a sample of 22 subjects (11 for each group) to detect a significant change with a power of 0.80 and an alpha of 0.05. To calculate the sample size, we used the GPower software (Universitat Dusseldorf-Germany).

4. Tools and Procedures

The internationally approved stabilometric parameters [35] we evaluated in this paper are: (1) Ellipse area (mm^2), contains 90% of the positions sampled of the center of pressure (CoP) and represents the dispersion of the oscillations and the precision of the system; and (2) CoP speed (mm/s), the average speed related to the CoP oscillations. The acquisition of stabilometric data was performed with the postural electronic multisensory baropodometer Diasu®, equipped with Milletrix® interface, which has previously been shown to be a valid and reliable tool [36] This tool features a scanning frequency of 100 frames per second in real time, acquisition surface of 40 cm^2 per module, accuracy of +/−5%, and maximum point pressure of 150 N/cm^2. The evaluations were carried out in six different gyms with a dedicated medical room, characterized by the absence of external perturbations, especially acoustic. Prior to the test, each dancer stretched and warmed up the muscles of the lower limbs via routine self-selected exercises for 5 min. Each dancer wore comfortable and adherent clothes, and a pair of cotton socks.

During the test, an expert podiatrist and a nurse were present in the room. The baropodometer was placed at a distance of two meters from a homogeneous color wall that the subjects faced during the whole time of examination. Each evaluation session was held in the early afternoon and each subject had to be at rest from training in the previous day. The subjects were evaluated with both eyes open and closed. To ensure a reference point to be observed during acquisitions, a mark was positioned on the wall at the same height and equidistant to the patient's eyes, and at a distance of 2 m. We acquired each measurement three times with eyes open and three times with eyes closed. The first try was considered as a demonstration and we did not record it. For each foot we tested, the patients in the following conditions both with eyes opened and closed.

Monopodalic stance with the contralateral limb slightly detached from the ground (5 s length) (Figure 1).

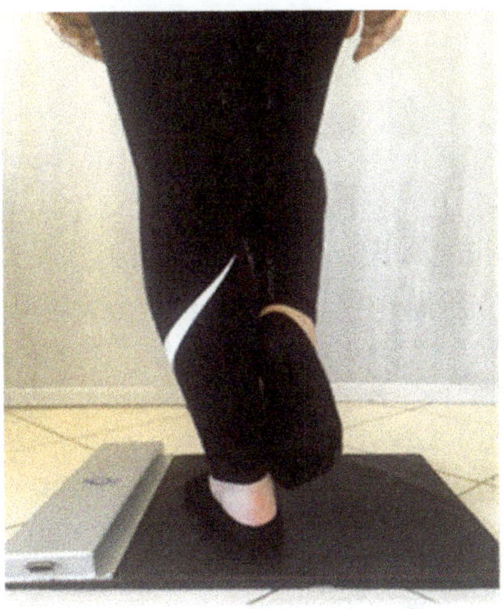

Figure 1. Monopodalic position.

Monopodalic with the limb in contact with the ground in "en dehors" position, and the contralateral in "arabesque" position, defining a 45° angle between them (5 s length) (Figure 2).

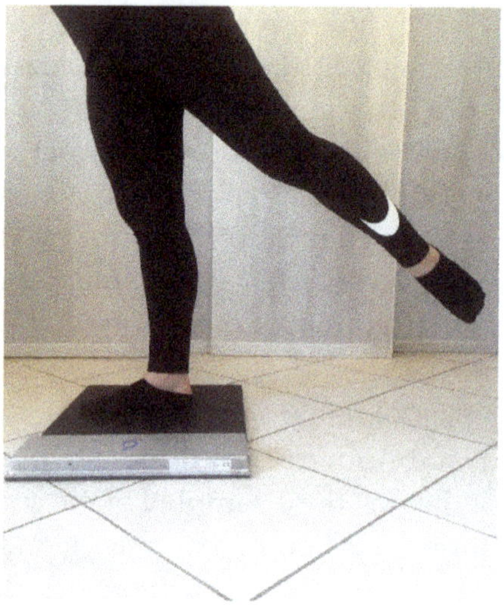

Figure 2. Arabesque.

Monopodalic with the limb in contact with the ground in "en dehors" position and the contralateral in "passé" position with a back "retiré" (5 s length) (Figure 3).

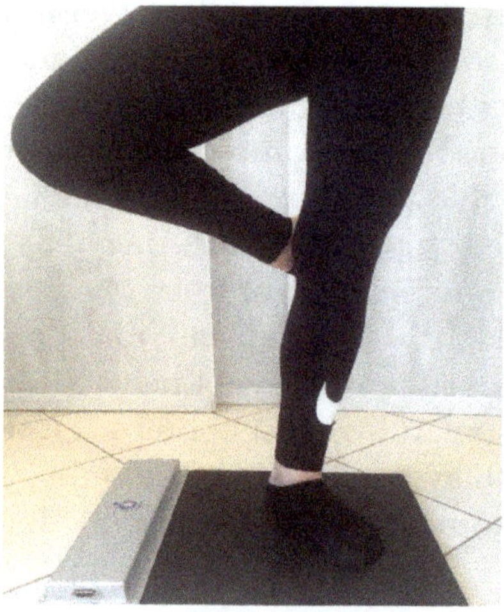

Figure 3. Passè.

5. Statistical Analysis

For each subject, parameters were determined by calculating the mean of the trials; subsequently, the grand average and the standard deviation over the subjects in each position were computed. Preliminary tests for normality (Kolmogorov-Smirnov test) and for equality of sample variances (Levene's test) provided the basis for using parametric statistics. All parameters were normally distributed. First, we checked if there were any significant statistical differences between the two groups as far as age, body mass index (BMI), years of dance practice, or age when they started practicing using an unpaired Student's *t*-test. Second, we compared stabilometric parameters, of each position, between the left and right foot in healthy subjects, and between injured and non-injured feet in the post-injury patients by the unpaired Student's *t*-test. Third, the difference between open and closed eyes in each condition, for each foot, was calculated; then, we checked if the differences in stabilometric parameters between closed and open eyes were larger in pathological vs. healthy feet using the unpaired Student's t-test. The level of significance was set to $p < 0.05$. Statistical analysis was performed using IBM SPSS 20.

6. Results

Demographical data of the study population are shown in Table 1. We could not find any statistical difference between the two groups for the parameters of age, BMI, years of dance practice, or age when they started practicing.

Table 1. Demographical data of participants.

	Post-Injury (N = 11)	Healthy (N = 11)	p-Values
Age (years)	16.36 ± 2.81	17.5 ± 3.37	>0.05
BMI (Kg/m^2)	19.85 ± 2.43	19.37 ± 2.33	>0.05
Years of Practice	11.91 ± 2.11	12.37 ± 4.07	>0.05
Age When They Started Practicing (years)	4.36 ± 1.23	5.18 ± 1.47	>0.05

Data are reported as Mean ± SD. Abbreviation: BMI, body mass index.

First, we analyzed the healthy subjects. We compared stabilometric parameters of the right and left feet for each parameter and no statistical differences for all parameters were detected (Table 2).

Table 2. Comparison between right and left foot in healthy subjects (N = 11) for stabilometric parameters acquired with open eyes.

	Right Foot	Left Foot	p-Values
Monopodalic Ellipse Area (mm^2)	105.91 ± 67.87	82.06 ± 47.43	>0.05
Monopodalic CoP Speed (mm/s)	13.84 ± 3.24	13.20 ± 5.34	>0.05
Arabesque Ellipse Area (mm^2)	274.40 ± 255.50	152.23 ± 87.54	>0.05
Arabesque CoP Speed (mm/s)	21.84 ± 8.46	19.65 ± 5.60	>0.05
Passè Ellipse Area (mm^2)	222.49 ± 130.06	133.26 ± 72.00	>0.05
Passè CoP Speed (mm/s)	22.22 ± 4.98	18.17 ± 5.58	>0.05

The pathological group was then analyzed. We compared stabilometric parameters between the injured feet and the healthy feet and no statistically significant differences were observed (Table 3).

Table 3. Comparisons between injured and healthy feet in pathological subjects (N = 11) for stabilometric parameters acquired with open eyes.

	Trauma	No Trauma	p-Values
Monopodalic Ellipse Area (mm^2)	128.25 ± 93.83	83.23 ± 49.15	>0.05
Monopodalic CoP Speed (mm/s)	14.23 ± 5.05	13.28 ± 5.55	>0.05
Arabesque Ellipse Area (mm^2)	165.17 ± 127.18	117.16 ± 59.89	>0.05
Arabesque CoP Speed (mm/s)	19.32 ± 4.38	18.54 ± 5.63	>0.05
Passè Ellipse Area (mm^2)	148.15 ± 82.43	119.66 ± 66.75	>0.05
Passè CoP Speed (mm/s)	20.75 ± 6.92	18.58 ± 5.97	>0.05

Data are reported as Mean ± SD. Abbreviation: CoP, Centre of Pressure.

We calculated the differences between open and closed eyes for all the parameters, and with reference to the pathological group, data collected with the feet that suffered a grade II ankle injury were compared with healthy contralateral limbs. As reported in Table 4, no significant differences between the sides were observed.

Lastly, we also compared right foot parameters of healthy and pathological subjects, both with open eyes (Table 5) and the difference between open and closed eyes (Table 6), and no significant differences were detected.

Table 4. Comparison between injured and healthy feet in pathological subjects (N = 11). Mean delta values (difference between open and closed eyes) of stabilometric parameters.

	Trauma	No Trauma	*p*-Values
Monopodalic Ellipse Area (mm^2)	321.47 ± 151.77	358.42 ± 310.67	>0.05
Monopodalic CoP Speed (mm/s)	15.77 ± 3.77	16.88 ±7.81	>0.05
Arabesque Ellipse Area (mm^2)	449.63 ± 203.33	440.82 ±378.02	>0.05
Arabesque CoP Speed (mm/s)	15.28 ± 9.60	15.29 ±9.60	>0.05
Passè Ellipse Area (mm^2)	330.93 ± 294.15	302.69 ± 216.10	>0.05
Passè CoP Speed (mm/s)	16.90 ± 9.22	12.66 ± 7.53	>0.05

Data are reported as Mean ± SD. Abbreviation: CoP, Centre of Pressure.

Table 5. Comparison between right feet of pathological and healthy subjects for stabilometric parameters acquired with open eyes.

	Right Foot Post-Injury (N = 11)	Right Foot Healthy (N = 11)	*p*-Values
Monopodalic Ellipse Area (mm^2)	105.91 ± 67.87	128.25 ± 93.83	>0.05
Monopodalic CoP Speed (mm/s)	13.84 ± 3.24	14.23 ± 5.05	>0.05
Arabesque Ellipse Area (mm^2)	274.40 ± 255.50	165.17 ± 127.18	>0.05
Arabesque CoP Speed (mm/s)	21.84 ± 8.46	19.32 ± 4.38	>0.05
Passè Ellipse Area (mm^2)	222.49 ± 130.06	148.15 ± 82.43	>0.05
Passè CoP Speed (mm/s)	22.22 ± 4.98	20.75 ± 6.92	>0.05

Data are reported as Mean ± SD. Abbreviation: CoP, Centre of Pressure.

Table 6. Comparison between right foot of pathological and healthy subjects. Mean delta values (difference between open and closed eyes) of stabilometric parameters.

	Right Foot POST-Injury (N = 11)	Right Foot Healthy (N = 11)	*p*-Values
Monopodalic Ellipse Area (mm^2)	321.47 ± 151.77	397.47 ± 252.87	>0.05
Monopodalic CoP Speed (mm/s)	15.77 ± 3.77	15.85 ± 5.29	>0.05
Arabesque Ellipse Area (mm^2)	449.63 ± 203.33	307.73 ± 252.13	>0.05
Arabesque CoP Speed (mm/s)	15.28 ± 9.60	14.64 ± 5.04	>0.05
Passè Ellipse Area (mm^2)	330.93 ± 294.15	294.46 ± 85.47	>0.05
Passè CoP Speed (mm/s)	16.90 ± 9.22	15.32 ± 7.14	>0.05

Data are reported as Mean ± SD. Abbreviation: CoP, Centre of Pressure.

7. Discussion

Our study showed that there is no ballet specific long-term balance deficit for grade II ankle injuries in ballet dancers. In order to have this specific conclusion, we checked if our sample of non-professional, but experienced, ballet dancers had any difference in balance while performing ballet specific positions on the dominant or non-dominant foot. We did not find any difference between the two sides. This finding is in contrast with a classic study performed by Leanderson et al. in 1996, where they tested professional athletes and non-athletes in the monopodalic position [15]. However, the study cited is 22 years older, so training techniques and materials such as shoes have changed, and are performed in a different, monocentric, and professional setting. This could very well explain the differences found. Moreover, the verified parameters of validity and reliability of the tools we used [36] and the power set at 80% for the sample size calculation, could be some of the reasons of the differences found between the outcomes of our study and the study published by Leanderson et al. Since the right and left foot were found to have no difference in the healthy group, we compared injured and non-injured side of our pathological group. We found out that, after six months, there was no significant difference in balance between the injured and non-injured sides. The internal (same subject) comparison is of the utmost importance, as any kind of difference in training could be an important bias [37]. In fact, using the contralateral healthy feet as a control, we were able to eliminate biases caused by potential differences in skills, body types, and other physical characteristics between athletes. Recently, a few studies pointed out that a crossover effect of injuries can exist, especially tendinitis, from one side to the other [38,39]. While it is not clear the mechanism of action of this crossover effect (e.g., central nervous system or anticipatory postural adjustments [40]), it still could be a possible confounder of our results as the pathological and healthy side could be similar because of it. Our study arrived to a different conclusion than a similar 2011 study [25]; however, we focused on a more selective group of subjects who had only grade II ankle injury. We supposed that patients with more severe ankle sprains could have long-term impairment in postural control.

One strength of our study was the use of stabilometry in a new way, comparing ballet-specific static positions for determining ankle injury effects. We found just two studies that examined ballet-specific positions; one examined the single-leg retiré position [37] and the other the passé en demi-pointe position [24]. However, neither of the studies focused on post-injury athletes. Another strength of the study was the comparison between healthy and injured feet in the same athletes that eliminate the role of possible differences in skills between different subjects, allowing us to better study the role of the previous ankle injury. Furthermore, we recruited the subjects in six different ballet schools. Different centers have different training strategies, so the results obtained are probably not linked to a peculiar type of training but to the natural history of grade II ankle injuries.

A limitation of our study is the small number of subjects involved; however, we enrolled 22 patients (11 for each group) as resulted with the sample size calculation. Our inclusion criteria were very strict to guarantee the internal validity of our study, and despite screening six different centers, we were able to find 11 patients meeting the required inclusion criteria for the pathological subjects group. Furthermore, because of our study design, we cannot exclude an important role of specific rehabilitation protocol in speeding up the recovery process, as we tested our patients long after their injury.

In the future, it could be important to study in a similar fashion different grades of ankle injuries, classified using imaging support, as well as different types of ankle injuries, such as inversion and eversion. Moreover, it could be interesting to evaluate the parameters used in our study in relevé, another ballet-specific position. One more possible future study could investigate the role of treatment (e.g., immobilization (functional or rigid) vs. no immobilization) and rehabilitation in the time to return to optimal performance as well as potential long-term effects in ankle injuries of higher clinical grading.

Our finding could encourage many dancers all over the world that suffered and will suffer ankle injuries [8]. Dancers with a grade II ankle injury should be reassured by clinicians that their functional ability as ballet dancers performing single-leg flat-foot stance will likely not be hindered in the long term.

8. Conclusions

Our findings show that grade II ankle injury does not compromise the ability of a ballet dancer, even if treated with just soft bandage applied for two weeks, even without a specific rehabilitation protocol.

Author Contributions: B.D.B., G.L., P.S., and F.N. designed the present study, checked the literature, and wrote the manuscript; J.A.V. performed the statistical analysis; L.B., J.A.V., A.S., and V.S. critically revised the manuscript; all authors gave the approval for the final version of the review submitted for publication. All authors have read and agreed to the published version of the manuscript.

References

1. Steinberg, N.; Tenenbaum, S.; Stern, M.; Zeev, A.; Siev-Ner, I. The association between menarche, intensity of training and passive joint ROM in young pre-professional female dancers: A longitudinal follow-up study. *Phys. Ther. Sport* **2018**, *32*, 59–66. [CrossRef]
2. Krityakiarana, W.; Jongkamonwiwat, N. Comparison of Balance Performance between Thai Classical Dancers and Non-Dancers. *J. Dance Med. Sci.* **2016**, *20*, 72–78. [CrossRef]
3. Tekin, D.; Agopyan, A.; Baltaci, G. Balance Training in Modern Dancers: Proprioceptive-Neuromuscular Training vs. Kinesio Taping. *Med. Probl. Perform. Art.* **2018**, *33*, 156–165. [CrossRef] [PubMed]
4. Bruyneel, A.V.; Mesure, S.; Paré, J.C.; Bertrand, M. Organization of postural equilibrium in several planes in ballet dancers. *Neurosci. Lett.* **2010**, *485*, 228–232. [CrossRef]
5. Yin, A.X.; Geminiani, E.; Quinn, B.; Owen, M.; Kinney, S.; McCrystal, T.; Stracciolini, A. The Evaluation of Strength, Flexibility, and Functional Performance in the Adolescent Ballet Dancer during Intensive Dance Training. *PM & R* **2019**, *11*, 722–730.
6. Krasnow, D.; Wilmerding, M.V.; Stecyk, S.; Wyon, M.; Koutedakis, Y. Biomechanical research in dance: A literature review. *Med. Probl. Perform. Art.* **2011**, *26*, 3–23. [PubMed]
7. da Silveira Costa, M.S.; de Sá Ferreira, A.; Felicio, L.R. Static and dynamic balance in ballet dancers: A literature review. *Fisioter. Pesqui.* **2013**, *20*, 299–305.
8. Vassallo, A.J.; Hiller, C.; Stamatakis, E.; Pappas, E. Epidemiology of Dance-Related Injuries Presenting to Emergency Departments in the United States, 2000-2013. *Med. Probl. Perform. Art.* **2017**, *32*, 170–175. [CrossRef]
9. Smith, T.O.; Davies, L.; de Medici, A.; Hakim, A.; Haddad, F.; Macgregor, A. Prevalence and profile of musculoskeletal injuries in ballet dancers: A systematic review and meta-analysis. *Phys. Ther. Sport* **2016**, *19*, 50–56. [CrossRef]
10. Smith, P.J.; Gerrie, B.J.; Varner, K.E.; McCulloch, P.C.; Lintner, D.M.; Harris, J.D. Incidence and Prevalence of Musculoskeletal Injury in Ballet: A Systematic Review. *Orthop. J. Sports Med.* **2015**, *3*. [CrossRef]
11. Lin, C.-W.; Su, F.-C.; Lin, C.-F. Influence of ankle injury on muscle activation and postural control during ballet grand plié. *J. Appl. Biomech.* **2014**, *30*, 37–49. [CrossRef] [PubMed]
12. Glencross, D.; Thornton, E. Position sense following joint injury. *J. Sports Med. Phys. Fitness* **1981**, *21*, 23–27. [PubMed]
13. Malliaropoulos, N.; Ntessalen, M.; Papacostas, E.; Longo, U.G.; Maffulli, N. Reinjury after acute lateral ankle sprains in elite track and field athletes. *Am. J. Sports Med.* **2009**, *37*, 1755–1761. [CrossRef] [PubMed]
14. Sousa, A.S.P.; Leite, J.; Costa, B.; Santos, R. Bilateral Proprioceptive Evaluation in Individuals with Unilateral Chronic Ankle Instability. *J. Athl. Train.* **2017**, *52*, 360–367. [CrossRef] [PubMed]
15. Leanderson, J.; Eriksson, E.; Nilsson, C.; Wykman, A. Proprioception in classical ballet dancers. A prospective study of the influence of an ankle sprain on proprioception in the ankle joint. *Am. J. Sports Med.* **1996**, *24*, 370–374. [CrossRef] [PubMed]
16. Attenborough, A.S.; Hiller, C.E.; Smith, R.M.; Stuelcken, M.; Greene, A.; Sinclair, P.J. Chronic ankle instability in sporting populations. *Sports Med. Auckl. NZ* **2014**, *44*, 1545–1556. [CrossRef]
17. Simon, J.; Hall, E.; Docherty, C. Prevalence of chronic ankle instability and associated symptoms in university dance majors: an exploratory study. *J. Dance Med. Sci.* **2014**, *18*, 178–184. [CrossRef]
18. Fusca, M.; Negrini, F.; Perego, P.; Magoni, L.; Molteni, F.; Andreoni, G. Validation of a Wearable IMU System for Gait Analysis: Protocol and Application to a New System. *Appl. Sci.* **2018**, *8*, 1167. [CrossRef]
19. Ghislieri, M.; Gastaldi, L.; Pastorelli, S.; Tadano, S.; Agostini, V. Wearable Inertial Sensors to Assess Standing Balance: A Systematic Review. *Sensors* **2019**, *19*. [CrossRef]
20. Lee, Y.-J.; Liang, J.N.; Wen, Y.-T. Characteristics of Postural Muscle Activity in Response to a Motor-Motor Task in Elderly. *Appl. Sci.* **2019**, *9*, 4319. [CrossRef]
21. McKeon, P.O.; Hertel, J. Systematic review of postural control and lateral ankle instability, part I: Can deficits be detected with instrumented testing. *J. Athl. Train.* **2008**, *43*, 293–304. [CrossRef] [PubMed]
22. Nardone, A.; Godi, M.; Grasso, M.; Guglielmetti, S.; Schieppati, M. Stabilometry is a predictor of gait performance in chronic hemiparetic stroke patients. *Gait Posture* **2009**, *30*, 5–10. [CrossRef] [PubMed]
23. Bruyneel, A.-V.; Humbert, A.; Bertrand, M. Comparison of balance strategies in mountain climbers during real altitude exposure between 1.500m and 3.200m: Effects of age and expertise. *Neurosci. Lett.* **2017**, *657*, 16–21. [CrossRef] [PubMed]

24. de Mello, M.C.; de Sá Ferreira, A.; Ramiro Felicio, L. Postural Control During Different Unipodal Positions in Professional Ballet Dancers. *J. Dance Med. Sci.* **2017**, *21*, 151–155. [CrossRef] [PubMed]
25. Lin, C.-W.; Lin, C.-F.; Hsue, B.-J.; Su, F.-C. A comparison of ballet dancers with different level of experience in performing single-leg stance on retiré position. *Motor Control* **2014**, *18*, 199–212. [CrossRef] [PubMed]
26. Witchalls, J.; Waddington, G.; Adams, R.; Blanch, P. Evaluation of the relative contribution of peripheral and focal vision to proprioceptive differentiation of underfoot inversion angles in young elite athletes. *Percept. Mot. Skills* **2013**, *117*, 923–934. [CrossRef]
27. Han, J.; Anson, J.; Waddington, G.; Adams, R.; Liu, Y. The Role of Ankle Proprioception for Balance Control in relation to Sports Performance and Injury. *BioMed Res. Int.* **2015**, *2015*, 842804. [CrossRef]
28. Marulli, T.A.; Harmon-Matthews, L.E.; Davis-Coen, J.H.; Willigenburg, N.W.; Hewett, T.E. Eyes-Closed Single-Limb Balance is Not Related to Hypermobility Status in Dancers. *J. Dance Med. Sci.* **2017**, *21*, 70–75. [CrossRef]
29. Casabona, A.; Leonardi, G.; Aimola, E.; La Grua, G.; Polizzi, C.M.; Cioni, M.; Valle, M.S. Specificity of foot configuration during bipedal stance in ballet dancers. *Gait Posture* **2016**, *46*, 91–97. [CrossRef]
30. Asseman, F.; Caron, O.; Crémieux, J. Is there a transfer of postural ability from specific to unspecific postures in elite gymnasts? *Neurosci. Lett.* **2004**, *358*, 83–86. [CrossRef]
31. Giboin, L.-S.; Gruber, M.; Kramer, A. Three months of slackline training elicit only task-specific improvements in balance performance. *PLoS ONE* **2018**, *13*, e0207542. [CrossRef] [PubMed]
32. Thalassinos, M.; Fotiadis, G.; Arabatzi, F.; Isableu, B.; Hatzitaki, V. Sport Skill-Specific Expertise Biases Sensory Integration for Spatial Referencing and Postural Control. *J. Mot. Behav.* **2018**, *50*, 426–435. [CrossRef] [PubMed]
33. Biernacki, J.L.; Stracciolini, A.; Fraser, J.; Micheli, L.J.; Sugimoto, D. Risk Factors for Lower-Extremity Injuries in Female Ballet Dancers: A Systematic Review. *Clin. J. Sport Med.* **2018**. [CrossRef] [PubMed]
34. Malliaropoulos, N.; Papacostas, E.; Papalada, A.; Maffulli, N. Acute lateral ankle sprains in track and field athletes: an expanded classification. *Foot Ankle Clin.* **2006**, *11*, 497–507. [CrossRef]
35. Scoppa, F.; Capra, R.; Gallamini, M.; Shiffer, R. Clinical stabilometry standardization: Basic definitions–acquisition interval–sampling frequency. *Gait Posture* **2013**, *37*, 290–292. [CrossRef]
36. Cuccia, A.M. Validity and reliability of spatio-temporal gait parameters in adolescents. *Iran. J. Pediatr.* **2013**, *23*, 610–611.
37. Lin, C.-W.; Chen, S.-J.; Su, F.-C.; Wu, H.-W.; Lin, C.-F. Differences of ballet turns (pirouette) performance between experienced and novice ballet dancers. *Res. Q. Exerc. Sport* **2014**, *85*, 330–340. [CrossRef]
38. Sansone, V.; Maiorano, E.; Applefield, R.C.; Gandola, M.; Negrini, F. Strength Reduction in Unilateral Shoulder Pain: Is the Healthy Side Really Healthy in Rotator Cuff Disease? *Am. J. Phys. Med. Rehabil.* **2019**, *98*, 382–386. [CrossRef]
39. Heales, L.J.; Lim, E.C.W.; Hodges, P.W.; Vicenzino, B. Sensory and motor deficits exist on the non-injured side of patients with unilateral tendon pain and disability–implications for central nervous system involvement: a systematic review with meta-analysis. *Br. J. Sports Med.* **2014**, *48*, 1400–1406. [CrossRef]
40. Cavallari, P.; Bolzoni, F.; Bruttini, C.; Esposti, R. The Organization and Control of Intra-Limb Anticipatory Postural Adjustments and Their Role in Movement Performance. *Front. Hum. Neurosci.* **2016**, *10*, 525. [CrossRef]

14

Effects of Whole-Body Vibration Exercises on Parameters Related to the Sleep Quality in Metabolic Syndrome Individuals

Claudia Figueiredo Azeredo [1,2], Patrícia de Castro de Paiva [1,2], Leandro Azeredo [3], Aline Reis da Silva [1,2], Arlete Francisca-Santos [2,4], Laisa Liane Paineiras-Domingos [2,4,5], Adriana Lírio Pereira da Silva [2], Camila Leite Bernardes-Oliveira [1,5], Juliana Pessanha-Freitas [2], Márcia Cristina Moura-Fernandes [2,6], Rubens Guimarães Mendonça [2], José Alexandre Bachur [7], Ygor Teixeira-Silva [2,5], Eloá Moreira-Marconi [2,6], Eliane de Oliveira Guedes-Aguiar [2,4,5], Bruno Bessa Monteiro de Oliveira [2,4], Mário Fritsch Neves [5], Luiz Felipe Ferreira-Souza [2], Vinicius Layter Xavier [8], Daniel Lago Borges [9], Ana Cristina Lacerda [10], Vanessa Amaral Mendonça [10], Anelise Sonza [11], Redha Taiar [12,*], Alessandro Sartorio [13], Mario Bernardo-Filho [2] and Danúbia da Cunha de Sá-Caputo [2,4,5]

1 Programa de Pós-graduação em Saúde, Medicina Laboratorial e Tecnologia Forense, Universidade do Estado do Rio de Janeiro, Rio de Janeiro, RJ 20950-003, Brazil; figueiredo.claudiaf@gmail.com (C.F.A.); patriciadecastrodepaiva@gmail.com (P.d.C.d.P.); fisioalinereis@gmail.com (A.R.d.S.); camilabernardes@hotmail.com (C.L.B.-O.)

2 Laboratório de Vibrações Mecânicas e Práticas Integrativas, Departamento de Biofísica e Biometria, Instituto de Biologia Roberto Alcântara Gomes e Policlínica Piquet Carneiro, Universidade do Estado do Rio de Janeiro, Rio de Janeiro, RJ 20950-003, Brazil; fisioarlete@gmail.com (A.F.-S.); laisanit@gmail.com (L.L.P.-D.); adrianaliriolavimpi@gmail.com (A.L.P.d.S.); ju.freitas.fisio@gmail.com (J.P.-F.); marciafernandesfisio@gmail.com (M.C.M.-F.); rubens_fisio@hotmail.com (R.G.M.); silvarogy@hotmail.com (Y.T.-S.); eloamarconi@gmail.com (E.M.-M.); ellianeguedes@gmail.com (E.d.O.G.-A.); bessa.oliveira@gmail.com (B.B.M.d.O.); lumadaragu@gmail.com (L.F.F.-S.); bernardofilhom@gmail.com (M.B.-F.); dradanubia@gmail.com (D.d.C.d.S.-C.)

3 Departamento de Fisioterapia, Hospital Central da Polícia Militar, Rio de Janeiro, RJ 20211-270, Brazil; azeredo.lm@gmail.com

4 Faculdade Bezerra de Araújo, Rio de Janeiro, RJ 23052-180, Brazil

5 Programa de Pós-Graduação em Ciências Médicas, Faculdade de Ciências Médicas, Universidade do Estado do Rio de Janeiro, Rio de Janeiro, RJ 20551-030, Brazil; mariofneves@gmail.com

6 Programa de Pós-Graduação em Fisiopatologia Clínica e Experimental, Instituto de Biologia Roberto Alcântara Gomes, Universidade do Estado do Rio de Janeiro, Rio de Janeiro, RJ 20550-900, Brazil

7 Cursos de Medicina e Fisioterapia da Universidade de Franca, Franca, SP 14401-426, Brazil; jabachur@hotmail.com

8 Departamento de Estatística, Instituto de Matemática e Estatística, Universidade do Estado do Rio de Janeiro, Rio de Janeiro, RJ 20550-900, Brazil; viniciuslx@ime.uerj.br

9 Hospital Universitário, Universidade Federal do Maranhão, São Luís do Maranhão, MA 65080-805, Brazil; dlagofisio83@hotmail.com

10 Faculdade de Ciências Biológicas e da Saúde, Universidade Federal dos Vales do Jequitinhonha e Mucuri, Diamantina, MG 39100-000, Brazil; lacerdaacr@gmail.com (A.C.L.); vaafisio@hotmail.com (V.A.M.)

11 Programa de Pós-graduação em Fisioterapia, Universidade do Estado de Santa Catarina, Florianópolis, SC 88080-350, Brazil; anelise.sonza@gmail.com

12 GRESPI, Université de Reims, 51100 Reims, France

13 Istituto Auxologico Italiano, IRCCS, Experimental Laboratory for Auxo-Endocrinological Research, Division of Metabolic Diseases & Auxology, 28824 Milan and Verbania, Italy; sartorio@auxologico.it

* Correspondence: redha.taiar@univ-reims.fr

Abstract: Metabolic syndrome (MetS) is an undesirable clinical condition with physiological, biochemical, clinical, and metabolic factors that contribute to increased cardiovascular risks (CR). A poor sleep quality might be found in obese and MetS individuals. Whole-body vibration (WBV) exercise has been used on the management of MetS individuals. This clinical trial investigated the effect of WBV exercise on parameters related to the sleep quality in MetS individuals. After randomization, nine individuals (seven women and two men) were exposed to a fixed frequency (FF) and ten individuals (eight women and two men) were exposed to a variable frequency (VF). Both groups performed the protocol twice a week, for 6 weeks. All of the evaluations were performed before the first and after the last sessions. Anthropometric and cardiovascular parameters were measured before and after the 6-week intervention. Pittsburgh Sleep Quality Index (PSQI), Epworth Sleepiness Scale (ESS), and Berlin Questionnaire were also used to evaluate the quality of the sleep. A significant ($p \leq 0.05$) reduction of the waist circumference in the VFG and an increase of the heart rate were found in the FFG and VFG group. The score of the PSQI of the both groups decreased significantly ($p = 0.01$). The score of the ESS decreased ($p = 0.04$) only in the VF group. The scores of the Berlin Questionnaire were not altered in both groups. In conclusion, WBV intervention was capable in interfering with physiological mechanisms with effects on the WC and HR, leading to the improvement of the quality of sleep in MetS individuals. WBV exercise might be an important clinical intervention to the management of some factors associated with poor quality of sleep (FFG and VFG) and in the daytime sleepiness in MetS individuals with variable frequencies (5–16 Hz) (VFG).

Keywords: metabolic syndrome; sleep quality; whole-body vibration exercise; Pittsburgh Sleep Quality Index; Epworth Sleepiness Scale; Berlin Questionnaire

---

1. Introduction

Metabolic syndrome (MetS) is an undesirable clinical condition with physiological, biochemical, clinical, and metabolic factors, including alterations on the level of the lipids on the plasma, arterial hypertension, central adiposity, insulin resistance (IR), and hyperglycemia. These conditions strongly contribute to increased cardiovascular risks (CR) [1], and they are interconnected by pathophysiological basis in low-grade chronic inflammation, increase of the risk of type 2 diabetes mellitus (T2DM), and all-cause mortality [2]. MetS is also related to the increased deposit of central adiposity and ectopic fat infiltration (muscle and liver) associated with overeating and/or sedentary lifestyles. These conditions are related to various deleterious consequences in late life [3,4].

Lian et al. [5], in a systematic review and meta-analysis, reported that the overall sleep quality as well as sleep complaints have significant positive associations with MetS. Massar et al. [6] and Tsai et al. [7] pointed out that this condition of the sleep is linked with cardiovascular disease. Massar et al. [6] reported in individuals with poor habitual sleep efficiency during the week before stress induction (Trier Social Stress Test) responded with higher stress-related elevations of blood pressure and cortisol levels as compared to subjects with high sleep efficiency. This relationship between poor sleep efficiency and elevated blood pressure persisted during the post-stress recovery period. In addition, poor sleep health is also associated with MetS and mental illness [8,9]. Iftikhar et al. [10], in a meta-analysis reported that some investigations demonstrated the association between sleep quality and MetS. It was verified that the poor sleep quality characterized by sleep fragmentation was related to impaired glucose metabolism, independent of sleep duration [11], however, the studies of the meta-analysis analyzed had not reached a consensus. Mesas et al. [12] reported that the difficulty falling asleep is associated with MetS and, in particular, with high blood pressure, and this association would be independent of sleep duration and would be not due to lifestyles related to poor sleep.

Ying et al. [5] reported in a systematic review and meta-analysis that the overall sleep quality, as well as sleep complaints have significant positive associations with MetS. Moreover, it is estimated [13,14] that 50% to 60% of obese and MetS individuals can present obstructive sleep apnea (OSA).

Some tools have been used to verify parameters (such as sleep duration, sleep inertia, sleep latency, snoring, disorientation or confusion during sleep, and daytime sleepiness) related to the quality of the sleep, such as the Pittsburgh Sleep Quality Index (PSQI) [15], Epworth Sleepiness Scale (ESS) [16] and the Berlin Questionnaire [17]. Moreover, the neck circumference (NC) [16] and waist circumference (WC) [18,19] have also been used.

There is moderate evidence supporting the use of physical exercise (PE) programs to counter MetS, although the optimal dose and type of PE is not well established. It is the main challenge for health care professionals to persuade individuals to have adherence to perform PE to the prevention and management of MetS [20]. In this case, it is relevant to consider the whole-body vibration (WBV) exercise, a modality of PE, an option. WBV exercise has been used as a clinical intervention in individuals with different clinical disorders, including MetS [21–26] and it can be considered a feasible, safe, and low-cost technique [27].

WBV exercise is generated in an individual who is on the base of a vibrating platform. It produces a mechanical vibration (MV) that is transmitted to the body inducing muscle contractions, with physiological responses like those produced by other types of PE, such as aerobic conditioning and strength training [28–30]. Biomechanical parameters, such as the frequency (f) and the peak-to-peak displacement (PPD) of the MV must be considered in the WBV exercise protocols [26,31,32].

As it is suggested that the sleep quality plays an important role in development of MetS [5] and putting together all of the previous considerations, to our knowledge, this is a first work aiming to study the effect of WBV exercise on the sleep quality of MetS individuals using the PSQI, ESS, and Berlin Questionnaire. It is hypothesized that the WBV exercise would be able in improving the sleep quality of MetS individuals.

2. Materials and Methods

2.1. Individuals

In this cross-sectional and randomized study, 31 subjects were recruited and 19 performed the protocol (58.79 ± 12.55 years old, 1.62 ± 0.09 m height, 86.27 ± 15.03 kg body mass). The recruitment of the participants occurred from January 2018 to January 2019, in the *Hospital Universitário Pedro Ernesto* (HUPE), in the *Universidade do Estado do Rio de Janeiro* (UERJ). The WBV protocol was performed in the *Laboratório de Vibrações Mecânicas e Práticas Integrativas* (LAVIMPI).

This project was approved by the Research Ethics Committee of HUPE-UERJ with the number CAAE 54981315.6.0000.5259, the registry in the Brazilian Registry of Clinical Trials (ReBEC) with the number RBR 2bghmh and UTN: U1111-1181-1177. The participants of both groups signed a consent form.

Consolidated Standards of Reporting Trials (CONSORT) was used to report all of the different steps of the interventions utilized in this work [33].

In the randomization, a blinded envelope was used for the cards with the name of the groups: fixed frequency group (FFG) (control group) or variable frequency group (VFG) (WBVE group).

The inclusion criteria were individuals of both sexes, over 18 years of age, with MetS according to the International Diabetes Federation.

The exclusion criteria were: (i) individuals with high blood pressure (BP) levels (systolic blood pressure (SBP) ≥ 180 mmHg and diastolic blood pressure (DBP) ≥ 110 mmHg); (ii) cardiovascular disease (CVD) clinically evident in the last 6 months, manifested by a myocardial infarction or a stroke; (iii) a neurological, muscular, or rheumatologic disease that difficulte the position of the individual on the vibrating platform; (iv) disabling clinical disease according to the evaluation; (v) speech therapy or respiratory physiotherapy in the last 3 months; (vi) body mass index (BMI) > 40 kg/m^2; (vii) orthodontic therapy with intraoral device; (viii) individuals who refuse to sign the consent form.

The participants declared that they were sedentary. They were instructed to continue their daily activities, dietary habits, and medications during the period of the investigation. The drugs used by the participants of both groups were diuretics, beta blockers, calcium channel blockers, angiotensin converting enzyme inhibitors, and angiotensin receptor antagonists.

2.2. Interventions

2.2.1. Fixed Frequency Group (Control Group)

After the randomization, nine individuals (seven women and two men) allocated in the FFG performed a protocol twice a week, for 6 weeks. In this protocol, the individuals were positioned in a squat position, barefoot and with 130° knee flexion (Figure 1A). The biomechanical parameters were 2.5, 5 and 7.5 mm (Figure 1B–D) of PPD and 5 Hz for 10 s of vibration and 110 s of non-vibration in each bout. From 1 to 4 weeks, were performed 3 bouts in each session, totaling 18 min of total time. From 5 to 8 weeks, were performed 4 bouts in each session, totaling 24 min of total time. From 9 to 12 weeks, were performed 5 bouts in each session, totaling 30 min of total time. The participants performed dynamic and static squats in the sessions.

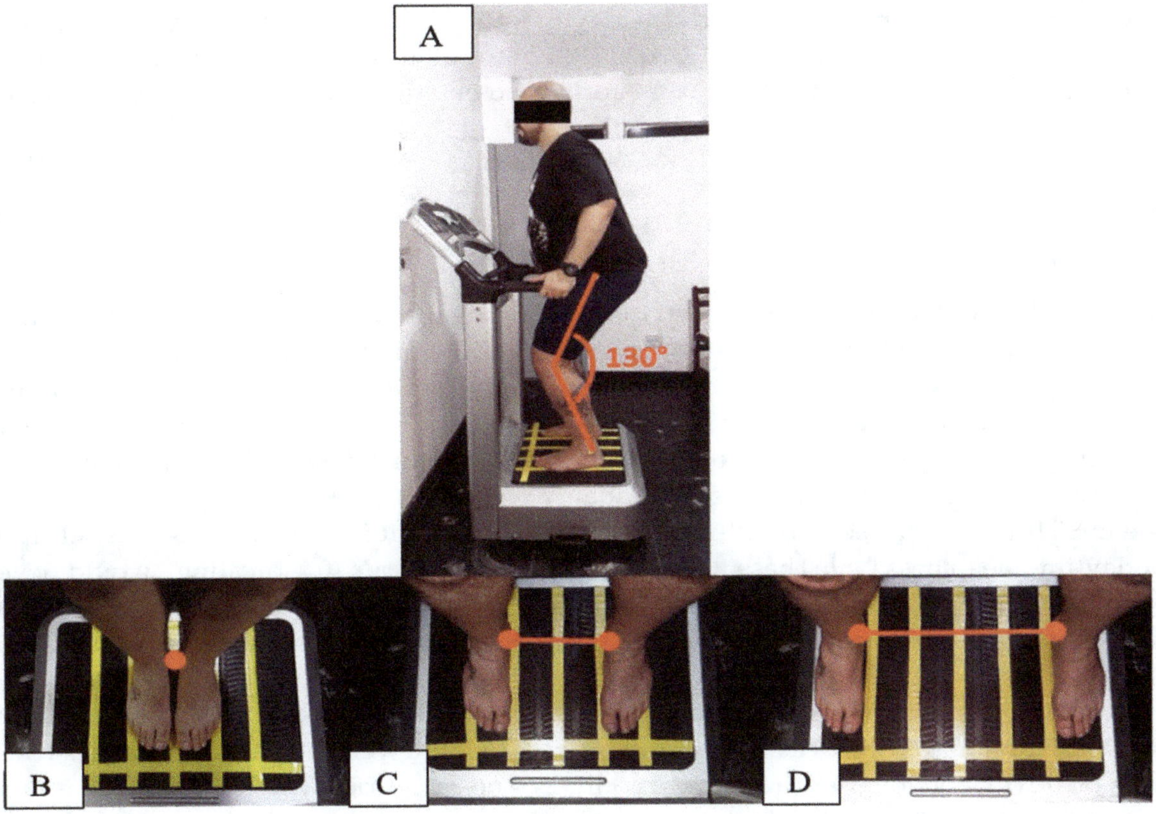

Figure 1. Biomechanical parameters during the intervention (fixed frequency (FF) and variable frequency (VF) groups) using the side alternating vibratory platform; (**A**) individual in a stand position, barefoot and with 130° knee flexion; (**B**) individual in 2.5 mm of peak-to-peak displacement (PPD) on the base of the vibrating platform with medial malleoli together; (**C**) individual in 5 mm of PPD on the base of the vibrating platform 21 cm apart between the medial malleoli; (**D**) individual in 7.5 mm of PPD on the base of the vibrating platform 38 cm apart between the medial malleoli.

2.2.2. Variable Frequency Group (WBVE Group)

After the randomization, ten individuals (eight women and two men) allocated in the VFG performed the protocol twice a week, for 6 weeks. In this protocol, the individuals were positioned in a squat position, barefoot and with 130° knee flexion (Figure 1) The biomechanical parameters of the MV were 2.5, 5 and 7.5 mm (Figure 1B–D) of the PPD; the frequency was 5 Hz in the first session and it increased by one Hz in each session, and it was 16 Hz in the last session. During the intervention, were performed 60 s of MV and 60 s of non-vibration in each bout. From 1 to 4 weeks were performed 3 bouts in each session, for a total time of 18 min. From 5 to 8 weeks, were performed 4 bouts in each session, for a total time of 24 min. From 9 to 12 weeks were performed 5 bouts in each session, for a total time of 30 min. Dynamic and static squats were performed in interspersed sessions.

2.3. Anthropometric Measurements and Physiological Parameters

All of the measurements were performed in the same location, at room temperature. Height and body mass were measured on a digital balance (MIC 200 PPA, Micheletti, São Paulo, Brazil). The BMI was calculated by dividing body mass (in kg) by square of height (in m) [34]. WC was obtained with a flexible measuring tape connecting the midpoints between the last costal arch and iliac crest, at the end of the soft exhalation and in the orthostatic position [34]. NC was obtained using a flexible metric tape just below the prominence of the larynx [35].

An automated device (OMRON, model HEM-7113, Dalian, China) was utilized to record the SBP and DBP (mm Hg), and the HR (beats/min) was measured on the left arm of seated patient after a 10-min rest. Three measurements were performed with 1 min of rest after each measurement. The mean of these 3 records of SBP and DBP and HR was used in the analyses of the WBV exercise group and the control group [36]. These evaluations were performed before and after the 6-week intervention in both groups.

The data of these parameters were expressed in mean and standard derivation and the Wilcoxon rank test was performed.

2.4. Questionnaires

The PSQI [15] was used to assess sleep quality and disturbances over a 1-month period. This questionnaire is composed of 19 self-rated questions and 5 questions that should be answered by bedmates or roommates. The 19 questions are separated into 7 categories and there is a score from 0 to 3. The components of this questionnaire are subjective sleep quality, sleep latency, sleep duration, habitual sleep efficiency, sleep disturbances, use of medication, and daytime dysfunction. The maximum PSQI score is 21 points. Higher scores indicate poor quality of sleep [37].

The ESS [16] is composed of 8 self-reported questions and it is used to assess the self-reported level of daytime sleepiness [38]. These items have a four-point scale (0 indicating "would never nod off" and 3 indicating a "strong chance of nodding off"). The questionnaire questions are related to daily activities. The questionnaire score ranges between 0 and 24. Higher total scores are related to more sleepiness [39].

The Berlin Questionnaire [17] has been proposed as a tool in screening OSA and validated in primary care. The subjects were classified into high risk (if there were 2 or more categories where the score was positive), and low risk (if there was only 1 or no categories where the score was positive). The percentage os individuals with high risk to OSA was calculated in both groups [40,41].

The PSQI, ESS, and Berlin Questionnaire were only measured before and after the 6-week intervention in both groups.

2.5. Statistical Analyses

For the sample size calculation, we used a standard deviation of 3.1, a margin of error of 2, the significance level of 5%, and a sample size of 9 individuals in each group, considering the PSQI [42].

The Wilcoxon signed-rank test with continuity correction was used in the analyses of the DBP, SBP, HR, WC, NC, the PSQI, and ESS. Descriptive statistics, median, and interquartile range (IQR) are also reported. Wilcoxon signed-rank test is a nonparametric test that was used to determine if paired samples, before and after intervention, have the same distribution. Fisher's exact test was applied to the qualitative variable, Berlin, to asses if the proportion of people in each class (high risk and low risk) have been affected by the experiment. In the analyses of the PSQI and ESS, the values are expressed in scores. The statistical analyses of the Berlin Questionnaire considered only the percentage of individuals with a high risk to OSA.

All statistical analysis was performed using R software, version 3.5.0 [43] and the R Librarie Table 1 [44]. Results are considered statistically significant if the p-value is under 0.05 ($p \leq 0.05$).

3. Results

The flow diagram with the enrolment of the study is shown in Figure 2. Thirty-one individuals were recruited, two individuals were excluded because they did not have risk of sleep apnea, three declined to participate, and seven individuals declined due to other reasons (economical problem related to the transportation).

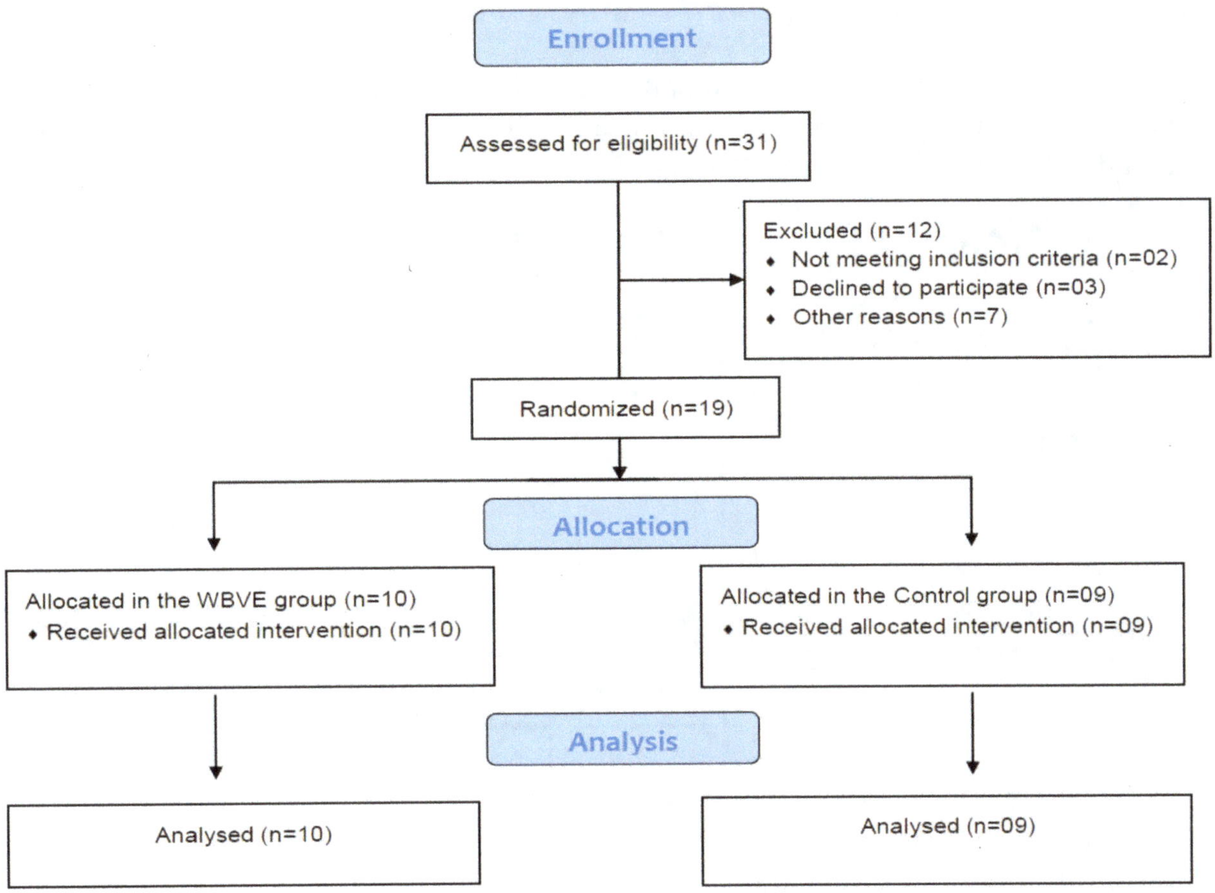

Figure 2. Flow diagram of the intervention.

Table 1 shows some anthropometric parameters of the individuals that were exposed to WBV exercise (FV group) and to only 5 Hz (FF group). An analysis is shown of both groups before and just after the treatments. It was verified that the BMI, NC, SBP, and DBP ($p > 0.05$) were not significantly altered in both groups. However, a significant increase in the HR ($p < 0.05$) was found in both groups exposed to mechanical vibration, only 5 Hz (FFG) and variable frequency 5–16Hz (VFG). Furthermore, a reduction was found in the group that was submitted to the variable frequency 5–16 Hz (VFG) in the WC.

Table 1. Anthropometrical parameters of the individuals exposed to variable frequency group (intervention 5–16 Hz) and to only 5 Hz (fixed frequency group).

	FFG before (Median [IQR])	FFG after (Median [IQR])	*p*	VFG before (Median [IQR])	VFG after (Median [IQR])	*p*
BMI (kg/m^2)	29.50 [29.0, 34.20]	29.60 [28.90, 34.10]	0.54	35.40 [32.40, 36.60]	34.70 [32.88, 36.08]	0.23
WC (cm)	105.00 [101.20, 106.30]	101.00 [100.00, 105.00]	0.23	108.90 [103.75, 116.10]	107.00 [102.17, 112.85]	0.02
NC (cm)	38.00 [36.40, 38.50]	36.60 [35.60, 39.50]	0.29	38.00 [37.58, 38.88]	38.30 [37.17, 39.00]	0.25
SBP (mm Hg)	129.00 [128.00, 130.00]	127.00 [121.00, 128.00]	0.12	130.00 [122.50, 132.50]	130.00 [120.00, 132.00]	0.76
DBP (mm Hg)	78.00 [75.00, 83.00]	75.00 [68.00, 87.00]	1.00	74.00 [72.25, 75.75]	70.00 [60.75, 74.75]	0.18
HR (bpm)	57.00 [56.00, 62.00]	62.00 [60.00, 66.00]	0.05	63.50 [59.75, 66.00]	72.00 [61.25, 83.00]	0.05

BMI—body mass index, WC—waist circumference, NC—neck circumference, SBP—systolic blood pressure, DBP—diastolic blood pressure, HR—heart rate, FF—fixed frequency group, VF—variable frequency group.

Figure 3 shows the values of the scores of the PSQI of the individuals of the group exposed only to mechanical vibration of 5 Hz (FFG-control). A significant decrease was found (p = 0.01) of the score (after and before) of the individuals of the FF group (exposure to 5 Hz).

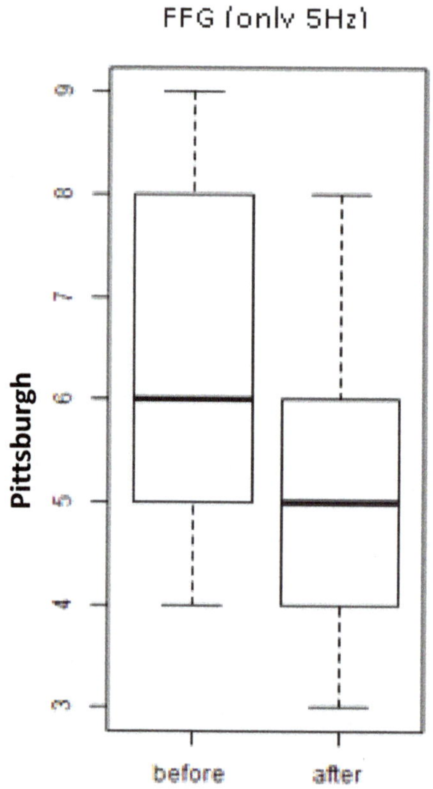

Figure 3. Scores of the Pittsburgh Sleep Quality Index (PSQI) of the individuals of the group exposed only to a mechanical vibration of 5 Hz (FFG) (before and after).

Figure 4 shows the values of the scores of the PSQI of the individuals of the groups exposed to the treatment with WBV exercises (VFG). It is observed that an important and significant ($p = 0.008$) decrease of score in the group after the exposure to various frequencies (intervention) was seen. This finding indicates an improvement of quality of the sleep.

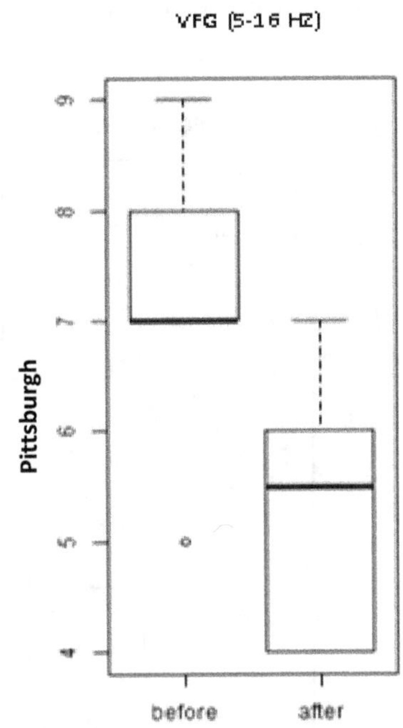

Figure 4. Scores of the PSQI of the individuals exposed to the whole-body vibration (WBV) intervention with variable frequency (VFG).

Figure 5 shows the values of the scores of the ESS of the individuals of the group exposed only to mechanical vibration of 5 Hz (FFG). It is observed that there was no significant decrease ($p = 1.0$) of the score (after and before) of the individuals. This finding indicates no reduction of daytime sleepiness.

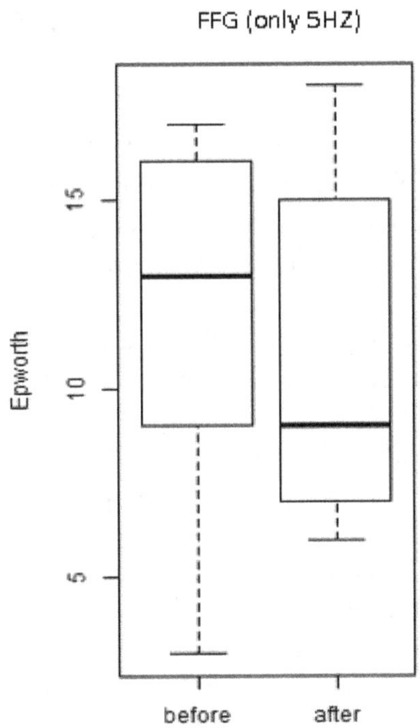

Figure 5. Scores of the Epworth Sleepiness Scale (ESS) of the individuals of the SG individuals of the FFG (before and after).

Figure 6 shows the values (before and after the interventions) of the scores of the ESS scale of the individuals of the groups exposed to the treatment with WBV exercises (VFG). It is observed that there was a significant ($p = 0.04$) decrease of the score in the group after the exposure to various frequencies (intervention). This finding indicates a reduction of daytime sleepiness.

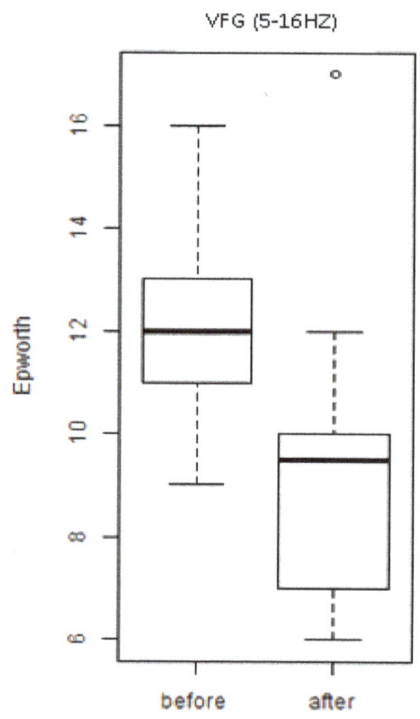

Figure 6. Scores of the ESS of the individuals of the group exposed to the intervention with WBV exercises (VFG).

Considering the Berlin Questionnaire, no alteration in ter percentage of individuals with risk to OSA were significantly found in both groups, the FF $p = 0.29$ and FVG $p = 1.00$.

4. Discussion

The underlying etiology of MetS is multifactorial, however, they are not well known, but sedentary lifestyles and unhealthy dietary habits favor the appearance of MetS [45]. Considering the high prevalence and strong and undesirable complications, early identifying and controlling the modified risk factors are key prevention methods to counter the development of MetS and its progression to CVD.

It is relevant to point out that, to our knowledge, this is the first work that was performed to evaluate the effect of WBV exercise in sleep quality of MetS individuals. As it was hypothesized that the WBV exercise would be able to improve the sleep quality of MetS individuals, the quality of sleep was improved (PSQI) and a reduction of daytime sleepiness (ESS) in the MetS was found due to a protocol with variable frequencies (5–16 Hz) of WBV. A protocol with fixed frequency (5 Hz) also improved the quality of sleep (PSQI).

It was shown (Table 1) that the 6-week intervention with WBV exercise with variable frequencies (from 5 up to 16 Hz) (VF group) did not alter significantly the BMI, NC, SBP, and DBP. The same finding was verified in the individuals with fixed frequency (5 Hz). These findings agree with other studies. Feairheller et al. [46], in a study of six months, have shown that aerobic exercise training is enough to elicit improvements in vascular structure and function in African Americans, even without alterations on BP measurements (SBP and DBP) in African Americans. Moreover, Sá-Caputo et al. [31] have reported that, in individuals with MetS exposed to acute WBV exercise, the SBP and DBP were not altered. Figueroa et al. [21] have reported that the BMI of overweight/obese women was not modified after 6 weeks of WBV exercises.

Considering the HR (Table 1), an increase was verified in FFG (only 5 Hz) and VFG (variable 5–16 Hz), and this is in agreement with Sunita et al. [47] that have also observed an increase of the HR in response to exercise. Moreover, Kang et al. [48] have described an association between resting HR and cardiorespiratory fitness with an elevated resting HR.

The findings presented in Table 1 indicated no alterations on SBP and DBP due to WBVE (a possible stressor), however, Massar et al. [6] reported that individuals with poor habitual sleep efficiency during the week before stress induction (Trier Social Stress Test) responded with higher stress-related elevations of blood pressure and cortisol levels as compared to subjects with high sleep efficiency.

In the current study, no alterations on the NC were found. However, a decrease on the WC was found (Table 1). Sîrbu et al. [49] have compared some anthropometric parameters in trained and sedentary healthy young students. It was found that in moderately aerobic trained students, the BMI and BP were not significantly different between the two groups. However, a significantly lower NC was found in the trained students. Considering the WC, in agreement with our results, King et al. [50] have verified that a 12-week supervised aerobic exercise intervention has reduced significantly the WC of overweight/obese men and women. But, Sîrbu et al. [49], have not found alteration in the WC due to exercise.

WBV exercise is an intervention with several improvements in populations with various diseases [23–25,31]. In this current study, it was verified that WBV exercise has improved the quality of the sleep in MetS when we used the PSQI (Figures 3 and 4) and ESS (Figure 6). This finding is partially in agreement with Souza et al. [51] who have evaluated, in a population of 16 individuals with OSA, the effectiveness of inspiratory muscle training (IMT) on sleep and functional capacity to exercise. It was a significant improvement in sleep quality was seen with PSQI values, but no significant changes were seen in daytime sleepiness (ESS) after the intervention. Furthermore, Reid et al. [52] have verified that moderate aerobic PE improved the sleep quality of sedentary adults considering the PSQI and the ESS. Brandão et al. [53] have reported that home exercise improves the quality of sleep and daytime sleepiness of elderlies considering, respectively, the PSQI and the ESS.

The findings of the current work have verified that the sleep quality was not altered when the Berlin Questionnaire was used. This result agrees with Brandão et al. [53] who have reported that home exercise does not alter the risk to OSA when the same questionnaire was used.

Kline et al. [54], evaluated the utility of PE for improving daytime functioning in adults with OSA. Sleepiness and functional impairment due to sleepiness also were improved following exercise versus control, though these changes were not statistically significant. It is suggested that PE may be helpful for improving aspects of daytime functioning of adults with OSA. Moreover, Yilmaz Gokmen et al. [55] have investigated the effects of Tai Chi and Qigong training on severity of OSA for 12-weeks. In the intervention group, there was a statistically significant decrease in the ESS. However, Itoh et al. [56], in a cross-sectional study among non-obese male workers in Japan, found no significant association between physical activity and the risk of sleep-disordered breathing.

Considering the MetS, not all forms of exercise are equally effective and safe; although aerobic exercise [57] or resistance training have been associated with decreased cardiovascular disease risk factors, obesity, or MetS severity [58,59]. Due to the pain or even the low physical fitness, most individuals are unable or unwilling to perform these exercises [60]. Given the limitations for some types of exercises that many individuals report, different forms of exercise are being suggested for MetS individuals [61]. WBV exercise has improved several parameters in MetS individuals [26,31,32] and in the current study a decrease of the WC was found (Table 1).

This study has some limitations, no control of daily activity, daily working, lifestyle habits, smoking, PE, and daily energy intake. The follow-up data were not available after the intervention. The external validity of this intervention considering its generalizability to other settings (like the everyday-living condition) was not explored and only a small sample was used. The big ratio of female to male would be also considered as a limitation of the study. Moreover, a sham group and a group of individuals without MetS were not used. Furthermore, the analysis of the questionnaires was not done in the weeks in which there were changes of the frequency and duration of the intervention in the VFG. Some points of the questionnaires are influenced by factors that are not taken into account in the current study, as categories of individuals (good-sleepers and bad-sleepers), sleep duration, sleep inertia, and sleep latency. In consequence, further investigations are required. However, putting together all the considerations, the strength was to verify that a WBV exercise might be suggested as an option to the management of MetS individuals with some important outcomes, and it would be expected that a WBV exercise might lead to responses that can reflect in improvements of the sleep quality.

5. Conclusions

In conclusion, WBV intervention was capable of interfering with physiological mechanisms with effects on the WC and HR, leading to the improvement of the quality of sleep in MetS individuals. Although the calculated sample size determined a study with a small number of individuals, WBV exercise might be an important clinical intervention to the management of some factors associated with poor quality of sleep (FFG and VFG) and in the daytime sleepiness in MetS individuals with variable frequencies (5–16Hz) (VFG). However, further investigations are necessary to try to understand the mechanisms that underlines this positive effect of the WBV exercise in the studied population, as well as with individuals with sleep disturbances without MetS.

Author Contributions: Conceptualization, R.T., A.S. (Alessandro Sartorio), M.B.-F., and D.d.C.d.C.D.S.-C.; data curation, C.F.A., J.A.B., V.L.X., and D.L.B.; formal analysis, J.A.B., V.L.X., D.L.B., A.C.L., V.A.M., A.S. (Anelise Sonza), and R.T.; funding acquisition, M.B.-F.; Investigation, C.F.A., P.d.C.d.P., L.A., A.R.d.S., A.F.-S., L.L.P.-D., A.L.P.d.S., C.L.B.-O., J.P.-F., M.C.M.-F., R.G.M., Y.T.-S., E.M.-M., E.d.O.G.-A., B.B.M.d.O., M.F.N., and L.F.F.-S.; methodology, C.F.A., P.d.C.d.P., L.A., A.R.D.S., A.F.-S., L.L.P.-D., A.L.P.d.S., C.L.B.-O., J.P.-F., M.C.M.-F., R.G.M., J.A.B., Y.T.-S., E.M.-M., E.d.O.G.-A., B.B.M.d.O., M.F.N., L.F.F.-S., and A.S.(Alessandro Sartorio); project administration, M.B.-F. and D.d.C.d.C.D.S.-C.; resources, C.F.A., P.d.C.d.P., L.A., A.R.d.S., R.G.M., and B.B.M.d.O.; software, V.L.X.; supervision, M.B.-F. and D.d.C.d.C.D.S.-C.; validation, V.L.X., M.B.-F., and D.d.C.d.C.D.S.-C.; visualization, A.S.(Anelise Sonza) and R.T.; writing—original draft, C.F.A.; Writing—review and editing, A.C.L., V.A.M., A.S. (Anelise Sonza), A.S. (Alessandro Sartorio), M.B.-F., and D.d.C.d.C.D.S.-C.

References

1. Kaur, J. Retracted: A Comprehensive Review on Metabolic Syndrome. *Cardiol. Res. Pract.* **2019**, *2019*, 4301528.
2. Seaman, D.R.; Palombo, A.D. An Overview of the Identification and Management of the Metabolic Syndrome in Chiropractic Practice. *J. Chiropr. Med.* **2014**, *13*, 210–219. [CrossRef]
3. Dominguez, L.J.; Barbagallo, M. The Biology of the Metabolic Syndrome and Aging:2006. *Curr. Opin. Clin. Nutr. & Metab. Care* **2016**, *9*, 5–11.
4. Alberti, K.G.M.M.; Zimmet, P.; Shaw, J. Metabolic syndrome-a new world-wide definition. A Consensus Statement from the International Diabetes Federation. *Diabet. Med.* **2006**, *23*, 469–480. [CrossRef]
5. Lian, Y.; Yuan, Q.; Wang, G.; Tang, F. Association between sleep quality and metabolic syndrome: A systematic review and meta-analysis. *Psychiatry Res.* **2019**, *274*, 66–74. [CrossRef]
6. Massar, S.A.A.; Liu, J.C.J.; Mohammad, N.B.; Chee, M.W.L. Poor habitual sleep efficiency is associated with increased cardiovascular and cortisol stress reactivity in men. *Psychoneuroendocrinology* **2017**, *81*, 151–156. [CrossRef]
7. Tsai, H.-J.; Kuo, T.B.J.; Lin, Y.-C.; Yang, C.C.H. The association between prolonged sleep onset latency and heart rate dynamics among young sleep-onset insomniacs and good sleepers. *Psychiatry Res.* **2015**, *230*, 892–898. [CrossRef]
8. Salo, P.; Sivertsen, B.; Oksanen, T.; Sjösten, N.; Pentti, J.; Virtanen, M.; Kivimäki, M.; Vahtera, J. Insomnia symptoms as a predictor of incident treatment for depression: Prospective cohort study of 40,791 men and women. *Sleep Med.* **2012**, *13*, 278–284. [CrossRef]
9. Wang, S.; Wu, Y.; Ungvari, G.S.; Ng, C.H.; Forester, B.P.; Gatchel, J.R.; Chiu, H.F.K.; Kou, C.; Fu, Y.; Qi, Y.; et al. Sleep duration and its association with demographics, lifestyle factors, poor mental health and chronic diseases in older Chinese adults. *Psychiatry Res.* **2017**, *257*, 212–218. [CrossRef]

10. Iftikhar, I.H.; Donley, M.A.; Mindel, J.; Pleister, A.; Soriano, S.; Magalang, U.J. Sleep Duration and Metabolic Syndrome. An Updated Dose–Risk Metaanalysis. *Ann. Am. Thorac. Soc.* **2015**, *12*, 1364–1372. [CrossRef]
11. Stamatakis, K.A.; Punjabi, N.M. Effects of Sleep Fragmentation on Glucose Metabolism in Normal Subjects. *Chest* **2010**, *137*, 95–101. [CrossRef]
12. Mesas, A.E.; Guallar-Castillón, P.; López-García, E.; León-Muñoz, L.M.; Graciani, A.; Banegas, J.R.; Rodríguez-Artalejo, F. Sleep quality and the metabolic syndrome: The role of sleep duration and lifestyle. *Diabetes. Metab. Res. Rev.* **2014**, *30*, 222–231. [CrossRef]
13. Resta, O.; Foschino-Barbaro, M.P.; Legari, G.; Talamo, S.; Bonfitto, P.; Palumbo, A.; Minenna, A.; Giorgino, R.; De Pergola, G. Sleep-related breathing disorders, loud snoring and excessive daytime sleepiness in obese subjects. *Int. J. Obes.* **2001**, *25*, 669–675. [CrossRef]
14. Drager, L.F.; Lopes, H.F.; Maki-Nunes, C.; Trombetta, I.C.; Toschi-Dias, E.; Alves, M.J.N.N.; Fraga, R.F.; Jun, J.C.; Negrão, C.E.; Krieger, E.M.; et al. The Impact of Obstructive Sleep Apnea on Metabolic and Inflammatory Markers in Consecutive Patients with Metabolic Syndrome. *PLoS ONE* **2010**, *5*, e12065. [CrossRef]
15. Kline, C.E.; Crowley, E.P.; Ewing, G.B.; Burch, J.B.; Blair, S.N.; Durstine, J.L.; Davis, J.M.; Youngstedt, S.D. The Effect of Exercise Training on Obstructive Sleep Apnea and Sleep Quality: A Randomized Controlled Trial. *Sleep* **2011**, *34*, 1631–1640. [CrossRef]
16. Soler, X.; Liao, S.-Y.; Marin, J.M.; Lorenzi-Filho, G.; Jen, R.; DeYoung, P.; Owens, R.L.; Ries, A.L.; Malhotra, A. Age, gender, neck circumference, and Epworth sleepiness scale do not predict obstructive sleep apnea (OSA) in moderate to severe chronic obstructive pulmonary disease (COPD): The challenge to predict OSA in advanced COPD. *PLoS ONE* **2017**, *12*, e0177289. [CrossRef]
17. Qu, X.-X.; Esangbedo, I.C.; Zhang, X.-J.; Liu, S.-J.; Li, L.-X.; Gao, S.; Li, M. Obstructive Sleep Apnea Syndrome is Associated with Metabolic Syndrome among Adolescents and Youth in Beijing. *Chin. Med. J.* **2015**, *128*, 2278–2283. [CrossRef]
18. Hoffstein, V.; Mateika, S. Differences in abdominal and neck circumferences in patients with and without obstructive sleep apnoea. *Eur. Respir. J.* **1992**, *5*, 377–381.
19. Horner, R.L.; Shea, S.A.; McIvor, J.; Guz, A. Pharyngeal size and shape during wakefulness and sleep in patients with obstructive sleep apnoea. *QJM* **1989**, *72*, 719–735.
20. Paley, C.A.; Johnson, M.I. Abdominal obesity and metabolic syndrome: Exercise as medicine? *BMC Sports Sci. Med. Rehabil.* **2018**, *10*, 7. [CrossRef]
21. Figueroa, A.; Kalfon, R.; Madzima, T.A.; Wong, A. Whole-body vibration exercise training reduces arterial stiffness in postmenopausal women with prehypertension and hypertension. *Menopause* **2014**, *21*, 131–136. [CrossRef]
22. Wong, A.; Alvarez-Alvarado, S.; Kinsey, A.W.; Figueroa, A. Whole-Body Vibration Exercise Therapy Improves Cardiac Autonomic Function and Blood Pressure in Obese Pre- and Stage 1 Hypertensive Postmenopausal Women. *J. Altern. Complement. Med.* **2016**, *22*, 970–976. [CrossRef]
23. Anwer, S.; Alghadir, A.; Zafar, H.; Al-Eisa, E. Effect of whole body vibration training on quadriceps muscle strength in individuals with knee osteoarthritis: A systematic review and meta-analysis. *Physiotherapy* **2016**, *102*, 145–151. [CrossRef]
24. Alev, A.; Mihriban, A.; Bilge, E.; Ayça, E.; Merve, K.; Şeyma, C.; Uğur, E.; Adnan, B.; Zeynel, K.; Mahmut, G.S. Effects of whole body vibration therapy in pain, function and depression of the patients with fibromyalgia. *Complement. Ther. Clin. Pract.* **2017**, *28*, 200–203. [CrossRef]
25. Zhou, J.; Pang, L.; Chen, N.; Wang, Z.; Wang, C.; Hai, Y.; Lyu, M.; Lai, H.; Lin, F. Whole-body vibration training-better care for COPD patients: A systematic review and meta-analysis. *Int. J. COPD* **2018**, *13*, 3243–3254. [CrossRef]
26. Sá-Caputo, D.; Paineiras-Domingos, L.L.; Francisca-Santos, A.; dos Anjos, E.M.; Reis, A.S.; Neves, M.F.T.; Oigman, W.; Oliveira, R.; Brandão, A.; Machado, C.B.; et al. Whole-body vibration improves the functional parameters of individuals with metabolic syndrome: An exploratory study. *BMC Endocr. Disord.* **2019**, *19*, 6. [CrossRef]
27. Braz, D.S.; de Andrade, A.D.; Teixeira, A.S.; Cavalcanti, C.A.; Morais, A.B.; Marinho, P.E.M. Whole-body vibration improves functional capacity and quality of life in patients with severe chronic obstructive pulmonary disease (COPD): A pilot study. *Int. J. COPD* **2015**, *10*, 125–132.

28. Rønnestad, B.R. Comparing the Performance-Enhancing Effects of Squats on a Vibration Platform With Conventional Squats in Recreationally Resistance-Trained Men. *J. Strength Cond. Res.* **2004**, *18*, 839–845.
29. Merkert, J.; Butz, S.; Nieczaj, R.; Steinhagen-Thiessen, E.; Eckardt, R. Combined whole body vibration and balance training using Vibrosphere®. *Z. für Gerontol. und Geriatr.* **2011**, *44*, 256–261. [CrossRef]
30. Cardim, A.B.; Marinho, P.E.; Nascimento, J.F.; Fuzari, H.K.; de Andrade, A.D. Does Whole-Body Vibration Improve the Functional Exercise Capacity of Subjects With COPD? A Meta-Analysis. *Respir. Care* **2016**, *61*, 1552–1559. [CrossRef]
31. Sá-Caputo, D.C.; Paineiras-Domingos, L.L.; Oliveira, R.; Neves, M.F.T.; Brandão, A.; Marin, P.J.; Sañudo, B.; Furness, T.; Taiar, R.; Bernardo-Filho, M. Acute Effects of Whole-Body Vibration on the Pain Level, Flexibility, and Cardiovascular Responses in Individuals With Metabolic Syndrome. *Dose-Response* **2018**, *16*, 155932581880213. [CrossRef]
32. Paineiras-Domingos, L.L.; da Cunha Sá-Caputo, D.; Reis, A.S.; Francisca Santos, A.; Sousa-Gonçalves, C.R.; dos Anjos, E.M.; dos Santos Pereira, M.J.; Sartorio, A.; Bernardo-Filho, M. Assessment Through the Short Physical Performance Battery of the Functionality in Individuals With Metabolic Syndrome Exposed to Whole-Body Vibration Exercises. *Dose-Response* **2018**, *16*, 155932581879453. [CrossRef]
33. Moher, D.; Hopewell, S.; Schulz, K.F.; Montori, V.; Gøtzsche, P.C.; Devereaux, P.J.; Elbourne, D.; Egger, M.; Altman, D.G. CONSORT 2010 explanation and elaboration: Updated guidelines for reporting parallel group randomised trials. *Int. J. Surg.* **2012**, *10*, 28–55. [CrossRef]
34. Casadei, K.; Kiel., J. *Anthropometric Measurement*; StatPearls Publishing LLC: Treasure Island, FL, USA, 2019. Available online: https://www.ncbi.nlm.nih.gov/books/NBK537315/ (accessed on 24 October 2019).
35. Gasa, M.; López-Padrós, C.; Monasterio, C.; Salord, N.; Mayos, M.; Vilarrasa, N.; Fernandez-Aranda, F.; Montserrat, J.M.; Dorca, J.; López-Padrós, C.; et al. Anthropometrical phenotypes are important when explaining obstructive sleep apnea in female bariatric cohorts. *J. Sleep Res.* **2019**, *28*, e12830. [CrossRef]
36. De Cardiologia, S.B. III Diretrizes Brasileiras Sobre Dislipidemias e Diretriz de Prevenção da Aterosclerose do Departamento de Aterosclerose da Sociedade Brasileira de Cardiologia. *Arq. Bras. Cardiol.* **2001**, *77*, 48.
37. Kim, T.Y.; You, S.E.; Ko, Y.S. Association between Sasang constitutional types with obesity factors and sleep quality. *Integr. Med. Res.* **2018**, *7*, 341–350. [CrossRef]
38. Schwab, R.J.; Pasirstein, M.; Pierson, R.; Mackley, A.; Hachadoorian, R.; Arens, R.; Maislin, G.; Pack, A.I. Identification of Upper Airway Anatomic Risk Factors for Obstructive Sleep Apnea with Volumetric Magnetic Resonance Imaging. *Am. J. Respir. Crit. Care Med.* **2003**, *168*, 522–530. [CrossRef]
39. Duarte, R.L.; Mello, F.C.; Magalhães-da-Silveira, F.J.; Oliveira-e-Sá, T.S.; Rabahi, M.F.; Gozal, D. Comparative performance of screening instruments for obstructive sleep apnea in morbidly obese patients referred to a sleep laboratory: A prospective cross-sectional study. *Sleep Breath.* **2019**, *23*, 1123–1132. [CrossRef]
40. Netzer, N.C.; Stoohs, R.A.; Netzer, C.M.; Clark, K.; Strohl, K.P. Using the Berlin Questionnaire to Identify Patients at Risk for the Sleep Apnea Syndrome. *Ann. Intern. Med.* **1999**, *131*, 485. [CrossRef]
41. Ng, S.S.; Tam, W.; Chan, T.O.; To, K.W.; Ngai, J.; Chan, K.K.P.; Yip, W.H.; Lo, R.L.; Yiu, K.; Ko, F.W.; et al. Use of Berlin questionnaire in comparison to polysomnography and home sleep study in patients with obstructive sleep apnea. *Respir. Res.* **2019**, *20*, 40. [CrossRef]
42. Cizza, G.; de Jonge, L.; Piaggi, P.; Mattingly, M.; Zhao, X.; Lucassen, E.; Rother, K.I.; Sumner, A.E.; Csako, G. Neck Circumference Is a Predictor of Metabolic Syndrome and Obstructive Sleep Apnea in Short-Sleeping Obese Men and Women. *Metab. Syndr. Relat. Disord.* **2014**, *12*, 231–241. [CrossRef] [PubMed]
43. Team, R. R Development Core Team. *R A Lang. Environ. Stat. Comput.* **2013**, *3*, 201.
44. Yoshida, K.; Bohn, J.; Yoshida, M.K. *Package 'Tableone'*; R Foundation for Statistical Computing: Vienna, Austria, 2016.
45. Rao, D.P.; Orpana, H.; Krewski, D. Physical activity and non-movement behaviours: Their independent and combined associations with metabolic syndrome. *Int. J. Behav. Nutr. Phys. Act.* **2016**, *13*, 26. [CrossRef] [PubMed]
46. Feairheller, D.L.; Diaz, K.M.; Kashem, M.A.; Thakkar, S.R.; Veerabhadrappa, P.; Sturgeon, K.M.; Ling, C.; Williamson, S.T.; Kretzschmar, J.; Lee, H.; et al. Effects of Moderate Aerobic Exercise Training on Vascular Health and Blood Pressure in African Americans. *J. Clin. Hypertens.* **2014**, *16*, 504–510. [CrossRef]
47. Mahajan, A.; Mishra, T.; Singh, N.; Jain, A. Heart rate and blood pressure response to exercise and recovery in subclinical hypothyroid patients. *Int. J. Appl. Basic Med. Res.* **2013**, *3*, 106. [CrossRef]

48. Kang, S.J.; Ha, G.C.; Ko, K.J. Association between resting heart rate, metabolic syndrome and cardiorespiratory fitness in Korean male adults. *J. Exerc. Sci. Fit.* **2017**, *15*, 27–31. [CrossRef]
49. Sîrbu, E.; Buzaș, R.; Mihăescu, R.; Suceava, I.; Lighezan, D. Influence of exercise training and eating behavior on arterial stiffness in young healthy students. *Wien. Klin. Wochenschr.* **2015**, *127*, 555–560. [CrossRef]
50. King, N.A.; Hopkins, M.; Caudwell, P.; Stubbs, R.J.; Blundell, J.E. Beneficial effects of exercise: Shifting the focus from body weight to other markers of health. *Br. J. Sports Med.* **2009**, *43*, 924–927. [CrossRef]
51. Souza, A.K.F.; de Andrade, A.D.; de Medeiros, A.I.C.; de Aguiar, M.I.R.; de Souza Rocha, T.D.; Pedrosa, R.P.; de Lima, A.M.J. Effectiveness of inspiratory muscle training on sleep and functional capacity to exercise in obstructive sleep apnea: A randomized controlled trial. *Sleep Breath.* **2018**, *22*, 631–639. [CrossRef]
52. Reid, K.J.; Baron, K.G.; Lu, B.; Naylor, E.; Wolfe, L.; Zee, P.C. Aerobic exercise improves self-reported sleep and quality of life in older adults with insomnia. *Sleep Med.* **2010**, *11*, 934–940. [CrossRef]
53. Brandão, G.S.; Gomes, G.S.B.F.; Brandão, G.S.; Callou Sampaio, A.A.; Donner, C.F.; Oliveira, L.V.F.; Camelier, A.A. Home exercise improves the quality of sleep and daytime sleepiness of elderlies: A randomized controlled trial. *Multidiscip. Respir. Med.* **2018**, *13*, 2. [CrossRef] [PubMed]
54. Kline, C.E.; Ewing, G.B.; Burch, J.B.; Blair, S.N.; Durstine, J.L.; Davis, J.M.; Youngstedt, S.D. Exercise Training Improves Selected Aspects of Daytime Functioning in Adults with Obstructive Sleep Apnea. *J. Clin. Sleep Med.* **2012**, *8*, 357–365. [CrossRef] [PubMed]
55. Yilmaz Gokmen, G.; Akkoyunlu, M.E.; Kilic, L.; Algun, C. The Effect of T'ai Chi and Qigong Training on Patients with Obstructive Sleep Apnea: A Randomized Controlled Study. *J. Altern. Complement. Med.* **2019**, *25*, 317–325. [CrossRef] [PubMed]
56. Itoh, H.; Yokoyama, K.; Matsukawa, T.; Kitamura, F. Association between physical activity and sleep-disordered breathing in male Japanese workers: A cross-sectional study. *BMC Res. Notes* **2017**, *10*, 37. [CrossRef]
57. Dixit, S.; Maiya, A.; Shastry, B. Effect of aerobic exercise on quality of life in population with diabetic peripheral neuropathy in type 2 diabetes: A single blind, randomized controlled trial. *Qual. Life Res.* **2014**, *23*, 1629–1640. [CrossRef]
58. Farias, D.L.; Tibana, R.A.; Teixeira, T.G.; Vieira, D.C.L.; Tarja, V.; Nascimento, D.D.C.; Silva, A.D.O.; Funghetto, S.S.; Coura, M.A.D.S.; Valduga, R.; et al. Elderly women with metabolic syndrome present higher cardiovascular risk and lower relative muscle strength. *Einstein* **2013**, *11*, 174–179. [CrossRef]
59. World Health Organization. *GLOBAL STATUS REPORT on Noncommunicable Diseases 2014—"Attaining the Nine Global Noncommunicable Diseases Targets; A Shared Responsibility"*; WHO Libr. Cat. Data: Geneva, Switzerland, 2014; p. 298.
60. Callaghan, B.C.; Xia, R.; Reynolds, E.; Banerjee, M.; Rothberg, A.E.; Burant, C.F.; Villegas-Umana, E.; Pop-Busui, R.; Feldman, E.L. Association Between Metabolic Syndrome Components and Polyneuropathy in an Obese Population. *JAMA Neurol.* **2016**, *73*, 1468. [CrossRef]
61. Sossa, C.; Delisle, H.; Agueh, V.; Sodjinou, R.; Ntandou, G.; Makoutodé, M. Lifestyle and dietary factors associated with the evolution of cardiometabolic risk over four years in West-African adults: The Benin study. *J. Obes.* **2013**, *2013*, 298024. [CrossRef]

15

Test-Retest Reliability of Kinematic Parameters of Timed Up and Go in People with Type 2 Diabetes

Francisco J. Dominguez-Muñoz [1], Miguel A. Hernández-Mocholi [1], Luis J. Manso [2], Daniel Collado-Mateo [3,*], Santos Villafaina [1,*], Jose C. Adsuar [4] and Narcis Gusi [1,5]

1 Physical Activity and Quality of Life Research Group (AFYCAV), Faculty of Sport Science, University of Extremadura, 10003 Cáceres, Spain; fjdominguez@unex.es (F.J.D.-M.); mhmocholi@unex.es (M.A.H.-M.); ngusi@unex.es (N.G.)

2 School of Engineering and Applied Sciences, Aston University, Birmingham B4 7ET, UK; l.manso@aston.ac.uk

3 Centre for Sport Studies, Rey Juan Carlos University, 28943 Fuenlabrada, Spain

4 Health Economy Motricity and Education (HEME), Faculty of Sport Science, University of Extremadura, 10003 Cáceres, Spain; jadssal@unex.es

5 CIBER de Fragilidad y Envejecimiento Saludable, 28029 Madrid, Spain

* Correspondence: danicolladom@gmail.com (D.C.-M.); svillafaina@unex.es (S.V.);

Abstract: Diabetes mellitus is a chronic disease defined as a state of hyperglycaemia in fasting or postprandial states. Patients with type 2 diabetes mellitus (T2DM) often show reduced physical function, including low levels of strength, balance or mobility. In this regard, the timed up and go (TUG) is a widely used physical fitness test in people with T2DM. However, there is a lack of studies evaluating the properties TUG in this population. The present study aimed to evaluate the test-retest reliability of kinetic and kinematic parameters obtained from TUG in the diabetic population with different levels of diabetic neuropathy. A total of 56 patients with T2DM participated in the study. They were divided into three groups according to the vibration threshold: (a) severe neuropathy, (b) moderate neuropathy and (c) normal perception. The TUG was performed using two force platforms to assess kinematic measurements. The results show that both kinetic and kinematic variables had good to excellent reliability. The reliability of TUG was excellent for the whole sample and the groups with non-severe neuropathy. However, it was just good for the group with severe neuropathy.

Keywords: forefoot; Gait; Heel; TUG; Type 2 diabetes mellitus

---

1. Introduction

Diabetes mellitus (DM) is a chronic disease defined as a state of hyperglycaemia in fasting or postprandial states [1]. DM is one of the largest global public health problems and affects approximately 415 million people in the world among adults aged 20–79 years-old. It is estimated that, in the year 2040, there will be 642 million persons (confidence interval 521–829 million) with DM in the world [2]. The International Diabetes Federation also estimates that, globally, 46.5% of people suffering from diabetes were still undiagnosed in 2015, which may markedly increase the reported prevalence. According with the American Diabetes Association (ADA), the total costs for diabetes care in the United States were approximately 245 billion dollars due to medical costs, lost productivity and disability [3]. Much of the burden of this disease comes from vascular complications, which include cardiovascular disease, retinopathy and nephropathy. Another complication is diabetic peripheral neuropathy, affecting more than 50% of long-term diabetic cases [4].

Diabetic neuropathy is characterised by progressive degeneration that primarily affects small-diameter cutaneous nociceptive fibres [5]. It may also affect motor fibres, which can cause muscular weakness. In this regard, persons with DM have a reduction of 17% and 14% in the strength of the flexor and extensor muscles of the knee, respectively [6]. Somatosensory feedback is a relevant factor to maintain balance and there is strong evidence showing that diabetic neuropathy affects this source of information, leading to alterations in postural and gait performance [7]. In this regard, previous studies have demonstrated that the main sources of deterioration in the balance in persons with type 2 DM (T2DM) are deficits in the proprioception of the foot and the ankle [8], or a loss of sensitivity in the feet [9].

The neurologic exam of the lower limb is the most important aspect in the clinical diagnosis of diabetic neuropathy [10]. The loss of foot vibration perception is associated with an increased risk of foot ulceration in people with diabetes [11]. In this regard, Abbott et al. [12] showed that each one-unit increment in the foot vibration threshold increases the risk of foot ulceration by more than 5% in a single year period. Therefore, the foot vibration threshold is a very relevant variable in the diabetic population.

Previous studies have demonstrated a relationship between the foot vibration threshold and the risk of falling [13], gait speed [14] and mobility disability [15]. Although balance and mobility tests are of great interest in DM studies due to the association with the risk of falling and the ability to perform activities of daily living, a recent systematic review showed that there is a lack of studies evaluating the properties of these tests when they are conducted in the diabetic population [16].

Therefore, the main objective of this study was to evaluate the test-retest reliability of the kinetic and kinematic parameters obtained from one of the most widely used tests for assessing balance and mobility, the timed up and go (TUG), in people suffering from T2DM. The second objective was to calculate the reliability of TUG according to the severity of peripheral neuropathy (assessed through an evaluation of the foot vibration threshold).

2. Materials and Methods

2.1. Participants

A total of 56 patients with DM participated in the study. Of these, 40 were men and 16 were women. The following inclusion criteria were: (a) diagnosed with T2DM, (b) affected by at least one risk factor of diabetic neuropathy: (1) being overweight, (2) a former smoker, (3) diagnosed with diabetic nephropathy and (4) diagnosed with diabetic retinopathy, (c) levels of glycated haemoglobin higher than 5.7%, and (d) have read and signed the written informed consent. In addition to these inclusion criteria, some exclusion criteria were defined: (a) pregnancy, (b) the use of psychotropic or chemotherapeutic medications, (c) affected by other diseases that may influence balance and gait, such as Parkinson's disease, and (d) patients with a high risk of non-diabetic neuropathy (HIV or uraemia). The protocol of the present study was approved by the Committee of Bioethics of the University and was developed in accordance with the updated Helsinki Declaration and the national legislation on bioethics, biomedical research and personal data confidentiality.

2.2. Procedure

After reading and signing the written informed consent, participants were measured and weighed. They were also asked about their age and years since diagnosis. Then, the vibration threshold was evaluated and, finally, the TUG was conducted after a light warm-up.

The foot vibration threshold was assessed using a Biothensiometer Vibratron II (Physitemp Instruments, Inc. Clifton; New Jersey; USA). This device drives vibration to modules A and B placed under the feet of the participant. Each module has a vibrating pole on the top, which vibrates at a frequency of 120 Hz. Therefore, the vibration threshold is determined by modifying the amplitude. These vibration units are related to the amplitude of the movement in microns according to the formula:

$A = x^2/2$ (where x is the vibration units (vu) and A is the amplitude in microns (μm)). The present study used the protocol the 'force two alternative choices procedure', which is one of the two methods suggested by the manufacturer. Participants were asked to place their first toe on the vibrating pole. The procedure started when the participant felt the vibration in the left or right toe. After that, the amplitude was reduced progressively until the participant was not able to tell which pole was vibrating. When the participant failed to detect vibration, the amplitude of the vibration was increased. The vibration threshold was then calculated using the last five rights and wrongs, but omitting the extreme low and high values. The average of the remaining eight values was then computed to calculate the vibration threshold [17].

TUG was performed three times, with a 5-min rest in between. The first repetition was for familiarisation, the second was the test measure and the third was the retest measure. All participants performed a light warm-up which included walking and joint mobility for 5 min. In the TUG, two force platforms (Kistler, NY, USA) were placed between the chair and the mark where participants had to turn around. Therefore, participants stepped on the platforms before and after reaching the mark placed at 3 m. The time required to complete the full test was assessed manually with a stopwatch by an expert rater.

Variables obtained from the force platforms included the duration of (a) the double support phase (both feet on the platforms), (b) left support (only the left foot on the platforms) and (c) right support (only the right foot on the platforms), as well as the left and right peak forces from the forefoot and the heel.

The results are presented for the whole sample (n = 56), and also according to the degree of neuropathy based on vibration perception, i.e., severe neuropathy (n = 22), moderate neuropathy (n = 22) and normal perception (n = 12). To classify patients into one of the three groups, the cut-off points suggested by normative values of the manual of the measuring device were considered.

2.3. Statistical Analysis

Descriptive statistics included mean and standard deviation (SD) of age, weight, glycated haemoglobin, years since T2DM diagnosis, body mass index and vibration threshold were calculated for the whole sample and divided into women or men. Parametric and non-parametric tests were conducted based on the results of Shapiro-Wilk and Kolmogorov-Smirnov tests.

Differences between test and retest were evaluated using the paired samples t-test or Wilcoxon signed rank test when appropriate. The time spent to complete the TUG, the duration of phases and the forces registered by the force platforms were included in those analyses to compare the test and retest results.

Reliability analyses were conducted in accordance with the recommendations of Weir [18]. An intraclass correlation coefficient (ICC) of 3.1 (two-way mixed, single measures) with a 95% CI for test and retest [19] was selected. Both absolute and relative reliability were computed. The standard error of measurement (SEM) was calculated as $SEM = SD\sqrt{1-ICC}$ where SD is the mean SD of the three repetitions, while the smallest real difference (SRD) was $SRD = 1.96 \times SEM \times \sqrt{2}$. These measures were converted into percentages (%SEM and %SRD, respectively) to enable comparisons with other investigations.

3. Results

3.1. Participant Characteristics

Table 1 summarises the participant characteristics. A total of 40 men and 16 women aged 64.52 (8.41) and 67.43 (8.86), respectively, participated in the present study. The mean weight of the whole sample was 80.08 (17.59) kg and the body mass index (BMI) was 28.81 (4.40) kg/m^2. The mean vibration threshold was 4.27 (1.90) for women and 5.75 (2.50) for men.

Table 1. Participant characteristics.

	All Participants (n = 56)	Men (n = 40)	Women (n = 16)
Age (years)	65.35 (8.56)	64.52 (8.41)	67.43 (8.86)
Weight (kg)	80.08 (17.59)	85.26 (18.03)	67.11 (6.14)
Glycated haemoglobin (%)	6.66 (0.91)	6.67 (0.90)	6.63 (0.94)
Years since diagnosis	9.10 (7.43)	9.07 (6.52)	9.18 (9.59)
BMI (kg/m^2)	28.81 (4.40)	29.24 (4.84)	27.73 (2.85
Vibration threshold (vu)	5.33 (2.42)	5.75 (2.50)	4.27 (1.90)

BMI: body mass index; vu: vibration units.

3.2. *Kinematic Variables of the Timed Up and Go*

Table 2 summarises the mean duration of the walking phases in the TUG. The results from the paired samples t-test or Wilcoxon signed rank test showed that there were significant differences between the test and retest values in some of the variables, including the time required to complete the TUG and the duration of the left support before reaching the mark for the whole sample. These differences were also observed in the group with severe neuropathy.

Table 2. Differences between test and retest on the duration of the walking phases in the entire sample and in participants with (a) severe neuropathy, (b) moderate neuropathy and (c) normal perception.

	Test Measurement	Test	Retest	p-Value [a]
GENERAL (n = 56)	TUG (S)	8.10 (1.37)	7.80 (1.28)	<0.001
	Double support phase duration (before reaching the mark)	0.09 (0.02)	0.09 (0.02)	0.341 [a]
	Double support phase duration (after reaching the mark)	0.10 (0.02)	0.10 (0.02)	0.483 [a]
	Right support duration (before reaching the mark)	0.62 (0.09)	0.60 (0.09)	0.047 [a]
	Left support duration (before reaching the mark)	0.62 (0.09)	0.60 (0.08)	0.005 [a]
	Right support duration (after reaching the mark)	0.62 (0.08)	0.61 (0.08)	0.261
	Left support duration (after reaching the mark)	0.63 (0.09)	0.63 (0.10)	0.399 [a]
SEVERE (n = 22)	TUG (S)	8.36 (1.40)	7.94 (1.10)	0.007
	Double support phase duration (before reaching the mark)	0.09 (0.02)	0.09 (0.02)	0.463 [a]
	Double support phase duration (after reaching the mark)	0.10 (0.02)	0.10 (0.02)	0.637 [a]
	Right support duration (before reaching the mark)	0.62 (0.09)	0.60 (0.08)	0.117 [a]
	Left support duration (before reaching the mark)	0.63 (0.08)	0.60 (0.06)	0.020 [a]
	Right support duration (after reaching the mark)	0.62 (0.06)	0.62 (0.06)	0.610
	Left support duration (after reaching the mark)	0.62 (0.06)	0.63 (0.08)	0.986 [a]
MODERATE (n = 22)	TUG (S)	7.92 (1.47)	7.69 (1.54)	0.016
	Double support phase duration (before reaching the mark)	0.09 (0.03)	0.09 (0.02)	0.930 [a]
	Double support phase duration (after reaching the mark)	0.10 (0.02)	0.10 (0.03)	0.974 [a]
	Right support duration (before reaching the mark)	0.61 (0.10)	0.60 (0.11)	0.443 [a]
	Left support duration (before reaching the mark)	0.60 (0.11)	0.60 (0.11)	0.750 [a]
	Right support duration (after reaching the mark)	0.61 (0.10)	0.61 (0.10)	0.697
	Left support duration (after reaching the mark)	0.64 (0.12)	0.64 (0.12)	0.650 [a]
NORMAL (n = 12)	TUG (S)	7.94 (1.16)	7.74 (1.15)	0.095
	Double support phase duration (before reaching the mark)	0.09 (0.01)	0.08 (0.01)	0.260 [a]
	Double support phase duration (after reaching the mark)	0.10 (0.01)	0.09 (0.02)	0.164 [a]
	Right support duration (before reaching the mark)	0.63 (0.09)	0.61 (0.07)	0.153 [a]
	Left support duration (before reaching the mark)	0.62 (0.06)	0.59 (0.06)	0.025 [a]
	Right support duration (after reaching the mark)	0.61 (0.05)	0.60 (0.06)	0.235
	Left support duration (after reaching the mark)	0.63 (0.08)	0.62 (0.09)	0.312 [a]

[a] p-values obtained from the Wilcoxon signed rank test.

Reliability parameters for the total time required to complete the TUG and duration of phases can be observed in Table 3. The ICC was good (0.70 to 0.90) or excellent (>0.90) for almost every variable and group. The best reliability was obtained for the time required to complete the TUG, which was excellent in the two groups with non-severe neuropathy, while it was just good in the group with severe neuropathy.

Table 3. Test-retest analyses of the duration of the walking phases in the entire sample and in participants with (a) severe neuropathy, (b) moderate neuropathy and (c) normal perception.

	Test Measurement	ICC (95% CI)	SEM (s)	SEM (%)	SRD (s)	SRD (%)
GENERAL (n = 56)	TUG (S)	0.927 (0.878–0.956)	0.36	4.52	0.99	12.55
	Double support phase duration (going)	0.760 (0.623–0.852)	0.01	14.07	0.03	39.02
	Double support phase duration (return)	0.801 (0.683–0.878)	0.01	10.73	0.03	29.74
	Right support duration (before reaching the mark)	0.865 (0.781–0.919)	0.03	5.74	0.09	15.93
	Left support duration (before reaching the mark)	0.845 (0.749–0.906)	0.03	5.80	0.09	16.08
	Right support duration (after reaching the mark)	0.876 (0.798–0.925)	0.02	4.71	0.08	13.05
	Left support duration (after reaching the mark)	0.860 (0.772–0.915)	0.03	5.77	0.10	16.01
SEVERE (n= 22)	TUG (S)	0.870 (0.714–0.944)	0.45	5.54	1.25	15.37
	Double support phase duration (going)	0.855 (0.684–0.937)	0.01	10.75	0.02	29.81
	Double support phase duration (return)	0.853 (0.678–0.936)	0.01	7.60	0.02	21.07
	Right support duration (before reaching the mark)	0.782 (0.544–0.903)	0.04	6.58	0.11	18.25
	Left support duration (before reaching the mark)	0.730 (0.454–0.879)	0.04	6.63	0.11	18.38
	Right support duration (after reaching the mark)	0.853 (0.678–0.936)	0.02	4.07	0.07	11.30
	Left support duration (after reaching the mark)	0.727 (0.448–0.877)	0.03	6.01	0.10	16.66
MODERATE (n = 22)	TUG (S)	0.963 (914–0.985)	0.29	3.727	0.80	10.31
	Double support phase duration (going)	0.723 (0.441–0.875)	0.01	18.06	0.04	50.07
	Double support phase duration (return)	0.861 (0.695–0.940)	0.01	10.83	0.03	30.03
	Right support duration (before reaching the mark)	0.914 (0.805–0.964)	0.03	5.37	0.09	14.90
	Left support duration (before reaching the mark)	0.923 (0.824–0.967)	0.03	5.11	0.08	14.17
	Right support duration (after reaching the mark)	0.903 (0.781–0.959)	0.03	5.43	0.09	15.06
	Left support duration (after reaching the mark)	0.912 (0.800–0.962)	0.03	5.71	0.10	15.83
NORMAL (n = 12)	TUG (S)	0.938 (0.800–0.982)	0.28	3.67	0.79	10.17
	Double support phase duration (going)	0.565 (0.018–0.852)	0.01	11.93	0.02	33.08
	Double support phase duration (return)	0.511 (0.059–0.829)	0.01	15.04	0.04	41.69
	Right support duration (before reaching the mark)	0.880 (0.636–0.964)	0.03	4.82	0.08	13.38
	Left support duration (before reaching the mark)	0.881 (0.639–0.964)	0.02	3.70	0.06	10.25
	Right support duration (after reaching the mark)	0.774 (0.387–0.929)	0.02	4.64	0.07	12.88
	Left support duration (after reaching the mark)	0.843 (0.543–0.952)	0.03	5.68	0.09	15.76

3.3. Peak Forces from the Heel and the Forefoot in the Timed Up and Go

Regarding the peak forces from the heel and the forefoot, differences between test and retest were only observed for the right heel and left forefoot forces in the group without neuropathy. For the rest of the variables, the retest was not significantly different than the test (see Table 4).

Table 4. Differences between the test and retest on the peak forces from the heel and the forefoot forces in the entire sample and in participants with (a) severe neuropathy, (b) moderate neuropathy and (c) normal perception.

	Test Measurement in Newtons	Test	Retest	p-Value
GENERAL (n = 56)	Right forefoot forces (before reaching the mark)	846.91 (185.68)	841.62 (192.78)	0.525 [a]
	Left forefoot forces (before reaching the mark)	827.33 (195.94)	828.06 (187.55)	0.562 [a]
	Right forefoot forces (after reaching the mark)	823.69 (181.65)	819.28 (174.34)	0.707 [a]
	Left forefoot forces (after reaching the mark)	773.50 (179.97)	767.44 (179.11)	0.458 [a]
	Right heel forces (before reaching the mark)	881.64 (201.23)	902.94 (209.41)	0.058 [a]
	Left heel forces (before reaching the mark)	934.64 (217.76)	944.97 (217.63)	0.098 [a]
	Right heel forces (after reaching the mark)	938.52 (226.32)	940.87 (211.95)	0.579 [a]
	Left heel forces (after reaching the mark)	937.35 (210.51)	943.70 (214.06)	0.458 [a]
SEVERE (n= 22)	Right forefoot forces (before reaching the mark)	868.77 (198.23)	867.59 (215.78)	0.833 [a]
	Left forefoot forces (before reaching the mark)	879.37 (208.31)	857.73 (204.77)	0.291 [a]
	Right forefoot forces (after reaching the mark)	855.99 (204.95)	849.56 (204.22)	0.615 [a]
	Left forefoot forces (after reaching the mark)	821.39 (199.56)	820.55 (194.15)	0.783 [a]
	Right heel forces (before reaching the mark)	937.91 (209.96)	958.33 (237.64)	0.485 [a]
	Left heel forces (before reaching the mark)	994.51 (229.16)	1004.19 (232.83)	0.338 [a]
	Right heel forces (after reaching the mark)	991.13 (263.60)	973.35 (237.58)	0.548 [a]
	Left heel forces (after reaching the mark)	983.31 (226.01)	979.73 (219.78)	0.783 [a]

Table 4. *Cont.*

	Test Measurement in Newtons	Test	Retest	*p*-Value
MODERATE (n = 22)	Right forefoot forces (before reaching the mark)	846.14 (212.30)	827.06 (207.90)	0.178 [a]
	Left forefoot forces (before reaching the mark)	809.70 (215.55)	819.77 (205.52)	0.638 [a]
	Right forefoot forces (after reaching the mark)	820.03 (187.24)	809.08 (174.89)	0.527 [a]
	Left forefoot forces (after reaching the mark)	747.40 (193.17)	741.54 (185.78)	0.200 [a]
	Right heel forces (before reaching the mark)	860.34 (204.46)	877.55 (202.41)	0.408 [a]
	Left heel forces (before reaching the mark)	919.46 (221.58)	934.12 (221.63)	0.168 [a]
	Right heel forces (after reaching the mark)	935.64 (208.33)	938.26 (211.80)	0.961 [a]
	Left heel forces (after reaching the mark)	929.66 (206.01)	947.18 (225.00)	0.200 [a]
NORMAL (n = 12)	Right forefoot forces (before reaching the mark)	808.24 (93.51)	820.69 (110.33)	0.136 [a]
	Left forefoot forces (before reaching the mark)	764.25 (100.23)	788.90 (107.78)	0.006 [a]
	Right forefoot forces (after reaching the mark)	771.20 (112.84)	782.47 (102.16)	0.388 [a]
	Left forefoot forces (after reaching the mark)	733.56 (83.56)	717.58 (113.36)	0.754 [a]
	Right heel forces (before reaching the mark)	817.53 (163.63)	847.94 (150.04)	0.099 [a]
	Left heel forces (before reaching the mark)	852.69 (167.82)	856.27 (153.98)	0.695 [a]
	Right heel forces (after reaching the mark)	847.34 (161.18)	886.09 (160.69)	0.034 [a]
	Left heel forces (after reaching the mark)	867.18 (182.55)	871.26 (178.58)	0.754 [a]

[a] *p*-values obtained from the Wilcoxon signed rank test.

Table 5 summarises the reliability analyses of the kinetic variables for the whole sample and according to the neuropathy classification. Reliability was excellent (ICC > 0.90) in almost every variable and group, except for the left forefoot forces after reaching the mark in the group with normal vibration perception.

Table 5. Test-retest analyses on the peak forces from the heel and the forefoot forces in the entire sample and in participants with (a) severe neuropathy, (b) moderate neuropathy and (c) normal perception.

	Test Measurement in Newtons	ICC (95% CI)	SEM (N)	SEM (%)	SRD (N)	SRD (%)
GENERAL (n = 56)	Right forefoot forces (before reaching the mark)	0.937 (0.894–0.962)	47.49	5.62	131.65	15.59
	Left forefoot forces (before reaching the mark)	0.944 (0.906–0.967)	45.37	5.48	125.77	15.19
	Right forefoot forces (after reaching the mark)	0.955 (0.925–0.974)	37.75	4.59	104.66	12.74
	Left forefoot forces (after reaching the mark)	0.942 (0.903–0.966)	43.23	5.61	119.85	15.55
	Right heel forces (before reaching the mark)	0.946 (0.910–0.968)	47.71	5.34	132.25	14.82
	Left heel forces (before reaching the mark)	0.941 (0.901–0.965)	52.87	5.62	146.57	15.59
	Right heel forces (after reaching the mark)	0.935 (0.892–0.961)	55.86	5.94	154.86	16.48
	Left heel forces (after reaching the mark)	0.955 (0.925–0.974)	45.03	4.78	124.82	13.27
SEVERE (n= 22)	Right forefoot forces (before reaching the mark)	0.952 (0.888–0.980)	45.35	5.22	125.71	14.48
	Left forefoot forces (before reaching the mark)	0.937 (0.854–0.973)	51.84	5.96	143.69	16.54
	Right forefoot forces (after reaching the mark)	0.968 (0.925–0.987)	36.59	4.29	101.44	11.89
	Left forefoot forces (after reaching the mark)	0.973 (0.936–0.989)	32.34	3.94	89.66	10.92
	Right heel forces (before reaching the mark)	0.947 (0.878–0.978)	51.52	5.43	142.81	15.06
	Left heel forces (before reaching the mark)	0.959 (0.903–0.983)	46.77	4.68	129.64	12.97
	Right heel forces (after reaching the mark)	0.933 (0.846–0.972)	64.86	6.60	179.79	18.30
	Left heel forces (after reaching the mark)	0.959 (0.904–0.983)	45.13	4.59	125.10	12.74
MODERATE- (n = 22)	Right forefoot forces (before reaching the mark)	0.925 (0.828–0.968)	57.53	6.87	159.49	19.06
	Left forefoot forces (before reaching the mark)	0.953 (0.890–0.980)	45.64	5.60	126.51	15.52
	Right forefoot forces (after reaching the mark)	0.944 (0.871–0.976)	42.84	5.26	118.77	14.58
	Left forefoot forces (after reaching the mark)	0.939 (0.858–0.974)	46.79	6.28	129.71	17.42
	Right heel forces (before reaching the mark)	0.947 (0.878–0.978)	46.83	5.38	129.81	14.93
	Left heel forces (before reaching the mark)	0.913 (0.803–0.963)	65.36	7.05	181.18	19.54
	Right heel forces (after reaching the mark)	0.945 (0.873–0.977)	49.26	5.25	136.55	14.57
	Left heel forces (after reaching the mark)	0.960 (0.906–0.983)	43.10	4.59	119.47	12.73
NORMAL (n = 12)	Right forefoot forces (before reaching the mark)	0.931 (0.778–0.980)	26.77	3.28	74.20	9.11
	Left forefoot forces (before reaching the mark)	0.976 (0.920–0.993)	16.11	2.07	44.66	5.75
	Right forefoot forces (after reaching the mark)	0.926 (0.765–0.978)	29.24	3.76	81.06	10.43
	Left forefoot forces (after reaching the mark)	0.697 (0.234–0.902)	54.20	7.47	150.24	20.70
	Right heel forces (before reaching the mark)	0.915 (0.732–0.975)	45.72	5.49	126.74	15.22
	Left heel forces (before reaching the mark)	0.934 (0.789–0.981)	41.33	4.83	114.57	13.40
	Right heel forces (after reaching the mark)	0.931 (0.778–0.980)	42.27	4.87	117.17	13.51
	Left heel forces (after reaching the mark)	0.928 (0.770–0.979)	48.45	5.57	134.30	15.45

4. Discussion

The present study aimed to evaluate the test-retest reliability of kinetic and kinematic parameters obtained from TUG in the diabetic population. The results were analysed according to the severity of neuropathy. The main finding was that almost each variable achieved good (ICC between 0.70 and 0.90) or excellent (>0.90) reliability considering the classification by Munro et al. [20].

The reliability of TUG seemed to be conditioned by the severity of neuropathy since the ICC was higher than 0.90 (excellent) for participants with moderate neuropathy and patients with normal foot vibration perception, but just good (0.70 to 0.90) for patients with severe neuropathy. Therefore, although the TUG is reliable in T2DM patients, changes in the duration of the phases (single and double support) must be taken with caution since the %SEM may be relatively high in some cases (over 10%). Furthermore, we can observe how the SRD of the required time to complete the TUG was higher in patients with severe neuropathy. These results must be considered by clinicians and researchers in order to interpret their results when using TUG in the T2DM population. This is relevant since a previous study showed that patients with diabetic neuropathy have worse health-related quality of life and lower functional status than patients without diabetic neuropathy [21]. Neuropathy leads to balance impairments [22], gait and mobility alterations [23,24] and an increased risk of falls [25]. In addition, patients with T2DM seem to be more susceptible to falls and consequently to bone fractures [26–28]. Due to the relevance of diabetic neuropathy in patients with T2DM, future studies aimed at improving physical conditioning variables should consider that the smallest clinically relevant improvement may be higher in T2DM patients with this complication.

To our knowledge, this is the first study to assess the reliability of TUG according to the severity of neuropathy. Only one previous study has evaluated the reliability of TUG in the diabetic population [29]. That study was conducted on a sample of 18 older adults with T2DM, and no classification of the participants was performed. Furthermore, that study only evaluated the time needed to complete the TUG and not any other measure such as the duration of walking phases or kinetic parameters. Comparing results from the present study with those obtained by Alfonso-Rosa, Del Pozo-Cruz, Del Pozo-Cruz, Sanudo and Rogers [29], both studies report excellent reliability. However, the ICC and %SEM from that study were 0.98 and 3.5%, respectively, whereas the present study reports an ICC of 0.927 and a %SEM of 4.52. Therefore, the reliability is slightly lower in this study, which may be linked to the greater heterogeneity of the sample in the current study. In this regard, it must be noted that the study by Alfonso-Rosa, Del Pozo-Cruz, Del Pozo-Cruz, Sanudo and Rogers [29] was conducted on 18 older adults with T2DM, while the current one was conducted with 56 adults aged 65.35 (8.56) years.

The current study reported not only the SEM but also the SRD, which is extremely relevant for clinicians and researchers since it indicates whether the differences obtained as a consequence of an intervention program could be considered clinically important [30]. A previous study in T2DM [29] established the SRD for the TUG at 9.8%, whereas in the present study the SRD was 12.55%. This difference could be also explained by the heterogeneity of the sample in the current study. In this regard, the results from the previous study were limited to older adults. Thus, those studies conducted with samples comprised of adults (but not limited older adults) had no information about the reliability and the minimal clinically important difference to interpret their results. Therefore, the current study was needed since it is the first to provide reliability information in a sample comprised of adults (not limited to older adults).

Test-retest analyses have been also reported in kinematic parameters, taking into account the heel and the forefoot forces during the TUG. The results revealed that the reliability of the heel and forefoot forces could be considered as excellent, so future studies can confidently use this as a measurement to evaluate gait patterns in T2DM patients. People with diabetic neuropathy often have balance problems while performing common activities such as walking or ascending/descending stairs [31]. Furthermore, the postural mechanisms at the ankle joints are impaired in diabetic neuropathy patients during quiet standing [32]. Thus, postural instability and gait imbalance in diabetic neuropathy may contribute to a high risk of fall incidence, especially in the geriatric population [7,31]. Therefore, future studies should be focused on the implementation of interventions aimed to modify gait parameters to reduce the risk of falling in T2DM patients. The current study provides useful information in order to interpret changes achieved after a specific program, stating the minimal clinically relevant change for kinetic and kinematic variables.

The present study has two main limitations. First, although the sample size ($n = 56$) was sufficient to conduct this test-retest reliability analysis, the group with no alteration in the foot vibration threshold was comprised of only 12 people. The second limitation may be related to the inclusion criteria and the difficulty in determining that peripheral neuropathy is caused by diabetes. Even though the inclusion and exclusion criteria were very restrictive (excluding people with other diseases and people who were taking drugs that may potentially affect balance and gait), there could be other non-diagnosed diseases, environmental factors or healthy/unhealthy habits that may increase or reduce neuropathy. In spite of these two limitations, this study succeeded at reporting reliability parameters according to the severity of neuropathy in patients with T2DM.

5. Conclusions

The reliability of TUG was excellent for the whole sample and the groups with non-severe neuropathy. However, it was just good for the group with severe neuropathy. Regarding the kinetic and kinematic parameters, the reliability was good or excellent for almost every variable and group. The present study reports the minimal change that may be considered real (SRD) and the SEM, which should be considered by future studies aimed to assess the effects of interventions on different variables related to the TUG.

Author Contributions: F.J.D.-M., J.C.A., M.A.H.-M. conceived the study. F.J.D.-M., S.V. and D.C.-M. collected the data. F.J.D.-M., N.G., L.J.M., D.C.-M. analysed the data. S.V., N.G. and D.C.-M. designed the figures and tables. F.J.D.-M., J.C.A. and D.C.-M. wrote the manuscript. S.V., M.A.H.-M., L.J.M., and N.G. provided critical revisions on successive drafts. All authors approved the manuscript in its final form.

Acknowledgments: The author SV is supported by a grant from the regional Department of Economy and Infrastructure of the Government of Extremadura and European Social Fund (PD16008). We are grateful to the Primary Care Centre "Manuel Encinas" in Cáceres for helping recruit the participants for this study. The funders had no role in study design, data collection and analysis, decision to publish, or preparation of the manuscript.

Abbreviations

ADA	American Diabetes Association
BMI	Body mass index
DM	Diabetes mellitus
ICC	Intraclass correlation coefficient
T2DM	Type 2 diabetes mellitus
TUG	Timed up and go
SEM	Standard error of measurement
SPSS	Statistical Package for Social Sciences
SRD	Smallest real difference

References

1. Alam, U.; Asghar, O.; Azmi, S.; Malik, R.A. General aspects of diabetes mellitus. *Handb. Clin. Neurol.* **2014**, *126*, 211–222. [CrossRef] [PubMed]
2. Ogurtsova, K.; da Rocha Fernandes, J.D.; Huang, Y.; Linnenkamp, U.; Guariguata, L.; Cho, N.H.; Cavan, D.; Shaw, J.E.; Makaroff, L.E. IDF Diabetes Atlas: Global estimates for the prevalence of diabetes for 2015 and 2040. *Diabetes Res. Clin. Pract.* **2017**, *128*, 40–50. [CrossRef] [PubMed]
3. ADA. American Diabetes Association: Economic costs of diabetes in the US in 2012. *Diabetes Care* **2013**, *36*, 1033–1046.
4. Boulton, A.J.; Malik, R.A.; Arezzo, J.C.; Sosenko, J.M. Diabetic somatic neuropathies. *Diabetes Care* **2004**, *27*, 1458–1486. [CrossRef]

5. Thomas, P.K. Classification, differential diagnosis, and staging of diabetic peripheral neuropathy. *Diabetes* **1997**, *46* (Suppl. 2), S54–S57. [CrossRef]
6. Andersen, H.; Nielsen, S.; Mogensen, C.E.; Jakobsen, J. Muscle strength in type 2 diabetes. *Diabetes* **2004**, *53*, 1543–1548. [CrossRef] [PubMed]
7. Mustapa, A.; Justine, M.; Mohd Mustafah, N.; Jamil, N.; Manaf, H. Postural control and gait performance in the diabetic peripheral neuropathy: A systematic review. *BioMed Res. Int.* **2016**, *2016*, 9305025. [CrossRef] [PubMed]
8. Van Deursen, R.; Simoneau, G.G. Foot and ankle sensory neuropathy, proprioception, and postural stability. *J. Orthop. Sports Phys. Ther.* **1999**, *29*, 718–726. [CrossRef]
9. Ducic, I.; Short, K.W.; Dellon, A.L. Relationship between loss of pedal sensibility, balance, and falls in patients with peripheral neuropathy. *Ann. Plast. Surg.* **2004**, *52*, 535–540. [CrossRef]
10. Boulton, A.J.M. Chapter 8—Diabetic neuropathy and foot complications. In *Handbook of Clinical Neurology*; Zochodne, D.W., Malik, R.A., Eds.; Elsevier: Amsterdam, The Netherlands, 2014; Volume 126, pp. 97–107.
11. Young, M.J.; Breddy, J.L.; Veves, A.; Boulton, A.J. The prediction of diabetic neuropathic foot ulceration using vibration perception thresholds. A prospective study. *Diabetes Care* **1994**, *17*, 557–560. [CrossRef]
12. Abbott, C.A.; Vileikyte, L.; Williamson, S.; Carrington, A.L.; Boulton, A.J. Multicenter Study of the Incidence of and Predictive Risk Factors for Diabetic Neuropathic Foot Ulceration. *Diabetes Care* **1998**, *21*, 1071–1075. [CrossRef]
13. Macgilchrist, C.; Paul, L.; Ellis, B.M.; Howe, T.E.; Kennon, B.; Godwin, J. Lower-limb risk factors for falls in people with diabetes mellitus. *Diabetic Med.* **2010**, *27*, 162–168. [CrossRef] [PubMed]
14. Allet, L.; Armand, S.; de Bie, R.A.; Golay, A.; Pataky, Z.; Aminian, K.; de Bruin, E.D. Clinical factors associated with gait alterations in diabetic patients. *Diabetic Med.* **2009**, *26*, 1003–1009. [CrossRef] [PubMed]
15. Ward, R.E.; Boudreau, R.M.; Caserotti, P.; Harris, T.B.; Zivkovic, S.; Goodpaster, B.H.; Satterfield, S.; Kritchevsky, S.B.; Schwartz, A.V.; Vinik, A.I.; et al. Sensory and motor peripheral nerve function and incident mobility disability. *J. Am. Geriatr. Soc.* **2014**, *62*, 2273–2279. [CrossRef] [PubMed]
16. Dixon, C.J.; Knight, T.; Binns, E.; Ihaka, B.; O'Brien, D. Clinical measures of balance in people with type two diabetes: A systematic literature review. *Gait Posture* **2017**, *58*, 325–332. [CrossRef] [PubMed]
17. Deng, H.; He, F.; Zhang, S.; Calleman, C.J.; Costa, L.G. Quantitative measurements of vibration threshold in healthy adults and acrylamide workers. *Int. Arch. Occup. Environ. Health* **1993**, *65*, 53–56. [CrossRef] [PubMed]
18. Weir, J.P. Quantifying test-retest reliability using the intraclass correlation coefficient and the SEM. *J. Strength Cond. Rres.* **2005**, *19*, 231–240. [CrossRef]
19. Shrout, P.E.; Fleiss, J.L. Intraclass correlations: Uses in assessing rater reliability. *Psychol. Bull.* **1979**, *86*, 420–428. [CrossRef]
20. Munro, B.; Visintainer, M.; Page, E. *Statistical Methods for Health Care Research*; Lippincott Williams & Wilkins: Philadelphia, PA, USA, 1986.
21. Riandini, T.; Wee, H.L.; Khoo, E.Y.; Tai, B.C.; Wang, W.; Koh, G.C.; Tai, E.S.; Tavintharan, S.; Chandran, K.; Hwang, S.W. Functional status mediates the association between peripheral neuropathy and health-related quality of life in individuals with diabetes. *Acta Diabetol.* **2018**, *55*, 155–164. [CrossRef]
22. Boucher, P.; Teasdale, N.; Courtemanche, R.; Bard, C.; Fleury, M. Postural stability in diabetic polyneuropathy. *Diabetes Care* **1995**, *18*, 638–645. [CrossRef]
23. Martinelli, A.R.; Mantovani, A.M.; Nozabieli, A.J.L.; Ferreira, D.M.A.; Barela, J.A.; de Camargo, M.R.; Fregonesi, C.E.P.T. Muscle strength and ankle mobility for the gait parameters in diabetic neuropathies. *Foot* **2013**, *23*, 17–21. [CrossRef]
24. Manor, B.; Li, L. Characteristics of functional gait among people with and without peripheral neuropathy. *Gait Posture* **2009**, *30*, 253–256. [CrossRef] [PubMed]
25. Richardson, J.K.; Hurvitz, E.A. Peripheral neuropathy: A true risk factor for falls. *J. Gerontol. Ser. A Biol. Sci. Med. Sci.* **1995**, *50*, M211–M215. [CrossRef] [PubMed]
26. Wongsurawat, N.; Armbrecht, H.J. Insulin modulates the stimulation of renal 1, 25-dihydroxyvitamin D3 production by parathyroid hormone. *Acta Endocrinol.* **1985**, *109*, 243–248. [CrossRef] [PubMed]
27. Pietschmann, P.; Schernthaner, G.; Woloszczuk, W. Serum osteocalcin levels in diabetes mellitus: Analysis of the type of diabetes and microvascular complications. *Diabetologia* **1988**, *31*, 892–895. [CrossRef] [PubMed]

28. Schwartz, A.V.; Sellmeyer, D.E.; Ensrud, K.E.; Cauley, J.A.; Tabor, H.K.; Schreiner, P.J.; Jamal, S.A.; Black, D.M.; Cummings, S.R.; Study of Osteoporotic Fractures Research Group. Older women with diabetes have an increased risk of fracture: A prospective study. *J. Clin. Endocrinol. Metab.* **2001**, *86*, 32–38. [CrossRef] [PubMed]

29. Alfonso-Rosa, R.M.; Del Pozo-Cruz, B.; Del Pozo-Cruz, J.; Sanudo, B.; Rogers, M.E. Test-retest reliability and minimal detectable change scores for fitness assessment in older adults with type 2 diabetes. *Rehabil. Nurs.* **2014**, *39*, 260–268. [CrossRef]

30. Beckerman, H.; Roebroeck, M.E.; Lankhorst, G.J.; Becher, J.G.; Bezemer, P.D.; Verbeek, A.L. Smallest real difference, a link between reproducibility and responsiveness. *Qual. Life Res.* **2001**, *10*, 571–578. [CrossRef]

31. Brown, S.J.; Handsaker, J.C.; Bowling, F.L.; Boulton, A.J.; Reeves, N.D. Diabetic peripheral neuropathy compromises balance during daily activities. *Diabetes Care* **2015**, *38*, 1116–1122. [CrossRef]

32. Lafond, D.; Corriveau, H.; Prince, F. Postural control mechanisms during quiet standing in patients with diabetic sensory neuropathy. *Diabetes Care* **2004**, *27*, 173–178. [CrossRef]

16

Patellofemoral Joint Loads during Running Immediately Changed by Shoes with Different Minimalist Indices

Chenhao Yang [1], Songlin Xiao [1], Yang Yang [1], Xini Zhang [1], Junqing Wang [1] and Weijie Fu [1,2,*]

[1] School of Kinesiology, Shanghai University of Sport, Shanghai 200438, China; chyang9610@163.com (C.Y.); xiao_songlin@126.com (S.X.); 18049922807@163.com (Y.Y.); zhangxini1129@163.com (X.Z.); wangjunqingray@163.com (J.W.)

[2] Key Laboratory of Exercise and Health Sciences of Ministry of Education, Shanghai University of Sport, Shanghai 200438, China

[*] Correspondence: fuweijie@sus.edu.cn or fuweijie315@163.com;

Abstract: Purpose: Given the high incidence of patellofemoral pain syndrome (PFPS) in runners, this study aimed to investigate the immediate effect of shoes with different minimalist indices (MI) on the mechanical loads of the patellofemoral joint. Methods: Fifteen healthy male rearfoot strike runners were recruited to complete overground running trials at 3.33 m/s (±5%) in two running shoe conditions (MI = 26% versus MI = 86%). The amount of ten Vicon infrared cameras (100 Hz) and two Kistler force plates (1000 Hz) were used to collect kinematic and ground reaction force (GRF) data simultaneously. Quadriceps strength, patellofemoral contact force, patellofemoral contact area, and patellofemoral contact stress were calculated. Results: No significant differences were observed in the impact force and the second peak of the vertical GRF between the two shoe conditions. Compared to wearing low-MI shoes, wearing high-MI shoes showed that the maximum flexion angle of the knee, the contact area of patellofemoral joint and the peak knee extension moment reduced significantly ($p < 0.01$), and the peak patellofemoral contact force and stress decreased significantly ($p < 0.05$). Conclusion: These findings suggest that wearing high-MI shoes significantly decreases the patellofemoral contact force and patellofemoral joint stress by reducing the moment of knee extension, thus effectively reducing the load of the patellofemoral joint during the stance phase of running and potentially lowering the risk of PFPS.

Keywords: minimalist index; patellofemoral contact force; patellofemoral contact stress; footwear; patellofemoral joint pain syndrome

---

1. Introduction

Hundreds of millions of citizens participate in sports, among which running is widely known. Injury remains high with the popularity of running, with 19.4% to 79.3% sustaining a running-related injury annually [1]; patellofemoral pain syndrome (PFPS) is one of the most common running injuries, exhibiting the highest incidence of 17% in the specific pathologies of running-related injuries [2]. Increased patellofemoral joint stress (PFJS) was determined as an important pathogenic factor [3]. The knee joint features a complex structure; the soft tissue and muscles maintain the stability of the tibia [4]. Thus, any change in mechanics may influence the force distribution around the patellofemoral joint. Studies have shown that patients with patellofemoral joint pain exhibit different biomechanical characteristics during running [5]. Therefore, changes in knee joint torque, patellofemoral contact force and stress during this activity may affect the risk of PFPS. Correspondingly, the mechanism of overwork injury is due to the cumulative effect of repeated high-load work of the muscles and bones [6];

therefore, reducing the knee load to a certain extent may considerably decrease the cumulative effect of long-term running on the knee joint.

With the development of technology, new materials and designs have been applied to sports shoes, especially midsole structures, to reduce the load on the lower extremities. The unique mechanical structures of different sports shoes can change the force characteristics of the human running gait [7]. For healthy runners, wearing different sneakers can affect the biomechanical characteristics of the lower extremities, such as stride frequency, ground contact angle, vertical load rate and joint force [8]. In recent years, barefoot running has become increasingly popular, and many runners have been opting for minimalist shoes, which provide basic protection but limited cushioning. The standardised definition of minimalist shoes, the Minimalist Index (MI), was developed to allow running shoes to be distinguished based on their degree of minimalism, and may help to decrease injuries related to footwear transition [9]. Numerous studies have verified [7,10,11] that minimalist shoes can change the landing posture of the lower limbs, mainly focusing on the adaptation of the ankle joints, that is changing the angle between the foot and the ground, the tendency of forefoot pattern strike and the adaptability of the calf triceps and the Achilles tendon. Relatively few studies have focused on knee load and this condition limits the understanding of the relationship between sneakers and knee joints, especially the patellofemoral joint.

This study aimed to determine the biomechanical characteristics of the patellofemoral joint during running. To achieve this the immediate effects of wearing running shoes with different minimalist indices on patellofemoral contact force (PFCF) and patellofemoral contact stress (PFJS) were explored. Based on the previous observations, it was hypothesized that PFCF and PFJS would decrease when wearing running shoes with high Minimalist Index (MI), e.g., minimalist shoes.

2. Materials and Methods

2.1. Participants

A total of fifteen recreational and healthy male runners (age: 31.4 ± 6.6 years; height: 174.7 ± 6.3 cm; body mass: 73.2 ± 9.8 kg; weekly running volume: 30.6 ± 9.5 km) were recruited. Inclusion criteria were as follows: 1) The weekly running volume in the past month was over 20 km; 2) rearfoot strikers and to be accustomed to wearing cushioned shoes; 3) no experience in barefoot running nor wearing minimalist shoes or special sneakers (e.g., five-finger shoes and racing spikes); 4) suffered no musculoskeletal injuries within three months prior to the tests. A two-tailed t-test was executed via the G*Power 3.1 software (Univ. Kiel, Kiel, Germany) to determine whether a sample size of 15 was sufficient to minimize the probability of type II error for all the variables ($P = 80\%$ at $\alpha = 0.05$).

This study, with detailed guidelines for participants' safety and experimental protocols, was approved by the Institutional Review Board of the Shanghai University of Sport (No. 2017007). The study was conducted in accordance with the declaration of Helsinki. Specifically, all procedures and potential hazards were clarified to the participants in nontechnical terms, and informed consent was signed prior to the tests. All participants had full knowledge of test procedures and requirements.

2.2. Shoe Conditions

A rating scale for the running shoes was developed in accordance with the work of Esculier et al. [9] and the MI was defined as the minimalism of different running shoes. Specifically, the MI of running shoes was calculated according to guidelines by weight, heel-to-toe drop, stack height, motion control/stability technologies and flexibility. The motion control/stability technologies included multi-density midsole, rigid heel counter, elevated medial insole under the foot arch, and tensioned medial upper. Flexibility included longitudinal and torsional flexibility. A high MI indicated high minimalism of running shoes.

In this experiment, the size of the experimental shoes ranged from EUR 41 to 43 based on the foot size of the participants. The used minimalist shoes were the INOV-8 Bare-XF 210 V2 series

(Figure 1). The outsole of the shoe was made of INOV Corp.'s patented viscous rubber, which measured approximately 3 mm in thickness, and the shoes contained no cushioning midsole. The upper was made of a mesh composite material, which was light, breathable, fitted the foot surface and was good for toe movement during running. The heel-to-toe drop of the shoe was 0 mm, the weight (EUR size 42) was 227 g, and the MI = 86%. The used cushioned shoes were the Nike Air Zoom Pegasus 34. EVA foam was used in the midsole of this brand, and a Zoom Air cushion was set in the heel and the forefoot. The heel-to-toe drop was 7 mm, the weight (EUR size 42) was 285 g, and the MI = 26%. The runners were required to wear uniform Nike Dri-FIT socks to eliminate interference. Table 1 shows the specific MI of the two experimental shoes.

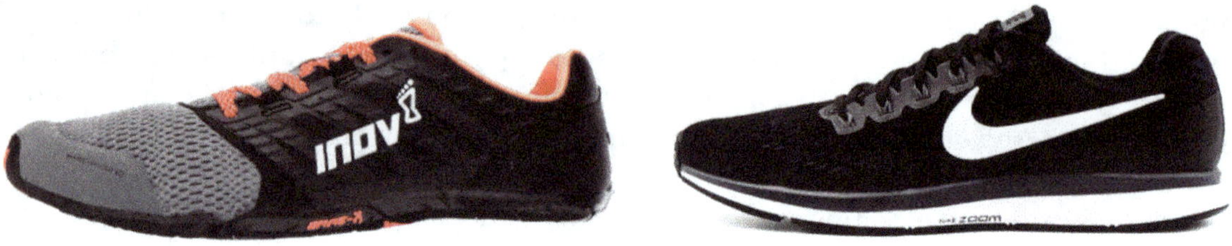

Figure 1. Shoes used in the experiment. Minimalist shoe: INOV-8 Bare-XF 210 V2 (**left**). Cushioned shoe: Nike Air Zoom Pegasus 34 (**right**).

Table 1. Detailed comparison of the Minimalist Index (MI) of the two shoes.

Shoe	Weight (g)	Stack Height (mm)	Heel-to-Toe Drop (mm)	Stability and Motion Control Technologies	Flexibility	MI (%)
INOV-8 Bare-XF 210 V2	227	3	0	None	longitudinal 360° torsional 360°	86
Subscore	2	5	5	5	4.5	
Nike Air Zoom Pegasus 34	285	30	7	Four devices	longitudinal 45°–90° torsional 0°–45°	26
Subscore	1	1	2	1	1.5	

Notes: Four stability and motion control technologies of the Nike Air Zoom Pegasus 34: multi-density midsole, rigid heel counter, supportive tensioned medial upper and medial flare. MI = sum of subscore × 4 × 100%.

2.3. Data Collection

First, the experimental process was explained to the participants and they signed the relevant questionnaire and informed consent. The same uniform sportswear was replaced, and forty infrared retroreflective markers (diameter: 14.0 mm) were attached bilaterally to both of the lower extremities to define hip, knee, and ankle joints according to the plug-in gait marker set [12]. Before the experiment, the participants performed a 5-min warm-up on a treadmill at an optional running speed only with cushioned shoes, followed by a 1-minute 3.33 m/s experimental speed adaptation. Meanwhile, it was the first time that they had worn minimalist shoes, which was considered as "immediately". After completing the preparation, the participants began the formal experimental tests.

Two 90 × 60 × 10 cm Kistler 3D force platforms (9287B, Kistler Corporation, Switzerland) were used to collect ground reaction force (GRF) data at a sampling rate of 1000 Hz. A 10-camera infrared 3D motion capture system (Vicon T40, Oxford Metrics, UK) was used to collect the trajectory markers (14.0 mm in diameter) of the bone landmarks of the lower extremities to define the knee joint at a sampling rate of 100 Hz (Figure 2). The participants randomly wore one of the shoes. A 5–10 minute break was provided between two shoe tests to eliminate the potential interference. Three running trials were collected per condition at 3.33 m/s (±5%). This target speed was common for recreational runners and all participants completed running trials without any discomfort. Running speed was monitored by the use of a Witty-Manual grating timing system (Micro gate, Italy) positioned 4 m apart along a 20 m runway. Meanwhile, the participants were required to run back and forth until three successful steps (trials) in which the foot of the dominant lower extremity (defined as preferred kicking leg [13]) was completely on the force plate were collected for each shoe condition. Each trial that met the following criteria was deemed successful: 1) The speed was 3.33 m/s (±5%) within the capture volume; 2) no relative sliding occurred between the shoes and the force plate.

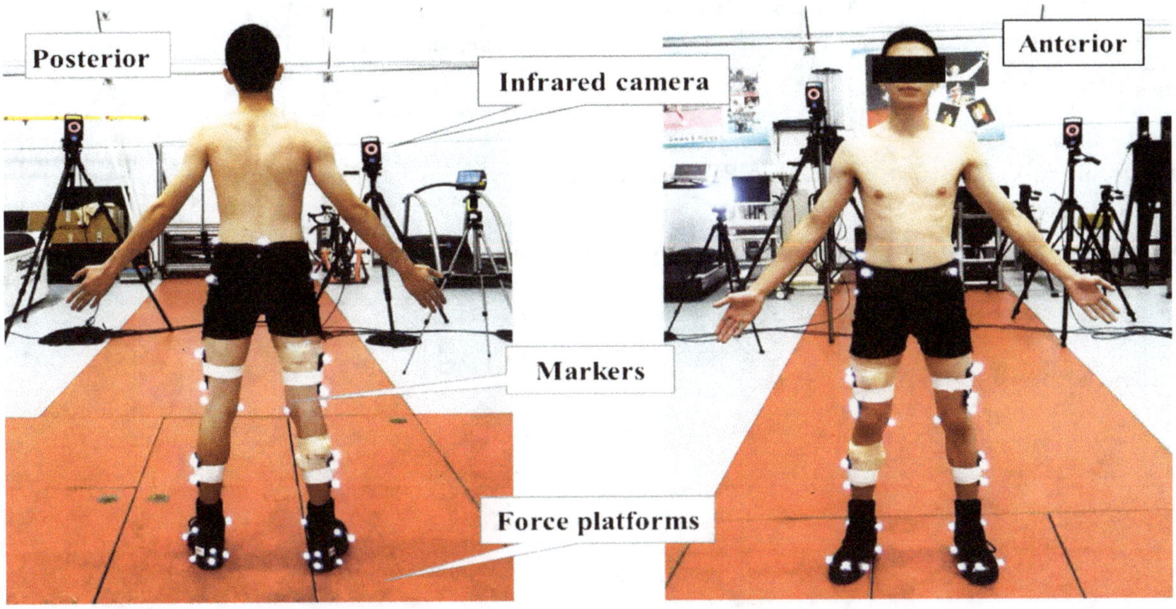

Figure 2. Set of reflective markers used in the study and the experimental setup.

2.4. Data Processing

Knee load during running was generally assessed by the peak torque of knee extension, patellofemoral contact force (PFCF) and patellofemoral contact stress (PFJS) [14,15]. First, marker trajectories were filtered with a cut-off frequency of 7 Hz via the gait analysis software Visual 3D (v5, C-Motion, Inc., Germantown, MD, USA). We established a 3D model in Visual 3D to calculate the GRF, knee flexion angle, torque of knee extension, angle of the knee joint when the runners touch the ground, angle of the ankle joint and the angle between the foot and the ground (foot inclination angle). The relevant parameters of the stance phase were standardised in time (0–100%), and a curve was plotted using the averages to identify the differences between the biomechanical parameters of the knee and various MI running shoes in the entire stand phase. In addition, PFCF, PFJS and related parameters were calculated by referring to previous studies. The details of the cited model were as follows.

The contact area (mm^2) between the patella and femur was a function of the sagittal knee angle and expressed as follows [16]:

$$S_{PFCA} = 0.0781 \times \theta_i{}^2 + 0.06763 \times \theta_i + 151.75 \tag{1}$$

where S_{PFCA} represents the contact area between the patella and the femur, and θ_i (°) was the sagittal angle of knee extension and flexion (Figure 3).

The effective arm of the quadriceps force (L_A, m) was a function of the sagittal knee angle and expressed as follows [17]:

$$L_A = \begin{cases} 0.036\theta_i + 3.0 \ (0 \leq \theta_i < 30°) \\ -0.043\theta_i + 5.4 \ (30 \leq \theta_i < 60°) \\ -0.027\theta_i + 4.3 \ (60 \leq \theta_i < 90°) \\ 2.0 \ (90 \leq \theta_i < 120°) \end{cases} . \tag{2}$$

Quadriceps force (N) was calculated as follows [14]:

$$F_Q(\theta_i) = M_{EXT}(\theta_i)/L_A(\theta_i) \quad (3)$$

where F_Q is the quadriceps force, and M_{EXT} is the extension moment (N·m).

The patellofemoral contact force (F_{PF}, N) was calculated as follows [17]:

$$F_{PF} = 2F_Q\sin(\beta/2) \quad (4)$$

where $\beta = 30.46 + 0.53(\theta_i)$, F_{PF} (N) is PFCF, and β (°) is the angle of the quadriceps line and patellar ligament (Figure 3).

The patellofemoral contact stress (MPa) was calculated as follows:

$$P_{PFS} = F_{PF}/S_{PFCA}(\theta_i) \quad (4)$$

where P_{PFS} is the PFJS.

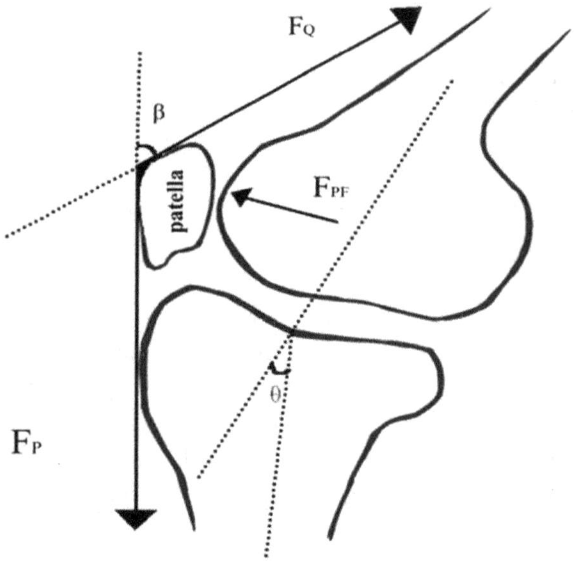

Figure 3. Free-body diagram of the patellofemoral joint. Notes: F_Q refers to the quadriceps muscle strength, F_{PF} denotes the patellofemoral contact force, F_P represents the patellar ligament tension line, β stands for the angle between the quadriceps muscle line and the patellar ligament tension line, and θ is the knee flexion angle.

2.5. Statistics

All the dependent variables were normally distributed, as indicated by the Shapiro–Wilk test. The paired t-test was used to determine the differences in all variables (GRF and joint mechanics) between the MI 86% and MI 26% of shoes (25.0, SPSS Inc., Chicago, IL, USA). The significance level was set as $\alpha = 0.05$.

3. Results

3.1. GRF

The vertical GRF (vGRF) of all the runners using both shoes exhibited two peaks. For the Minimal Index (MI) 86% and MI 26% shoes, no significant differences were observed between the impact force (first peak, FP) and the peak vGRF (second peak, SP) during the stance phase ($p > 0.05$) (Table 2).

3.2. Kinematics

The foot inclination angle at foot strike was positive regardless of shoe conditions, indicating that all the runners ran with a rearfoot strike. No statistical differences were identified between the knee flexion angle and the ankle plantar flexion angle at the moment of foot strike ($p > 0.05$). However, with the MI 86% shoes, the foot inclination angle significantly reduced by 35.6% ($p < 0.05$). Moreover, the peak knee flexion angle and the peak contact area of the patellofemoral joint were significantly lower than those with the MI 26% shoes, in which the peak knee flexion angle decreased by 6.5% and the peak contact area of the patellofemoral joint reduced by 5.4% ($p < 0.05$) (Table 2). The curve of the entire stance phase with the minimalist shoes indicated a considerably lower knee flexion angle than that with the cushioned shoes in the middle and late phases (Figure 4A).

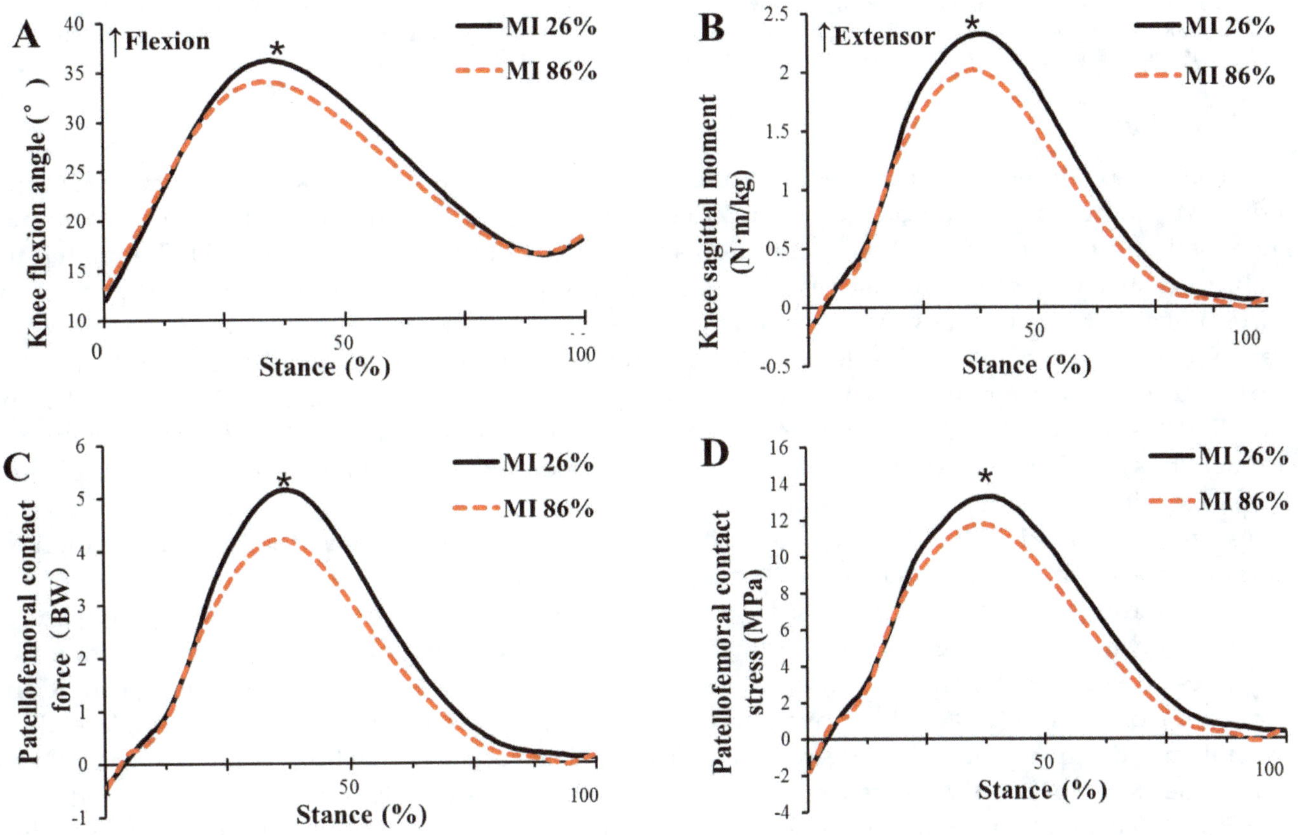

Figure 4. Comparison of the mean values of knee kinematics and kinetics from all participants between shoe conditions (MI 26%: cushioned shoes; MI 86%: minimalist shoes). (**A**) knee flexion angle during stance phase; (**B**) knee sagittal moment during stance phase; (**C**) patellofemoral contact force during stance phase; (**D**) patellofemoral contact stress during stance phase. *$P < 0.05$.

3.3. Kinetics

At the peak knee extension moment, the peaks of PFCF and PFJS were significantly lower with the MI 86% shoes than with the MI 26% shoes, in which, at the peak knee extension moment, the peaks of PFCF and PFJS reduced by 12.3%, 17.0% and 10.4%, respectively ($p < 0.05$) (Table 2). Consistent with the knee flexion angle curve, the curves of the abovementioned knee loading parameters were lower under the MI 86% shoe condition during the middle- and late-stance phases than those under the MI 26% shoe condition (Figure 4B–D).

Table 2. Sagittal plane kinematics and kinetics during running with two different shoe conditions ($\bar{x} \pm$ SD.

Phase	Parameters	MI 26%	MI 86%	p
Touch-down	Knee flexion angle (°)	12.64 ± 4.56	13.56 ± 5.60	0.637
	Ankle plantar flexion angle (°)	0.13 ± 7.92	0.13 ± 4.29	0.835
	Foot inclination angle (°)	12.54 ± 2.18	8.07 ± 4.64	<0.001
Stance phase	FP (BW)	1.74 ± 0.23	1.78 ± 0.16	0.701
	SP (BW)	2.59 ± 0.31	2.61 ± 0.25	0.559
	Peak knee flexion angle (°)	36.29 ± 3.41	33.93 ± 1.74	0.008
	Peak patellofemoral joint contact area (mm^2)	280.10 ± 21.96	265.08 ± 10.20	0.008
	Peak knee extension moment (N × m/kg)	2.36 ± 0.41	2.07 ± 0.47	<0.001
	Peak patellofemoral contact force (BW)	5.23 ± 1.12	4.34 ± 0.97	<0.001
	Peak patellofemoral contact stress (MPa)	13.48 ± 2.64	12.08 ± 3.27	0.015

Notes: Foot inclination angle is the angle between the foot and the ground. The FP (the first peak of the vGRF) and SP (the second peak of the vGRF), knee extension moment and patellofemoral contact force are standardised by body weight (BW). MI 86%: minimalist shoes. MI 26%: cushioned shoes.

4. Discussion

This study aimed to determine the immediate effects of wearing shoes with different Minimal Index (MI) on the patellofemoral joints and to explore whether directly changing shoes can reduce knee load and the risk of patellofemoral pain syndrome (PFPS). The conventional belief is that the cushioned structure of running shoes can reduce the impact force during running and protect the lower limbs. In this study, however, the MI 26% shoes caused no change in the impact force during the stance phase and the ankle/knee flexion angle at touchdown compared with those with the MI 86% shoes. Moreover, during the transition and propulsive phases of the stance phase (20–100%), wearing the MI 86% shoes can effectively reduce the patellofemoral contact force (PFCF) and patellofemoral contact stress (PFJS) by changing the parameters of knee loads, such as the knee flexion angle and knee extension moment. The mechanism of PFPS is that the patellofemoral joints are subjected to excessively high loads [14,18,19]. Therefore, the results of this study suggest that running in high-MI running shoes might be beneficial for reducing the risk of PFPS.

This finding is consistent with those in previous studies [20,21]. Sinclair and Esculier [7,8] reported that the body actively changed the lower limb strategy while wearing minimalist shoes, i.e., increased step rates, lowered foot inclination angle at foot strike and reduced knee maximum flexion angle and joint range of motion (ROM). Moreover, according to the equation for the knee joint angle and the patellofemoral joint contact area, a decreased knee ROM decreased the patellofemoral joint contact area during the stance phase of runners wearing minimalist shoes; this condition is adverse to the reduction of PFJS. By contrast, runners with high-MI shoes showed a considerably smaller knee extension moment during the propulsive phase, which substantially reduced PFCF and, eventually, the PFJS decreased by 10.4%. Furthermore, we explored the characteristics of PFCF and PFJS during the entire stance phase with minimalist shoes. Findings showed that in the 0–20% stance phase (braking phase), the curves were coincident on different shoe conditions (Figure 4), and the differences between the two shoes mostly occurred from 20% to 100% of the stance phase. First, the initial 20% of the stance phase is the braking phase. At this phase, the lower limbs were subjected to the impact of the ground, and the vGRF reached the FP (impact force). The results of the current study showed no significant difference in the impact or propulsive force (SP of vGRF) between the low- and high-MI shoes. The braking phase accounts for 1/4 of the entire stance phase, and this study suggests that wearing high-MI shoes is beneficial for decreasing knee load in the propulsive phase (20–100%). According to recent research supporting barefoot running, running shoes not only reduce the impact force and loading rate and filter high-frequency impact signals [22] but also provide different neural inputs to the lower limbs, resulting in different responses and changes in the lower limb strategy [23]. As shown in this study, the lower limbs actively changed the knee flexion angle and extension moment when the runner was wearing minimalist shoes during the propulsive phase. This phase accounts for a large proportion and may be important for reducing the patellofemoral joint loads.

Using the rating scale for minimalist shoes, this study compared minimalist shoes (MI = 86%) with cushioned shoes (MI = 26%) to further explore the relationship between knee joint load and the MI. Esculier [8] tested shoes with different MI with regards to running mechanics and observed that a higher MI shoe indicates a low foot inclination angle at foot strike and a low peak PFCF. Sinclair [7] compared minimalist, cushioned and maximalist shoes in terms of patellofemoral kinetics and observed that the knee ROM decreased when the runner was wearing minimalist shoes. Interestingly, the patellofemoral joint loads were greater with the low-MI shoes, i.e., maximalist shoes, than with the others. The above findings are similar to the results of this study. Shoes with low MI caused no reduction in the patellofemoral joint loading despite the thick midsole. By contrast, the neural inputs caused by the cushioning midsole resulted in a reduced limb movement strategy with increased knee flexion angle and knee extension moment, which may increase the risk of knee joint load and PFPS.

In previous studies, subjects were recruited regardless of their foot strike patterns and researchers failed to rule out runners who had experience with wearing minimalist shoes [13]. More than 70% of long-distance runners adopt the heel strike pattern [24,25]. Horvais noted that heel strikers use the midfoot or forefoot strike pattern during the adaptation process when wearing minimalist shoes for the first time [26]. In the current study, the vGRF graph showed two peaks, and the foot inclination angle at the point of foot strike was positive. Therefore, the runners still used the heel strike pattern after wearing the minimalist shoes [27], but the foot inclination angle at the point of foot strike still reduced by 35.6%.

Furthermore, adopting the heel strike pattern while wearing minimalist shoes on hard ground would cause heel pain. The runners who are used to rearfoot running have difficulties in switching to forefoot strike immediately when wearing minimalist shoes for a short distance. Correspondingly, runners will actively attempt to use the midfoot or forefoot strike pattern to avoid pain (various reasons lead to changes in foot strike patterns when transitioning to minimalist shoes) during longer running distances [28]. Numerous studies have shown that the reduced PFCF and PFJS in forefoot strike running can also reduce knee loads and PFPS [16,21,29]. Therefore, the analysis of the long-term effects of switching to high-MI running shoes on patellofemoral joint loads still needs to be confirmed.

In general, an adaptive process occurs when we first wear high-MI shoes. Wearing high-MI shoes, e.g., minimalist shoes, is similar to barefoot running, which has certain requirements (increased strength of the plantar muscles) [30]. Lieberman [31] stated that the function of the foot in human evolution is to adapt to barefoot walking or running, and humans began wearing cushioned shoes only in the last hundred years. Thus, the biomechanical characteristics of the foot may not be fully adapted to current cushioned shoes. The plantar muscles of runners who are accustomed to wearing cushioned shoes may lack strength to wear minimalist shoes for a long period, consequently resulting in fatigue and foot injury. Meanwhile, minimalist shoes change the runner's strike patterns to the forefoot, which requires increased calf triceps strength [32]. Therefore, in switching to high-MI shoes, the runner should gradually increase the duration of running in minimalist shoes based on previous running time and distances, thereby gradually improving the related muscle strength and the lower limb/foot adaptability.

Several limitations should be considered in this investigation that could be addressed in follow-up studies. First, we only considered the immediate shoe influence on patellofemoral joint loads. Therefore, the assessment of knee muscle forces or activation was warranted to provide further evidence of neuro-musculoskeletal reactions. Second, a long-term effect of wearing different MI shoes and the gender effects should ideally be taken into account. Finally, one should be cautioned that the differences in leg length were not considered in this study.

5. Conclusions

Patellofemoral joint loads during running were immediately changed by wearing shoes with different Minimalist Index (MI). In particular, while maintaining similar running velocity, wearing high-MI shoes significantly decreased patellofemoral contact force (PFCF) and patellofemoral contact stress (PFJS)—compared with those with low-MI shoes—by reducing the knee extension moment. This condition effectively reduced the loads on the patellofemoral joint during the mid-stance phase of running, thereby possibly reducing the risk of patellofemoral pain syndrome (PFPS).

Author Contributions: C.Y., S.X., contributed equally. Conceptualization, W.F.; methodology, C.Y., S.X.; formal analysis, C.Y., Y.Y., X.Z., J.W. and S.X.; investigation, C.Y., S.X., Y.Y., X.Z., J.W. and W.F.; resources, W.F.; data curation, X.Z.; writing—original draft preparation, C.Y., S.X.; writing—review and editing, W.F.; project administration, W.F.; funding acquisition, W.F.

References

1. Van Gent, R.N.; Siem, D.; van Middelkoop, M.; van Os, A.G.; Bierma-Zeinstra, S.M.; Koes, B.W. Incidence and determinants of lower extremity running injuries in long distance runners: A systematic review. *Br. J. Sports Med.* **2007**, *41*, 469–480. [CrossRef] [PubMed]
2. Ceyssens, L.; Vanelderen, R.; Barton, C.; Malliaras, P.; Dingenen, B. Biomechanical Risk Factors Associated with Running-Related Injuries: A Systematic Review. *Sports Med.* **2019**, *49*, 1095–1115. [CrossRef] [PubMed]
3. Dutton, R.A.; Khadavi, M.J.; Fredericson, M. Patellofemoral Pain. *Phys. Med. Rehabil. Clin. N. Am.* **2016**, *27*, 31–52. [CrossRef] [PubMed]
4. Jordan, M.J.; Aagaard, P.; Herzog, W. A comparison of lower limb stiffness and mechanical muscle function in ACL-reconstructed, elite, and adolescent alpine ski racers/ski cross athletes. *J. Sport Health Sci.* **2018**, *7*, 416–424. [CrossRef]
5. Neal, B.S.; Barton, C.J.; Gallie, R.; O'Halloran, P.; Morrissey, D. Runners with patellofemoral pain have altered biomechanics which targeted interventions can modify: A systematic review and meta-analysis. *Gait Posture* **2016**, *45*, 69–82. [CrossRef] [PubMed]
6. Del Coso, J.; Herrero, H.; Salinero, J.J. Injuries in Spanish female soccer players. *J. Sport Health Sci.* **2018**, *7*, 183–190. [CrossRef]
7. Sinclair, J.; Richards, J.; Selfe, J.; Fau-Goodwin, J.; Shore, H. The Influence of Minimalist and Maximalist Footwear on Patellofemoral Kinetics During Running. *J. Appl. Biomech.* **2016**, *32*, 359–364. [CrossRef]
8. Esculier, J.F.; Dubois, B.; Bouyer, L.J.; McFadyen, B.J.; Roy, J.S. Footwear characteristics are related to running mechanics in runners with patellofemoral pain. *Gait Posture* **2017**, *54*, 144–147. [CrossRef]
9. Esculier, J.F.; Dubois, B.; Dionne, C.E.; Leblond, J.; Roy, J.S. A consensus definition and rating scale for minimalist shoes. *J. Foot Ankl. Res.* **2015**, *8*, 42. [CrossRef]
10. Squadrone, R.; Rodano, R.; Hamill, J.; Preatoni, E. Acute effect of different minimalist shoes on foot strike pattern and kinematics in rearfoot strikers during running. *J. Sports Sci.* **2015**, *33*, 1196–1204. [CrossRef]
11. Rice, H.M.; Jamison, S.T.; Davis, I.S. Footwear Matters: Influence of Footwear and Foot Strike on Load Rates during Running. *Med. Sci. Sports Exerc.* **2016**, *48*, 2462–2468. [CrossRef] [PubMed]
12. Xia, R.; Zhang, X.; Wang, X.; Sun, X.; Fu, W. Effects of Two Fatigue Protocols on Impact Forces and Lower Extremity Kinematics during Drop Landings: Implications for Noncontact Anterior Cruciate Ligament Injury. *J. Healthc. Eng.* **2017**, *2017*, 5690519. [CrossRef] [PubMed]
13. Sun, X.; Yang, Y.; Wang, L.; Zhang, X.; Fu, W. Do Strike Patterns or Shoe Conditions have a Predominant Influence on Foot Loading? *J. Hum. Kinet.* **2018**, *64*, 13–23. [CrossRef] [PubMed]
14. Heino Brechter, J.; Powers, C.M. Patellofemoral stress during walking in persons with and without patellofemoral pain. *Med. Sci. Sports Exerc.* **2002**, *34*, 1582–1593. [CrossRef] [PubMed]
15. Dos Santos, A.F.; Nakagawa, T.H.; Serrao, F.V.; Ferber, R. Patellofemoral joint stress measured across three different running techniques. *Gait Posture* **2019**, *68*, 37–43. [CrossRef] [PubMed]

16. Vannatta, C.N.; Kernozek, T.W. Patellofemoral joint stress during running with alterations in foot strike pattern. *Med. Sci. Sports Exerc.* **2015**, *47*, 1001–1008. [CrossRef] [PubMed]
17. Bressel, E. The influence of ergometer pedaling direction on peak patellofemoral joint forces. *Clin. Biomech.* **2001**, *16*, 431–437. [CrossRef]
18. LaBella, C. Patellofemoral pain syndrome: Evaluation and treatment. *Prim. Care* **2004**, *31*, 977–1003. [CrossRef]
19. Besier, T.F.; Gold, G.E.; Beaupre, G.S.; Delp, S.L. A modeling framework to estimate patellofemoral joint cartilage stress in vivo. *Med. Sci. Sports Exerc.* **2005**, *37*, 1924–1930. [CrossRef]
20. Sinclair, J. Effects of barefoot and barefoot inspired footwear on knee and ankle loading during running. *Clin. Biomech.* **2014**, *29*, 395–399. [CrossRef]
21. Kulmala, J.P.; Avela, J.; Pasanen, K.; Parkkari, J. Forefoot strikers exhibit lower running-induced knee loading than rearfoot strikers. *Med. Sci. Sports Exerc.* **2013**, *45*, 2306–2313. [CrossRef] [PubMed]
22. Nigg, B.M.; Baltich, J.; Hoerzer, S.; Enders, H. Running shoes and running injuries: Mythbusting and a proposal for two new paradigms: 'preferred movement path' and 'comfort filter'. *Br. J. Sports Med.* **2015**, *49*, 1290–1294. [CrossRef]
23. Holowka, N.B.; Wynands, B.; Drechsel, T.J.; Yegian, A.K.; Tobolsky, V.A.; Okutoyi, P.; Mang'eni Ojiambo, R.; Haile, D.W.; Sigei, T.K.; Zippenfennig, C.; et al. Foot callus thickness does not trade off protection for tactile sensitivity during walking. *Nature* **2019**, *571*, 261–264. [CrossRef] [PubMed]
24. Hasegawa, H.; Yamauchi, T.; Kraemer, W.J. Foot strike patterns of runners at the 15-km point during an elite-level half marathon. *J. Strength Cond. Res.* **2007**, *21*, 888–893. [CrossRef] [PubMed]
25. Kasmer, M.E.; Liu, X.C.; Roberts, K.G.; Valadao, J.M. Foot-strike pattern and performance in a marathon. *Int. J. Sports Physiol. Perform.* **2013**, *8*, 286–292. [CrossRef]
26. Bonacci, J.; Hall, M.; Saunders, N.; Vicenzino, B. Gait retraining versus foot orthoses for patellofemoral pain: A pilot randomised clinical trial. *J. Sci. Med. Sport* **2018**, *21*, 457–461. [CrossRef]
27. Lieberman, D.E.; Venkadesan, M.; Werbel, W.A.; Daoud, A.I.; D'Andrea, S.; Davis, I.S.; Mang'eni, R.O.; Pitsiladis, Y. Foot strike patterns and collision forces in habitually barefoot versus shod runners. *Nature* **2010**, *463*, 531–535. [CrossRef]
28. Perl, D.P.; Daoud, A.I.; Lieberman, D.E. Effects of footwear and strike type on running economy. *Med. Sci. Sports Exerc.* **2012**, *44*, 1335–1343. [CrossRef]
29. Roper, J.L.; Harding, E.M.; Doerfler, D.; Dexter, J.G.; Kravitz, L.; Dufek, J.S.; Mermier, C.M. The effects of gait retraining in runners with patellofemoral pain: A randomized trial. *Clin. Biomech.* **2016**, *35*, 14–22. [CrossRef]
30. Ervilha, U.F.; Mochizuki, L.; Figueira, A., Jr.; Hamill, J. Are muscle activation patterns altered during shod and barefoot running with a forefoot footfall pattern? *J. Sports Sci.* **2017**, *35*, 1697–1703. [CrossRef]
31. Holowka, N.B.; Wallace, I.J.; Lieberman, D.E. Foot strength and stiffness are related to footwear use in a comparison of minimally- vs. conventionally-shod populations. *Sci. Rep.* **2018**, *8*, 3679. [CrossRef] [PubMed]
32. Takabayashi, T.; Edama, M.; Nakamura, M.; Nakamura, E.; Inai, T.; Kubo, M. Gender differences associated with rearfoot, midfoot, and forefoot kinematics during running. *Eur. J. Sport Sci.* **2017**, *17*, 1289–1296. [CrossRef] [PubMed]

17

Simple Assessment of Height and Length of Flight in Complex Gymnastic Skills: Validity and Reliability of a Two-Dimensional Video Analysis Method

Christoph Schärer [1,2,*], Luca von Siebenthal [1], Ishbel Lomax [1], Micah Gross [1], Wolfgang Taube [2] and Klaus Hübner [1]

1 Department of Elite Sport, Swiss Federal Institute of Sport (SFISM), 2532 Magglingen, Switzerland; lvsiebenthal@gmail.com (L.v.S.); ishbel.lomax@gmail.com (I.L.); micah.gross@baspo.admin.ch (M.G.); huebner@baspo.admin.ch (K.H.)

2 Department of Neuroscience and Movement Science, University of Fribourg, 1700 Fribourg, Switzerland; wolfgang.taube@unifr.ch

* Correspondence: christoph.schaerer@baspo.admin.ch;

Abstract: In artistic gymnastics, the possibility of using 2D video analysis to measure the peak height (h_{peak}) and length of flight (L) during routine training in order to monitor the execution and development of difficult elements is intriguing. However, the validity and reliability of such measurements remain unclear. Therefore, in this study, the h_{peak} and L of 38 vaults, performed by top-level gymnasts, were assessed by 2D and 3D analysis in order to evaluate criterion validity and both intrarater and interrater reliability of the 2D method. Validity calculations showed higher accuracy for h_{peak} (±95% LoA: ±3.6% of average peak height) than for L (±95% LoA: ±7.6% of average length). Minor random errors, but no systematic errors, were observed in the examination of intrarater reliability (h_{peak}: $CV\% = 0.44\%, p = 0.81$; L: $CV\% = 0.87\%, p = 0.14$) and interrater reliability (h_{peak}: $CV\% = 0.51\%, p = 0.55$; L: $CV\% = 0.72\%, p = 0.44$). In conclusion, the validity and reliability of the 2D method are deemed sufficient (particularly for h_{peak}, but with some limitations for L) to justify its use in routine training of the vault. Due to its simplicity and low cost, this method could be an attractive monitoring tool for gymnastics coaches.

Keywords: two-dimensional video analysis; validity; reliability; quantitative biomechanical parameters; artistic gymnastics

---

1. Introduction

Video analysis is common in elite sports and covers different areas of application. In individual sports, especially acrobatic sports, video analysis is used to compare and improve complex skills [1]. For quantifying biomechanical aspects of such skills, such as score-relevant kinematic variables of vaults in artistic gymnastics, 3D motion capture (3D video analysis) is used. [2,3]. By means of video analyses, Brehmer and Naundorf [4] created reference values for kinematic parameters, indicating the safe execution of vaults. To make use of such reference values, measuring certain kinematic parameters in routine training becomes crucial, so that gymnasts' performances can be compared with the requirements of certain vaults. In regard to monitoring training progress, using video analysis during routine training is intriguing [2,3].

The gold standard for complex kinematic analyses is 3D motion capture, with which movements can be analyzed in sagittal, frontal, and transversal planes simultaneously [5]. However, precise 3D motion capture is associated with considerable financial, spatial, and temporal issues, and is therefore uncommon in routine training settings [6]. Two-dimensional video analysis (2D analysis), if sufficiently accurate, could offer a more practical alternative for measuring kinematics during training, especially since advancements in smartphone and tablet technology are continually making high-definition video capture and analysis more convenient. Aside from convenience while capturing motion, 2D video is faster, cheaper, and requires less prior knowledge compared to 3D analysis [1,7]. Nonetheless, although multiple studies showed moderate validity compared to 3D motion capture and high intrarater reliability of 2D analysis when examining joint angles during simple movements, such as single-leg squats and running [1,5–7], the validity and reliability of 2D video analysis for complex skills in acrobatic sports are unclear and must be scientifically assessed before this method can be recommended for gymnastics. The validity and reliability of 2D analysis were deemed sufficient for measuring the flight time and height of vertical jumps, when compared to optical measurement systems (Opto Jump, Microgate, I) [8] or to a force plate [9]. Further, 2D analysis was deemed valid (ICC = 0.8) and reliable (ICC > 0.85) for measuring joint angles during the more complex skill of baseball pitching, as long as the camera was placed properly [1], so the possibility of it being useful in gymnastics seems worthy of investigation.

In summary, the studies mentioned above offer justification for using simple, time-saving, and cost-effective 2D analysis for simple lower-extremity movements based on good validity and reliability compared to gold-standard methods. However, in contrast to movements in previous studies, artistic gymnastics involve highly complex movements that are performed with high accelerations and velocities. Therefore, the aim of this study was to investigate criterion validity (comparison of 2D to 3D analysis) and both intrarater (test-retest) and interrater (equivalence of two assessors) reliability of 2D video analysis for the peak height (h_{peak}) and length of flight (L) of vaults in artistic gymnastics.

2. Materials and Methods

Twenty-two junior and international elite gymnasts (female: n = 5; male: n = 17) volunteered to participate in the study. All subjects gave written informed consent before participating in the study. All study procedures were approved by the ethics committee Bern (17.01.2017; Project-ID: 2016-01970) and conducted in accordance with the current version of the Declaration of Helsinki, the ICH-GCP, ISO EN 14155, and all national legal and regulatory requirements.

In total, 38 vaults were used for assessment. These included vaults from the three most important vault categories (handspring, Tsukahara, and Yurchenko) and comprised a variety of different sagittal plane rotations (tuck/double tuck, pike/double pike, and layout), which were combined with up to three turns around the longitudinal axis. These vaults were simultaneously recorded with conventional 2D video and a 3D motion capture system (Vicon Motion System, Denver, CO, USA) and analyzed to determine h_{peak} and L in the second flight phase.

For 2D analysis, vaults were filmed using an iPad (iPad Pro 9.7", Apple Corporation, Cupertino, CA, USA) at 100 frames/s. The lens of the iPad was placed at a height of 1.55 m and at a distance of 10 m from the vaulting table, so that the take-off, first and second flight phases, and landing were all visible. The height and width of the image were calibrated within the analytical software (Dartfish SA, Fribourg, CH) by using a rod of known length (2.78 m) that was held vertically and horizontally along the landing zone (Figure 1). With the Dartfish software, h_{peak} was measured as the vertical distance between the landing mat and the gymnast's center of gravity at its highest point during the second flight phase of the vault. For this, the gymnast's center of gravity was estimated visually in the video frame at which the maximal height was deemed to have occurred. L was determined as the horizontal distance between the ankle at the foot's first contact with the mat upon landing and the end of the vaulting table (Figure 2). The software then automatically calculated h_{peak} and L by using the reference height and length.

For the 3D analysis, all vaults were captured by 14 Vicon Vantage Cameras (Vicon Motion System, Denver, CO, USA) that were arranged in two planes: eight cameras were placed at a height of 5.50 m and six were placed at a height of 1.70 m (Figure 3) above ground level. Forty-three reflective markers were placed on the gymnasts' bodies, according to the Vicon Plug-in Gait model [10] (Figure 4). For capturing and, afterward, determining h_{peak} and L, Vicon Nexus, version 2.6, Vicon Motion System, Denver, CO, USA) software was used.

The 2D videos were analyzed by a first-time assessor and an experienced assessor. The first-time assessor was only briefly introduced to the relevant functions of the software (reference measurements) and the important aspects of the measurement of h_{peak} and L (e.g., determination of the center of gravity at the maximum height of flight) before evaluating the trials.

The parameters determined by the first-time assessor ($2D_1$) were compared to those obtained by 3D analysis to assess criterion validity of 2D analysis ($2D_1$ vs. 3D). Further, the parameters were determined with Dartfish (Dartfish SA, Fribourg, CH) by the same assessor at two different points in time (first measurement: $2D_1$; second measurement: $2D_2$) and by an experienced assessor ($2D_e$) to verify intrarater ($2D_1$ vs. $2D_2$) and interrater reliability ($2D_1$ vs. $2D_e$).

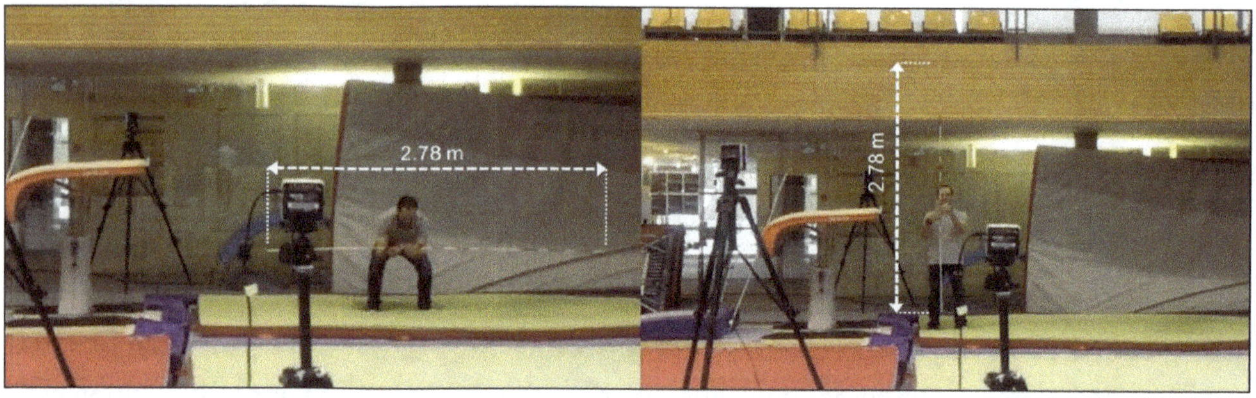

Figure 1. 2D calibration: calibration of measuring range by definition of reference height and width with the calibration rod (2.78 m) in the 2D-video software Dartfish (Dartfish SA, Fribourg, CH).

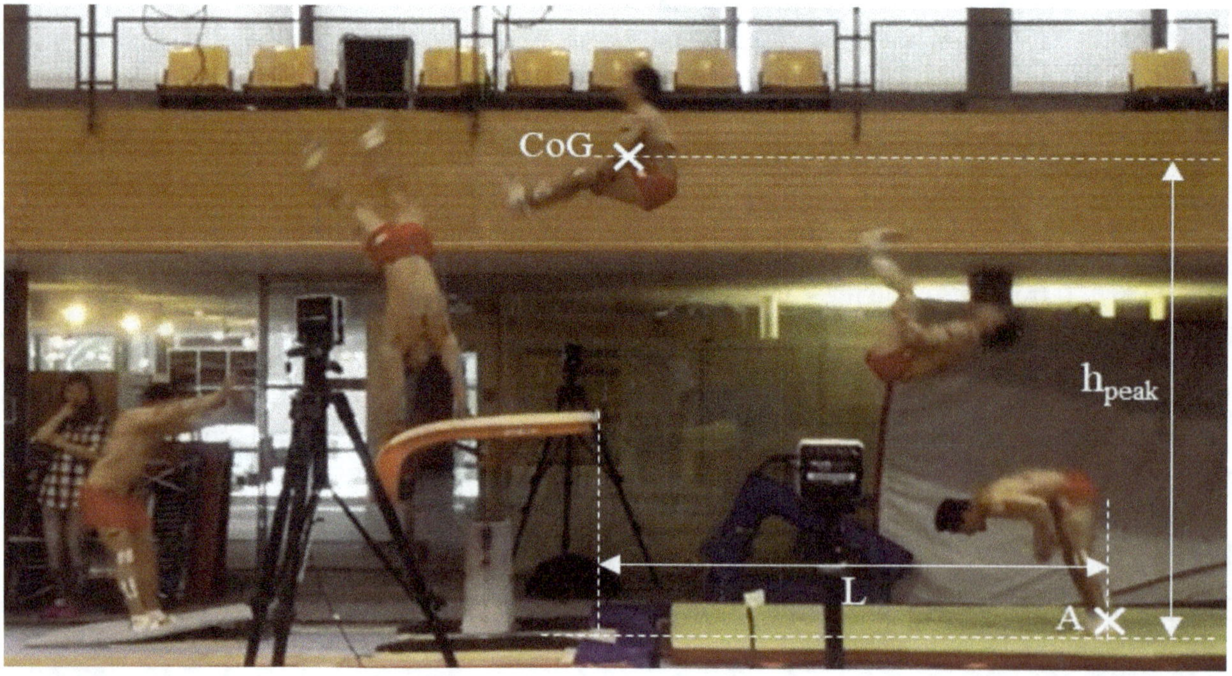

Figure 2. 2D measurements: determination of peak height (h_{peak}) and length of flight (L) for a "Yeo" Vault (CoG: position of center of gravity at the highest point of the second flight phase; A: position of the ankle at first foot contact).

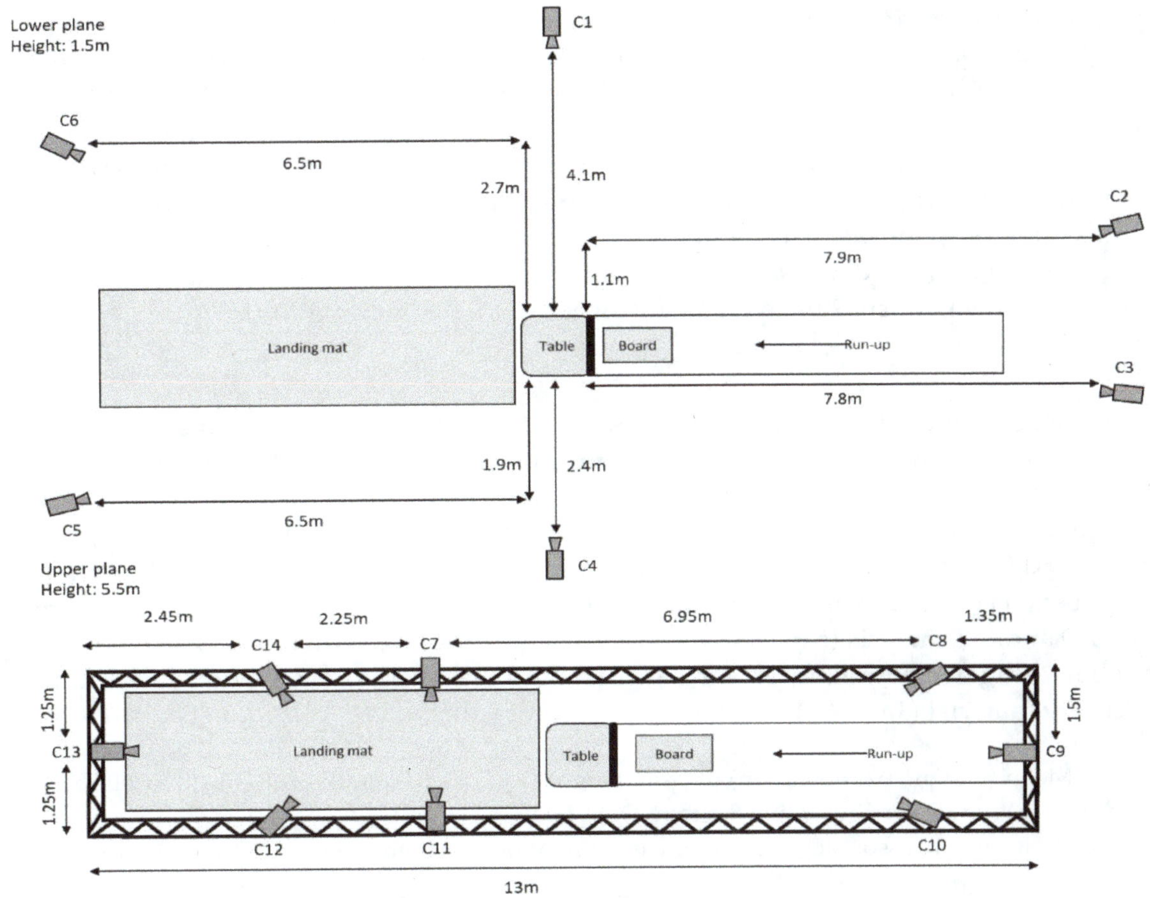

Figure 3. Placement of 3D cameras: positioning of the 14 Vicon Vantage Cameras (C1–C14) in an upper and lower plane for three-dimensional recording of vaults.

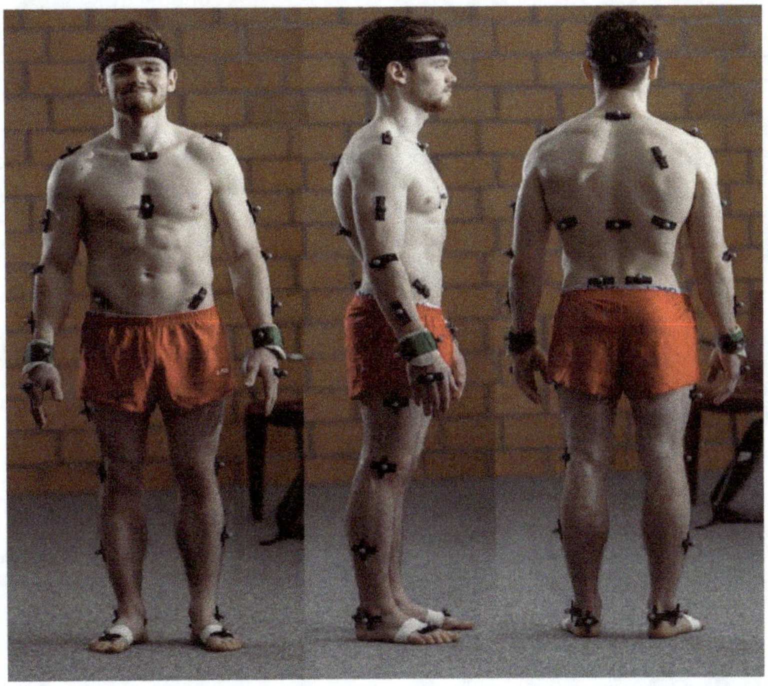

Figure 4. Plug-in Gait model: positioning of 43 markers for 3D analysis, attached to the athlete according to Vicon Plug-in Gait model [10].

Mean, standard deviation, Pearson's correlation coefficient (r), random error (*CV*%), typical error (*TE*), and systematic error (t-test: p) of h_{peak} and L measurements were calculated to determine criterion validity (3D vs. $2D_1$) and both intrarater ($2D_1$ vs. $2D_2$) and interrater reliability ($2D_1$ vs. $2D_e$), according to Hopkins et al. [11]. The comparison between the 3D and $2D_1$ measurements (criterion validity) is displayed in a Bland–Altman diagram [12]. In order to determine the influence of lateral displacement at landing on the accuracy of the 2D measurements, the relationship between the difference in L (2D–3D measurement) and displacement along the x axis (to the left or right) was calculated. The level of statistical significance was set to $p < 0.05$. Data analysis was conducted using Microsoft Excel spreadsheets (Microsoft Excel 2016, Microsoft Corporation, Redmond, WA, USA).

3. Results

Two-dimensional analysis ($2D_1$) showed small differences in mean compared to 3D analysis (Table 1). The ±95% limits of agreement corresponded to measurement errors of ±3.6% for h_{peak} and ±7.6% for L (Figure 5). Regarding the validity and reliability of 2D analysis, high correlation coefficients and minor random errors for the h_{peak} and L of vaults were found (Table 2). In contrast, there was a tendency for a systematic error for h_{peak} with 2D compared to 3D analysis. Further, we found a significant correlation between the lateral displacement (x axis) at landing and the difference in L between 2D and 3D analysis ($r = 0.58$; $p < 0.01$). The ex post facto power analysis revealed a power of ~1 for all investigated correlations. The data of all measurements in this study can be found in the supplementary material (Table S1).

Table 1. Mean (± standard deviation) of peak height (h_{peak}) and length of flight (L) of all recorded vaults (n = 38) for 3D (Vicon Motion System, Denver, USA) and 2D analyses (Dartfish SA, Fribourg, CH; $2D_1$: first-time assessor; $2D_2$: second measurement of first-time assessor; $2D_e$: expert assessor).

	h_{peak} ± SD (m)	L ± SD (m)
3D	2.73 ± 0.24	2.29 ± 0.49
$2D_1$	2.75 ± 0.24	2.28 ± 0.51
$2D_2$	2.75 ± 0.24	2.27 ± 0.51
$2D_e$	2.75 ± 0.24	2.27 ± 0.52

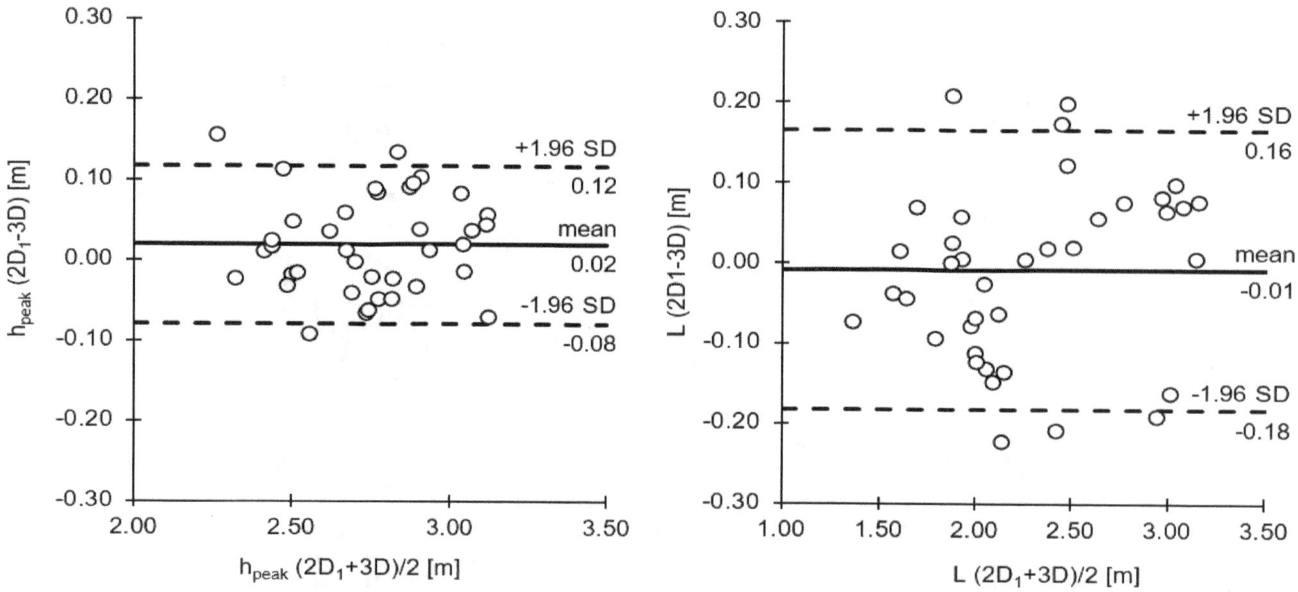

Figure 5. Validity: Bland–Altman diagrams comparing 2D and 3D analyses of peak height (h_{peak}) and length of flight (L) of vaults (n = 38). $2D_1$: two-dimensional video analysis with Dartfish SA of a first-time assessor); 3D: three-dimensional motion capture with Vicon Motion System).

Table 2. Random error (CV%), typical error (TE), correlation coefficient, and systematic error (p) of peak height (h_{peak}) and length of flight (L) of vauls, when comparing first 2D video analysis ($2D_1$) evaluations to 3D motion capture (validity) and to second 2D analysis (intrarater reliability), as well as second 2D video analysis ($2D_2$) and expert 2D video analysis ($2D_e$) (interrater reliability).

	h_{peak}				L			
	CV%	TE (cm)	r	p	CV%	TE (cm)	r	p
Validity	2.24	6.16	0.97	0.06	4.64	10.59	0.98	0.43
Intrarater reliability	0.44	1.21	0.99	0.81	0.87	1.98	0.99	0.14
Interrater reliability	0.51	1.40	0.99	0.55	0.72	1.63	0.99	0.44

4. Discussion

This paper is the first to evaluate the validity and reliability of 2D video analysis of the h_{peak} and L of vaults in artistic gymnastics. Compared to 3D analysis (validity), 2D analysis showed smaller ±95% limits of agreement for h_{peak} (±3.6%) than for L (±7.6%). Further, we found smaller random errors for h_{peak} (CV% = 2.24%) than for L (CV% = 4.64%). In contrast, there was a tendency toward a systematic error of h_{peak} ($p = 0.06$), but not for L ($p = 0.43$). Regarding reliability, the h_{peak} and L of vaults can be repeatedly (intrarater reliability: h_{peak}: CV% = 0.44%, $r = 0.99$; L: CV% = 0.87%, $r > 0.99$) and independently (interrater reliability: h_{peak}: CV% = 0.51%, $r = 0.99$; L: CV% = 0.72%, $r > 0.99$) determined by 2D analysis.

The results support 2D video analysis as a valid measurement tool—particularly for determining the h_{peak}, but slightly less so for the L, of vaults in gymnastics. Our findings are in line with those of Balsalobre-Fernandez, Tejero-Gonzalez, del Campo-Vecino, and Bavaresco [9], who have shown that 2D analysis is a valid technique for accurately measuring the flight height of vertical jumps. Thus, under the described measurement conditions, an increase of at least 6.16 cm in h_{peak} or of at least 10.59 cm in L, measured by 2D video analysis, can be considered a true performance increase.

Differences in the validity between the h_{peak} and L of vaults, as shown in the Bland–Altman diagram, may have several reasons. The most obvious is that 2D analysis measures the height and length of flight in the sagittal plane only. Accordingly, lateral displacement at the landing cannot be detected by 2D analysis and presents a possible confounding factor. This was shown by the significant relationship between lateral displacement upon landing and the difference between 2D and 3D determinations of L. This result supports research by Oyama, Sosa, Campbell, and Correa [1], who compared 2D to 3D analysis of joint angles during complex movements. They found that 2D analysis is a valid measure only when cameras are placed perpendicular to the segment of interest. This limitation of 2D analysis was less important for the measurement of h_{peak}, because the lateral displacement is at its maximum at landing, long after the attainment of h_{peak}. Further, since L was determined as the distance between the vaulting table and the ankle, even straddled legs at landing may result in a lateral displacement and may lead to a measurement error of 2D analysis. In contrast, h_{peak} was measured vertically from the landing mat to the center of gravity. Therefore, the determination of h_{peak} did not depend on the position of one single extremity but on the highest point on the center of gravity's smooth trajectory.

Another reason for the less accurate measurement of L could be the quality of the 2D videos (resolution and frame rate). The still frame at landing was often slightly blurred due to the velocity of the recorded movement. Therefore, it was difficult in some cases to determine the position of the ankle precisely, and, for this reason, small measurement errors may have occurred. In contrast, the slightly blurred image did not affect the determination of the center of gravity for the measurement of h_{peak}, since the determination of the center of gravity depends on a global view of the body and not on a small single part of the body.

One more reason for the larger inaccuracy in the determination of L may be the slight bend in the calibration rod when it was held horizontally to scale the image width (Figure 1). This would have caused the reference length to be slightly too long, although this effect was too small to be apparent in our results (nonsignificant p-value).

In this study, we observed a tendency toward a systematic underestimation of h_{peak} with 2D analysis. Since the measurements of the experienced assessor were not statistically different from the values of the first-time assessor, it can be assumed that both assessors encountered the same basic problem that may have led to this tendency. In particular, it was difficult to determine the zero-point on the landing mat vertically underneath the highest point of the center of gravity during the second flight phase. We assume that this was the reason for the (almost significant) underestimation of h_{peak}. Nonetheless, considering the small measurement error when determining h_{peak}, 2D analysis may be considered a valid method. This knowledge is especially worthwhile since the height of flight dictates the potential to perform somersaults and twists during the second flight phase, and it is therefore an important performance-determining factor for vaults.

When comparing 2D analysis at two consecutive points in time, the variation coefficients of the h_{peak} and L of vaults were very low. For instance, the differences of 2D analysis were only 1.21 cm (h_{peak}) and 1.98cm (L), at a mean height of 2.75 m and a mean length of 2.28 m. These minor random errors are likely due to slightly different definitions of the zero-points (on the landing mat or at the end of the vaulting table), or of the gymnast's center of gravity (h_{peak}) or ankle (L), rather than a different determination of the frame at which h_{peak} or L were determined. Therefore, the almost perfect correlation of the first and second 2D analysis and the low variation coefficient values demonstrate a very high intrarater reliability. Thus, 2D analysis using Dartfish (Dartfish SA, Fribourg, CH) is a reliable and reproducible measure for the h_{peak} and L of vaults. This result is in line with the findings of Maykut, Taylor-Haas, Paterno, DiCesare, and Ford (2015), who, among other things, examined intrarater reliability of 2D analyses of joint angles during running. They measured kinematic variables during running on a treadmill with the same video analytical software we used (Dartfish SA, Fribourg, CH), and they reported excellent intrarater reliability [7]. Other studies have also shown 2D analyses to be reliable for measuring joint angles [6] and flight height [9].

Lastly, we compared the values of h_{peak} and L evaluated by an experienced assessor with those evaluated by a first-time assessor. Our results show that the h_{peak} and L of vaults are similar, as the coefficients of variance are low and the correlations are high. In this context, it should be mentioned that a brief introduction to the measurement software and determination of center of gravity is sufficient but indispensable. Therefore, 2D analysis is a straightforward measurement tool, where values of an inexperienced assessor, for example, those evaluated by a coach, are comparable to those of an expert. Therefore, our results show good interrater reliability with 2D analysis.

When evaluating data-collection procedures, it is important to evaluate practicality and not only validity and reliability. As there are few studies regarding the validity and reliability of 2D analysis, comparisons are difficult. Nevertheless, our results are similar to the results reached by Brehmer and Naundorf [4], as well as Schurr, Marshall, Resch, and Saliba [5], in regard to validity. As such, 2D analysis seems to be a reasonable, inexpensive, and portable alternative to 3D motion capture analysis. Furthermore, 2D analysis is time efficient, as video analysis of the h_{peak} and L of complex skills only takes about one minute for practiced evaluators. Additionally, the equipment needed for 2D analysis (video camera, tripod, analytical software, and calibration rod) is normally readily available in an artistic-gymnastics facility, making the described method an easy and cost-effective analytical tool. Lastly, even first-time assessors can precisely determine the important parameters of complex skills if they are briefly introduced to the measurement method. Thus, 2D analysis is a useful analytical tool for practical use in training and for scientific research, as the financial, spatial, and temporal costs are minimal.

5. Conclusions

This study evaluated the validity and reliability of 2D video analysis of the h_{peak} and L of vaults in artistic gymnastics. We conclude that 2D video analysis is a valid and reliable alternative to 3D motion capture, particularly for determining the h_{peak}, but slightly less so for the assessment of the L, of vaults. Thus, the ease of use and cost-effectiveness of 2D analysis, along with the results from this study, support the use of 2D analysis in routine training and scientific research.

Author Contributions: Conceptualization, C.S. and L.v.S.; methodology, C.S. and L.v.S.; formal analysis, C.S. and L.v.S.; investigation, C.S., L.v.S., and M.G.; data curation, C.S., L.v.S., and M.G.; writing—original-draft preparation, C.S. and I.L.; writing—review and editing, K.H. and W.T.; supervision, K.H. and W.T.; project administration, C.S.

References

1. Oyama, S.; Sosa, A.; Campbell, R.; Correa, A. Reliability and validity of quantitative video analysis of baseball pitching motion. *J. Appl. Biomech.* **2017**, *33*, 64–68. [CrossRef] [PubMed]
2. Farana, R.; Uchytil, J.; Zahradnik, D.; Jandacka, D. The "akopian" vault performed by elite male gymnasts: Which biomechanical variables are related to a judge's score? *Acta. Gymnica.* **2015**, *45*, 33–40. [CrossRef]
3. Farana, R.; Vaverka, F. The effect of biomechanical variables on the assessment of vaulting in top-level artistic female gymnasts in world cup competitions. *Acta. Univ. Palacki. Olomuc. Gymn.* **2012**, *42*, 49–57. [CrossRef]
4. Brehmer, S.; Naundorf, F. Key parameters of the 2nd flight phase of the tsukahara with salto backward piked. In Proceedings of the 32nd International Conference of Biomechanics in Sports, Johnson City, TN, USA, 13 July 2014.
5. Schurr, S.A.; Marshall, A.N.; Resch, J.E.; Saliba, S.A. Two-dimensional video analysis is comparable to 3d motion capture in lower extremity movement assessment. *Int. J. Sports. Phys. Ther.* **2017**, *12*, 163–172. [PubMed]
6. Gribble, P.; Hertel, J.; Denegar, C.; Buckley, W. Reliability and validity of a 2-d video digitizing system during a static and a dynamic task. *J. Sport Rehabil.* **2005**, *14*, 137–149. [CrossRef]
7. Maykut, J.N.; Taylor-Haas, J.A.; Paterno, M.V.; DiCesare, C.A.; Ford, K.R. Concurrent validity and reliability of 2d kinematic analysis of frontal plane motion during running. *Int. J. Sports Phys. Ther.* **2015**, *10*, 136–146. [PubMed]
8. Balsalobre-Fernandez, C.; Tejero-Gonzalez, C.M.; del Campo-Vecino, J.; Bavaresco, N. The concurrent validity and reliability of a low-cost, high-speed camera-based method for measuring the flight time of vertical jumps. *J. Strength Cond. Res.* **2014**, *28*, 528–533. [CrossRef] [PubMed]
9. Balsalobre-Fernandez, C.; Glaister, M.; Lockey, R.A. The validity and reliability of an iphone app for measuring vertical jump performance. *J. Sports Sci.* **2015**, *33*, 1574–1579. [CrossRef] [PubMed]
10. Vicon. Vicon plug-in gait product guide—foundation notes revision. Vicon Motion Systems Ltd.: Oxford, UK, 2010.
11. Hopkins, W.G.; Schabort, E.J.; Hawley, J.A. Reliability of power in physical performance tests. *Sports Med.* **2001**, *31*, 211–234. [CrossRef] [PubMed]
12. Bland, J.M.; Altman, D.G. Statistical methods for assessing agreement between two methods of clinical measurement. *Lancet* **1986**, *1*, 307–310. [CrossRef]

18

Shoe Cushioning Effects on Foot Loading and Comfort Perception during Typical Basketball Maneuvers

Xini Zhang [1], Zhen Luo [1], Xi Wang [1], Yang Yang [1], Jiaxin Niu [1] and Weijie Fu [1,2,*]

1 School of Kinesiology, Shanghai University of Sport, Shanghai 200438, China; zhangxini1129@163.com (X.Z.); 15621573815@163.com (Z.L.); zwx252@163.com (X.W.); 18049922807@163.com (Y.Y.); jfhou_sus@163.com (J.N.)

2 Key Laboratory of Exercise and Health Sciences of Ministry of Education, Shanghai University of Sport, Shanghai 200438, China

* Correspondence: fuweijie@sus.edu.cn or fuweijie315@163.com;

Abstract: Purpose: This study aimed to explore the relationship between foot loading and comfort perception in two basketball shoes during basketball-specific maneuvers. Methods: Twelve male collegiate basketball players were required to complete three basketball maneuvers (i.e., side-step cutting, 90° L-direction running, and lay-up jumping) in two basketball shoe conditions (shoe L and shoe N, with different midsole cushioning types). Two Kistler force plates and a Medilogic insole plantar pressure system were used to collect kinetic data (i.e., impact force, peak loading rate, and plantar pressure variables). Perception scales were used to evaluate comfort perception. Results: No significant difference was observed between the two shoes during maneuvers in terms of ground reaction force. However, the plantar pressure of shoe L in the midfoot and lateral foot regions was significantly greater than that of shoe N during side-step cutting and lay-up jumping. Shoe N was significantly superior to shoe L, especially in dynamic scale in terms of the perception of comfort. The plantar pressure and perception characteristics in the two shoes were significantly different but inconsistent with each other. Conclusion: The biomechanical characteristics of the shoes themselves and the perception evaluation of the athletes should be considered in comprehensive shoe-cushioning design and evaluation.

Keywords: basketball shoe; comfort perception; foot loading; plantar pressure; maneuver

1. Introduction

In basketball, the lower limbs of athletes are subjected to large impact forces during each landing [1]. Players complete 70 jumps/landings in a single game and attenuate impacts of up to nine times their body weight every time [2], which increases the risk of knee and ankle injuries [3]. Reducing impact forces (which includes both magnitude and loading rate characteristics) may help prevent foot injuries [4]. The shock absorption characteristics and comfort of basketball shoes, as core equipment of the sport, have important influences not only on the performance of the players but also on the prevention of lower extremity injuries [5]. The impact force and pressure distribution characteristics between the feet and the shoes must be understood to effectively optimize the technical movements, reduce foot injuries, and improve the design of specialized shoes [6]. However, the existing studies on foot loading have mainly focused on common gait characteristics, such as walking and running [7,8], and studies on specific sports maneuvers, such as cross-over running and lay-up jumping [9–11], are limited.

Meanwhile, comfort and stability have been identified as the principal factors of specialized sports shoes [12], in addition to meeting the functional requirements of specific sports and strengthening the foot protection function [13]. However, these factors are easily neglected. The comfort of basketball shoes is closely related to the performance of basketball athletes, as well as to ankle injury and its prevention [2]. The subjective perception scale has been proven to be an effective and credible method for assessing the aforementioned variables [14,15]. Hennig et al. [16] found that a close relationship exists between runners' subjective perception of shoes' cushioning performance and their impacts on plantar pressure during running. Meanwhile, foot comfort is also closely related to the impact load on the lower limbs at initial contact [17]. Thus, the functionality and comfort of basketball shoes for typical maneuvers in basketball must be explored through both the subjective perception and foot biomechanical tests [18].

Therefore, the current study aims to determine the effect of different basketball shoes on the ground reaction force (GRF) and plantar pressure characteristics in three typical basketball maneuvers and to further understand foot loading characteristics in basketball and their relationship with comfort through the subjective perception scale evaluation of basketball shoes. It was hypothesized that wearing different shoes would affect comfort perception, and correspondingly change GRF and plantar pressure characteristics during basketball maneuvers.

2. Materials and Methods

2.1. Participants

Twelve healthy male collegiate basketball players (age: 23.1 ± 2.0 years; height: 176.3 ± 4.5 cm; body mass: 70.5 ± 7.5 kg) with an average of 8.4 years of experience in basketball events were recruited for this experiment. An observational cross-sectional research design according to the Strengthening The Reporting of OBservational Studies in Epidemiology (STROBE) criteria [19,20]. The inclusion criteria were: (1) at least five years of experience in basketball events; (2) none has suffered musculoskeletal injuries of the lower extremity over the last six months; (3) none has engaged in strenuous training within 24 h. A two-tailed *t*-test was executed via the G*Power 3.1 software to determine whether a sample size of 12 was sufficient to minimize the probability of type II errors for all the variables (P = 80% at $\alpha = 0.05$). All the participants signed an informed consent form, and ethical approval was granted by the Institutional Review Board of Shanghai University of Sports prior to the study (2017007).

2.2. Shoes and Instrumentations

Two types of U.S. size nine basketball shoes were used in this study. One of the shoes was a new sample provided by a local sports science laboratory (hereinafter referred to as shoe L), and the other (Figure 1) was a commercially available type with a popular international brand (hereinafter referred to as shoe N). The following are some details of the property of Shoe N: (1) upper: Black synthetic leather and Phyposite technology—Breathable tongue inner sleeve with a traditional lacing system; (2) midsole: Phylon midsole design that minimizes weight while maximizing cushioning with animpact absorption system; (3) outsole: Non-traditional outsole to reduce weight and optimize traction. Overall, the two types of shoes were similar in the abovementioned materials, design, color, weight (≈530 g), and so on, and only differed in the impact absorption systems of the midsole.

Two 90 cm × 60 cm three-dimensional force plates (9287B, Kistler Corporation, Switzerland) were utilized to collect GRF data, with a sampling rate of 1200 Hz.

The insole measurement system (Medilogic Corporation, Germany) was used to capture the plantar pressure of different regions. This system has been validated [21]. Each insole was calibrated using the manufacturer's calibration device (T&T medilogic Medizintechnik GmbH, Schönefeld, Germany) prior to the study. The size of the pressure insole was 8/9 according to the participants' foot size. The pressure insole consisted of 225 pressure sensors (0.6 cm × 0.4 cm), with a pressure range of

0-64 N/cm^2 and a maximum sampling rate of 300 Hz (Figure 2a). The plantar regions were divided into five parts, namely, the forefoot, the midfoot, the heel, the lateral, and the medial (Figure 2b).

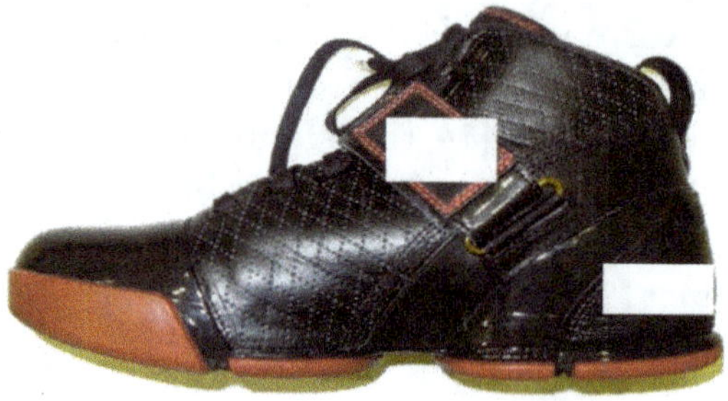

Figure 1. Basketball shoes (shoe N) from a famous international manufacturer.

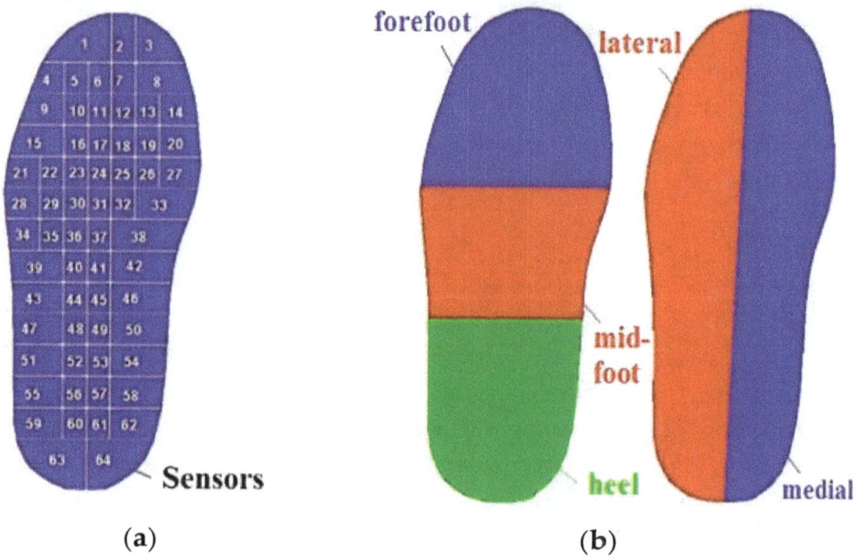

Figure 2. (**a**) Composition of insole pressure sensors with a pressure range of 0–64 N/cm^2; (**b**) region division of plantar pressure, including the forefoot, the midfoot, the heel, the lateral, and the medial parts.

2.3. Experimental Protocol

Three typical maneuvers, which are the most frequently used in basketball games according to the video observation and the coach interview, were selected, namely, side-step cutting (SS), 90° L-direction running (90° LR), and lay-up toe-off (LU_{TO}) and touch-down (LU_{TD}). The sports surface used in this study is the most common wooden floor used in basketball games. The participants first set their pace according to their personal movement habits and then tried their best to complete the movements. They were required to achieve the three typical maneuvers (SS, 90° LR, and lay-up) in the two different shoes in random order. Five successful trials were obtained for each condition. The pressure insoles were placed flat in the shoes before the experiment, and data were transmitted to the computer in real-time via a wireless receiver. The participants were required to familiarize themselves with the maneuvers before the formal tests began. The familiarization period for each participant was 10–15 min. To avoid the influence of fatigue on the results, 1–2 min breaks were given between each trial [22].

The perception-comfort scale used in this experiment was adapted from the perception scale provided by a famous shoe research center in the US. The scale includes two parts, namely, general fit and dynamic scale (Figure 3). The indices of the general fit test include the toe-box height, the toe-box width, the ball girth, the waist/instep, the elasticity at the heel, and the shoe length. The index scores range from 1 to 9: 1 means too low (toe-box height), too narrow (toe-box width), too tight (ball girth, waist/instep, heel), or too short (length); 9 means too high, too wide, too loose, or too long; and 5 means just right (Figure 3a). A dynamic scale was used to evaluate the fit of the basketball shoes during the maneuvers, including overall liking, heel cushioning, heel responsiveness, heel stability, heel-to-toe transition, and forefoot cushioning, which were also scored 1–9 points (1 for extremely dislike, 5 for neutral, and 9 for extremely like). In addition to overall liking, the intensity aspects were also rated 1–9: 1 means soft (heel and forefoot cushioning), no response (heel responsiveness), very unstable (heel stability), no smoothness (heel-toe transition), and so on; and 9 means hard, very reactive, very stable, very smooth, and so on (Figure 3b). The experiment process included a 10-minute regular-intensity basketball maneuver practice (including SS, 90° LR, and lay-up). The tongue and logos of the basketball shoes were completely covered before testing to avoid the brand effect and the influence of other factors on the scoring results.

	FIX			JUST RIGHT				FIX	
Toebox Height	1 Too Low	2	3	4	5 JR	6	7	8	9 Too High
Toebox Width	1 Too Narrow	2	3	4	5 JR	6	7	8	9 Too Wide
Ball Girth	1 Too Tight	2	3	4	5 JR	6	7	8	9 Too Loose
Waist / Instep	1 Too Tight	2	3	4	5 JR	6	7	8	9 Too Loose
Heel	1 Too Tight	2	3	4	5 JR	6	7	8	9 Too Loose
Length	1 Too Short	2	3	4	5 JR	6	7	8	9 Too Long

(a)

Overall Liking	○ Dislike Extremely	○ Dislike Very Much	○ Dislike Moderately	○ Dislike Slightly	○ Neither Like nor Dislike	○ Like Slightly	○ Like Moderately	○ Like Very Much	○ Like Extremely

ATTRIBUTE	LIKING									INTENSITY								
Heel Cushioning	○ Dislike Extremely	○ Dislike Very Much	○ Dislike Moderately	○ Dislike Slightly	○ Neither Like nor Dislike	○ Like Slightly	○ Like Moderately	○ Like Very Much	○ Like Extremely	○ Soft	○	○	○	○	○	○	○	○ Hard
Heel Responsiveness	○ Dislike Extremely	○ Dislike Very Much	○ Dislike Moderately	○ Dislike Slightly	○ Neither Like nor Dislike	○ Like Slightly	○ Like Moderately	○ Like Very Much	○ Like Extremely	○ Not Responsive	○	○	○	○	○	○	○	○ Very Responsive
Heel Stability	○ Dislike Extremely	○ Dislike Very Much	○ Dislike Moderately	○ Dislike Slightly	○ Neither Like nor Dislike	○ Like Slightly	○ Like Moderately	○ Like Very Much	○ Like Extremely	○ Very Unstable	○	○	○	○	○	○	○	○ Very Stable
Heel-to-toe transition	○ Dislike Extremely	○ Dislike Very Much	○ Dislike Moderately	○ Dislike Slightly	○ Neither Like nor Dislike	○ Like Slightly	○ Like Moderately	○ Like Very Much	○ Like Extremely	○ Not Smooth	○	○	○	○	○	○	○	○ Very Smooth
Forefoot cushioning	○ Dislike Extremely	○ Dislike Very Much	○ Dislike Moderately	○ Dislike Slightly	○ Neither Like nor Dislike	○ Like Slightly	○ Like Moderately	○ Like Very Much	○ Like Extremely	○ Soft	○	○	○	○	○	○	○	○ Hard

(b)

Figure 3. (**a**) General fit scale includes the toe-box height, the toe-box width, the ball girth, the waist/instep, the elasticity at the heel, and the shoe length. The index scores range from 1 to 9 points; (**b**) dynamic scale includes overall liking, heel cushioning, heel responsiveness, heel stability, heel-to-toe transition, and forefoot cushioning, which were scored 1–9 points.

2.4. Data Processing and Analysis

The main variables of the GRF included the following: (1) peak vertical GRF (Fz) and appearance time (t_F) and (2) peak loading rate (G_Z) and appearance time (t_G). Fz and Gz were normalized by bodyweight (BW).

According to Bontrager's study on the settings of the insole area and the structure of the pressure insoles [20], the peak pressure (normalized by BW) and the peak pressure distribution (contact area) were measured for six plantar areas, namely, the entire sole, the forefoot, the midfoot, the rearfoot, the medial, and the lateral (Figure 2).

The shoe comfort characteristics included (1) general fit: toe-box height, toe-box width, ball girth, waist/instep, heel, and length; and (2) dynamic fit: overall liking, heel cushioning, heel responsiveness, heel stability, heel-to-toe transition, and forefoot cushioning. Liking and intensity were involved in each dynamic fit variable.

2.5. Statistics

All data were normally distributed based on the Shapiro–Wilk test. The paired sample t-test was used to determine the effects of different basketball shoe cushioning on the GRF and the plantar pressure characteristics. The comfort perception variables were determined by the Wilcoxon rank-sum test (SPSS 19.0, SPSS Inc., Chicago, IL, USA). The significance level was set at 0.05.

3. Results

3.1. Vertical GRF

The passive impact phase in SS and 90° LR occurred within 100 ms after ground contact, with the Fz approximately twice that of the BW (Figure 4a). The vertical GRF increased rapidly in LUTO and LUTD during contact, that is, the Fz during the push-off phase and after landing could be as large as four and eight-times the BW, respectively (Figure 4b). However, no significant differences in Fz, G_Z, t_F, and t_G were observed between the two basketball shoes during SS, 90° LR, LU_{TO}, and LU_{TD} (Table 1).

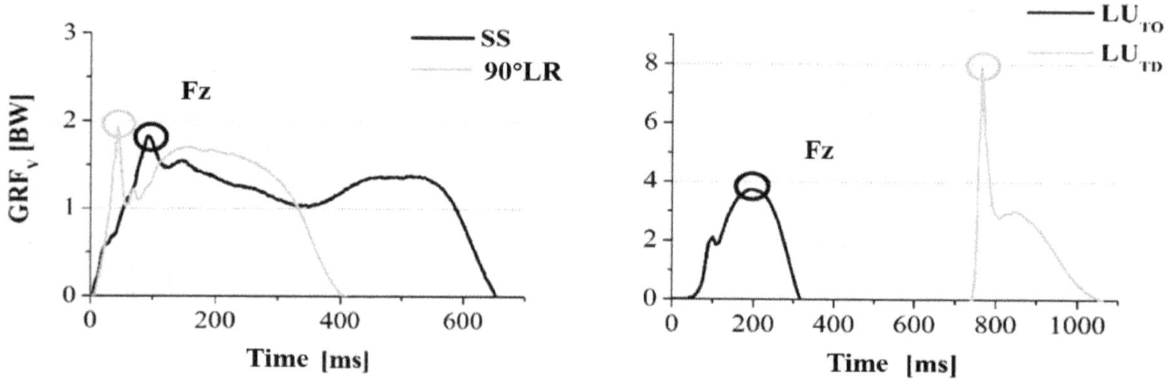

(a) (b)

Figure 4. (**a**) Vertical ground reaction force-time curves during side-step cutting (SS) and 90° L-direction running (90° LR) maneuvers; (**b**) vertical ground reaction force-time curves during lay-up toe-off (LU_{TO}) and lay-up touch-down (LU_{TD}) maneuvers. Notes: GRF is ground reaction force, Fz is peak vertical GRF, and BW is bodyweight.

Table 1. Effect of different basketball shoes on ground reaction force during side-step cutting, 90° L-direction running, and lay-up toe-off and lay-up touch-down maneuvers.

Maneuvers	Shoes	Fz (BW)	t_F (ms)	G_Z (BW/ms)	t_G (ms)
SS	L	1.92 ± 0.32	74.4 ± 30.2	0.26 ± 0.18	27.2 ± 21.8
	N	2.02 ± 0.43	63.3 ± 28.1	0.17 ± 0.06	19.7 ± 11.4
90° LR	L	2.47 ± 0.61	55.4 ± 25.6	0.35 ± 0.08	13.4 ± 12.6
	N	2.25 ± 0.71	54.8 ± 26.4	0.21 ± 0.07	13.2 ± 9.7
LU_{TO}	L	3.53 ± 0.43	130.7 ± 47.6		
	N	3.55 ± 0.67	124.8 ± 42.1		
LU_{TD}	L	6.33 ± 3.10	26.4 ± 9.7	1.13 ± 0.87	10.3 ± 4.2
	N	9.72 ± 3.42	28.6 ± 13.8	0.93 ± 0.32	11.9 ± 4.8

Notes: GRF is ground reaction force, Fz is peak vertical GRF, G_Z is peak loading rate, tF is time to peak vertical GRF, t_G is time to peak loading rate, BW is bodyweight, SS is side-step cutting, 90° LR is 90° L-direction running, LU_{TO} is lay-up toe-off, and LU_{TD} is lay-up touch-down.

3.2. Maximum Plantar Pressure

Shoe L showed a lower maximum pressure in the entire sole ($p < 0.05$) and midfoot ($p < 0.01$) regions during SS (Table 2) compared with shoe N. Although shoe L showed a low plantar pressure in the entire sole and in the forefoot, the heel, the medial, and in the lateral regions, no significant differences were observed between the two shoes during 90° LR.

Table 2. Effect of different basketball shoes on maximum pressure of each plantar region during side-step cutting, 90° L-direction running, and lay-up toe-off and lay-up touch-down maneuvers.

Maneuvers	Shoe	Maximum Pressure of Each Plantar Region (N/kg/cm^2)					
		Entire	Forefoot	Midfoot	Heel	Lateral	Medial
SS	L	0.028 ± 0.008 *	0.037 ± 0.018	0.011 ± 0.012 **	0.024 ± 0.014	0.026 ± 0.013	0.033 ± 0.005
	N	0.032 ± 0.006	0.043 ± 0.022	0.023 ± 0.016	0.029 ± 0.014	0.031 ± 0.015	0.035 ± 0.008
90° -LR	L	0.028 ± 0.018	0.048 ± 0.031	0.020 ± 0.015	0.026 ± 0.018	0.026 ± 0.018	0.033 ± 0.023
	N	0.030 ± 0.019	0.051 ± 0.034	0.023 ± 0.021	0.025 ± 0.017	0.027 ± 0.019	0.035 ± 0.024
LU_{TO}	L	0.061 ± 0.008	0.098 ± 0.014	0.048 ± 0.009 **	0.080 ± 0.018	0.072 ± 0.009	0.054 ± 0.010
	N	0.063 ± 0.012	0.093 ± 0.018	0.061 ± 0.014	0.082 ± 0.020	0.075 ± 0.014	0.053 ± 0.012
LU_{TD}	L	0.064 ± 0.011	0.081 ± 0.019	0.050 ± 0.017 **	0.093 ± 0.038	0.063 ± 0.011 **	0.067 ± 0.019
	N	0.071 ± 0.012	0.082 ± 0.022	0.064 ± 0.017	0.099 ± 0.038	0.070 ± 0.011	0.076 ± 0.023

Notes: SS is side-step cutting, 90° LR is 90° L-direction running, LU_{TO} is lay-up toe-off, and LU_{TD} is lay-up touch-down. * $p < 0.05$; ** $p < 0.01$.

Notably, shoe L showed a lower maximum pressure in the midfoot and in the lateral regions during LU_{TO} ($p < 0.01$) and LU_{TD} ($p < 0.01$) compared with shoe N. Although no statistical differences were observed in plantar pressure on the rest of the regions, the maximum pressure was evidently lower in shoe L than in shoe N.

3.3. Foot Pressure Distribution

In general, the overall pressure distribution in the two shoes was similar but wider in shoe L than in shoe N, and the pressure value of each region was lower in shoe L than in shoe N. Specifically, less fore-lateral pressure distribution was noted in shoe L during SS; a wide heel pressure distribution was observed in shoe L during 90° LR, with pressure concentrated at the first metatarsal head, the first phalanges, and the fifth metatarsal head (Figure 5a); the foot pressure of each region in shoe L was smaller than that in shoe N during LU_{TO}; and a smaller pressure at the first phalanges and a wider heel pressure distribution were noted in shoe N compared with shoe L during LU_{TD} (Figure 5b).

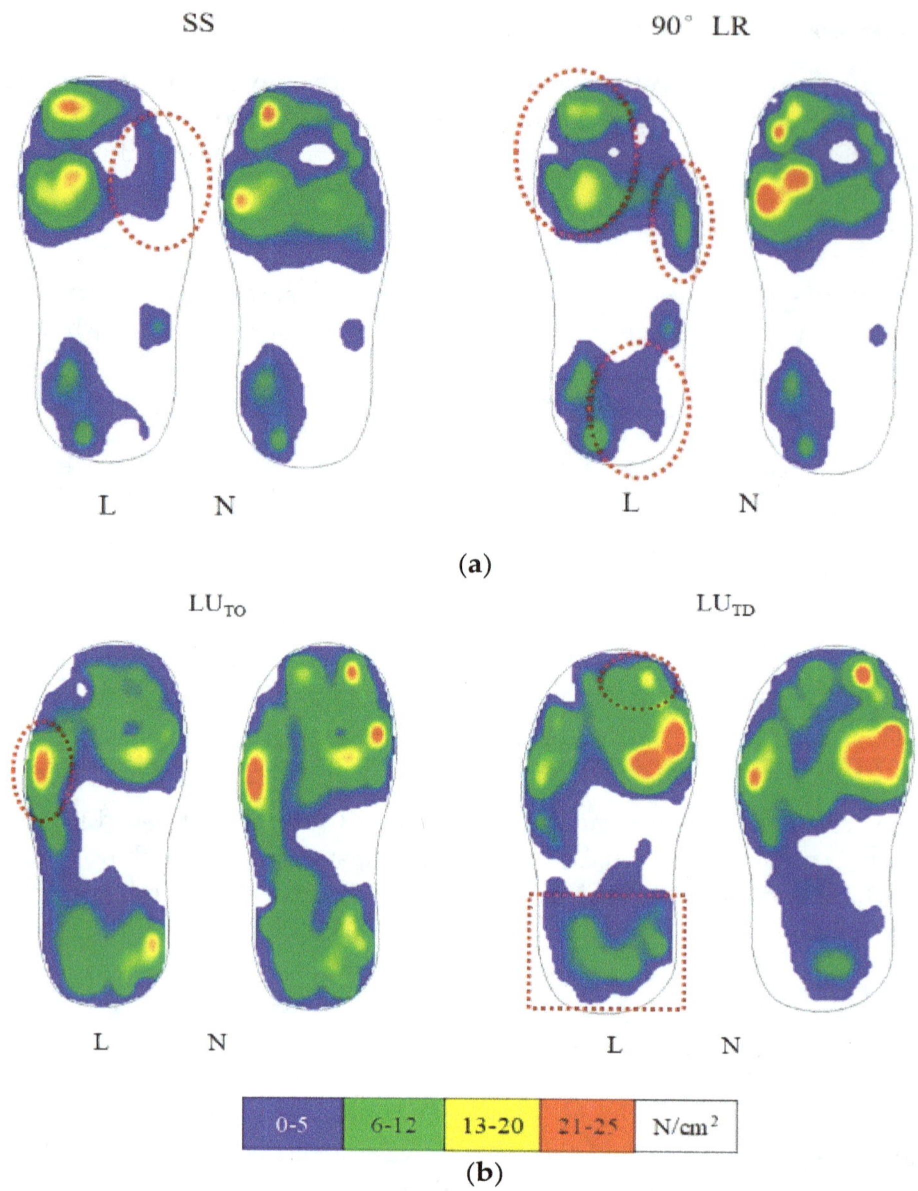

Figure 5. (**a**) Effect of different basketball shoes (L vs. N) on plantar pressure distribution during side-step cutting (SS) and 90° L-direction running (90° LR) maneuvers; (**b**) effect of different basketball shoes (L vs. N) on plantar pressure distribution during lay-up toe-off (LU_{TO}), and lay-up touch-down (LU_{TD}) maneuvers. Different colors represented different pressure values. The pressure values from small to large were blue, green, yellow and red.

3.4. Comfort Perception

No significant differences were observed in the general fit between shoe L and shoe N (Figure 6).

From the dynamic comfort scale perspective, the overall liking of shoe N was significantly higher than that of shoe L ($p < 0.01$) owing to forefoot and heel cushioning ($p < 0.01$). The heel responsiveness and stability of shoe N were greater than those of shoe L ($p < 0.05$), but no significant differences were observed in the heel-to-toe transition between the two shoes (Figure 7). The forefoot and heel cushioning of shoe L were significantly higher than those of shoe N ($p < 0.05$) (Figure 7) in terms of dynamic intensity. Meanwhile, no significant difference was observed in the heel-to-toe transition, heel response, and heel stability between the two types of shoes.

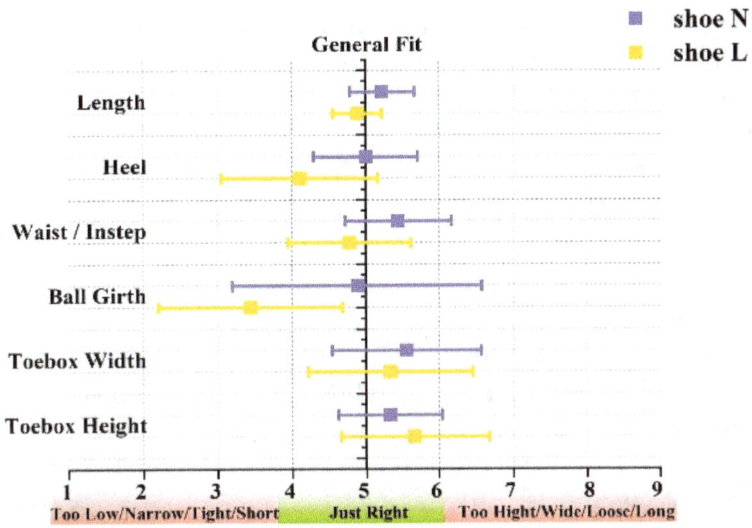

Figure 6. Effect of different basketball shoes (N vs. L) on general fit.

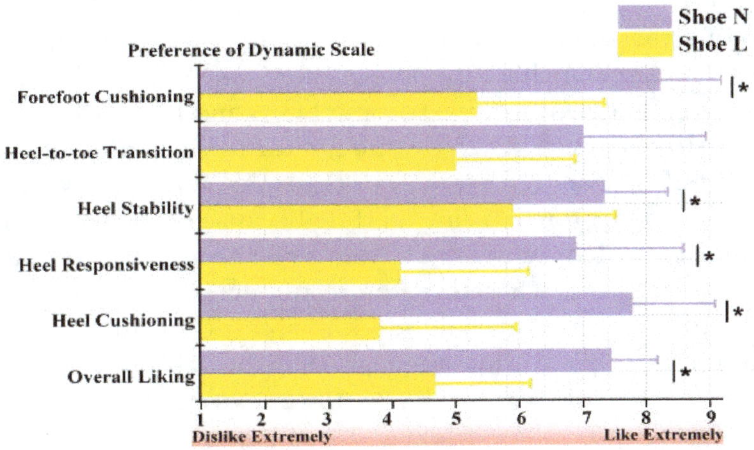

(**a**)

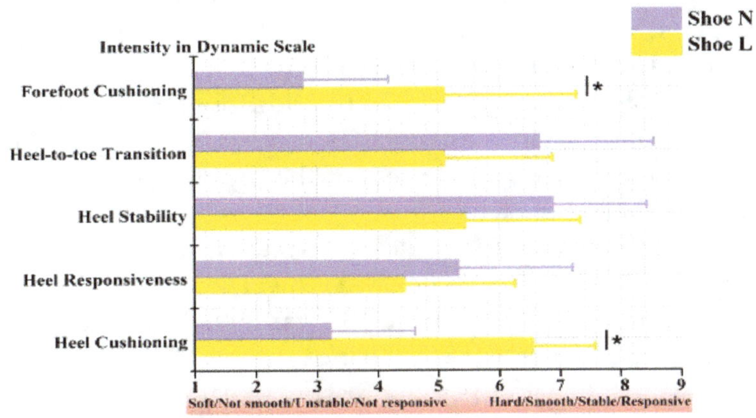

(**b**)

Figure 7. (**a**) Effect of different basketball shoes (N vs. L) on preference of dynamic scale; (**b**) effect of different basketball shoes (N vs. L) on intensity in dynamic scale.

4. Discussion

This study aimed to investigate the effect of two different shoe cushionings on foot loading (GRF and plantar pressure) and the perception of comfort during three basketball-specific maneuvers (i.e., SS, 90° LR, and LU_{TO}/LU_{TD}). Consistent with our hypothesis, compared to shoe N, shoe L showed a lower maximum pressure in the entire and midfoot regions during SS and a lower maximum pressure in the midfoot and lateral regions during LU_{TO} and LU_{TD}. The overall pressure distribution was wider in shoe L than in shoe N. In terms of the perception of comfort, shoe N was significantly superior to shoe L, especially in the dynamic scale. However, contrary to our hypothesis, no significant differences in Fz, G_Z, t_F, and t_G were noted between the two basketball shoes during SS, 90° LR, LU_{TO}, and LU_{TD}.

4.1. Vertical GRF

In general, two peaks appeared in the vertical GRF on the lower limbs when running or jumping, namely, the impact force (first peak) and the active force (second peak). The impact force is closely related to sports injuries [2,23]. This study analyzed the characteristics of GRF during three kinds of basketball-specific maneuvers, namely, side-step cutting (SS), 90° varied-direction running (90° LR), and lay-up toe-off (LU_{TO}) and lay-up touch-down (LU_{TD}). Notably, the impact forces, which were approximately twice the BW, were identified as passive forces that appeared within 100 ms at the initial contact during SS and 90° LR, and the active forces were regarded as the principal components. However, the results indicated that no significant differences in GRF existed between the two pairs of shoes during SS and 90° LR.

Among the numerous basketball maneuvers, the lay-up is one of the most representative and relatively complex movements that include the acceleration, take-off, and landing phases. The results of the present study showed that the GRF curves during LU_{TO} and LU_{TD} were very similar to the those when running with a heel strike pattern [24,25]. Although the force would not cause impact damage to the lower extremity at take-off, which was nearly four times the BW, the participants were subjected to up to eight times of the BW impact force during landing because of the high jumps performed in this study. The repeated impacts loaded on the lower limbs can easily lead to injuries, especially when high impacts cannot be loaded [26]. Therefore, the results indicated that the high impacts during LU_{TD} caused overuse injuries. However, we found no significant differences in Fz, G_Z, t_F, and t_G regardless of shoe conditions. This finding suggests that though the two midsole materials were different, the impacts of the active movements on the lower extremities made a small difference.

4.2. Plantar Pressure Characteristics

We found that shoe L exhibited a significantly lower maximum pressure on the entire sole and on the midfoot regions compared with shoe N. Although shoe L showed a lower plantar pressure on the entire sole and on the forefoot, the heel, the medial, and the lateral regions, no significant differences were noted between the two shoes during 90° LR. In addition, shoe L showed a lower maximum pressure on the midfoot and lateral regions during LU_{TO} and LU_{TD} compared with shoe N. Although no statistical differences were observed in the rest of the plantar pressure regions, the maximum pressure was lower in shoe L than in shoe N.

The overall plantar pressure distribution in the two shoes was similar but wider in shoe L than in shoe N, and the pressure value of each region was lower in shoe L than in shoe N. Specifically, the fore-lateral pressure distribution of shoe L during SS was low; the heel pressure distribution of shoe L during 90° LR was wide, with the pressure was concentrated at the first metatarsal head, the first phalanges, and the fifth metatarsal head; the foot pressure of each region of shoe L was smaller than that of shoe N during LU_{TO}; the pressure was smaller at the first phalanges; and the heel pressure distribution was wider for shoe N than those for shoe L during LU_{TD}. At present, plantar pressure distribution has been measured for efficiency in studies on the characteristics and biomechanical mechanism of plantar pressure in various sports. These studies have provided key technologies for sports shoes of different events, especially in terms of individualized design and manufacturing. The material of the sole and its structure for energy absorption and release are important factors in attenuating impacts and protecting the lower extremity from injury [27].

A significant difference was noted in the present study on the plantar pressure of the two shoes during the different maneuvers. However, no significant differences were observed in the GRF or loading rates, which suggests that the mechanical relationship between the foot and the ground became an indirect one owing to the intervention of shoe conditions. This change was mainly due to the special medium of the midsole. A special patented cushioning material was used in the midsole of shoe L. The materials and structures of the midsoles differed in the two shoes, thereby resulting in significant differences in plantar pressure during the three maneuvers despite the similar GRF. This finding suggests that the mechanical performance of shoes and feet and the relationship between feet and shoes caused by different midsole materials should be considered when exploring the function of sports shoes [28]. These factors should then be combined with plantar pressure to create a comprehensive design and to improve sports shoes effectively.

4.3. Comfort Perception

In addition to meeting the functional requirements of specific sporting events and strengthening foot protection, the most important element in specialized sport's shoes is comfort [12,29]. At present, subjective scoring is still the most frequently applied method for internationally applicable comfort testing; however, the scales and questionnaires used in each study differ. The perception test which was used in this experiment mainly includes two parts, namely, the general fit and the dynamic scale, which have been proven reliable.

For the general fit, the two shoes provided comfort with no significant differences. However, shoe N outperformed shoe L significantly on each index for liking in the dynamic scale, especially in heel stability, heel response, heel cushioning, forefoot cushioning, and overall impression. Moreover, shoe N had above five scores in all the indices. The other feedback from the participants regarding shoe L included poor appearance, dehumanized overall design, thick sponge behind the shoes, and lack of details. In terms of dynamic comfort intensity, shoe L was insufficiently stable at the heel, while shoe N was not only stable but also responsive. Although the cushioning of shoe N was softer at the forefoot, the forefoot and heel cushioning of shoe L were better than those of shoe N, based on the participants' feedback. This finding is probably due to the fact that shoe N was too soft to provide sufficient cushioning. The general fit in the perceptual test was preferred for assessing the appropriateness of the shoes, while the dynamic scale was preferred for evaluating the perceptual likings and performance of the two shoes from a functional aspect. The deficiency of shoe L was mainly due to its lack of ergonomic design for fit or may be related to the materials and structural design.

Notably, the results of plantar pressure were inconsistent with the perceptual comfort of shoe L and shoe N in the above-mentioned plantar pressure and perceptual comfort scale tests [30]. Although shoe L has a lower plantar pressure on the forefoot, it is not as comfortable as shoe N. The results of plantar pressure indicated the advantage of the forefoot cushioning performance of shoe L. However, the midsole structure of shoe L should be improved to avoid excessive force concentration under intense impact from the pressure distribution. Che et al. [31] found that the plantar pressure index affects comfort assessment. Similarly, the midsole material and structure could affect individual comfort assessment [32]. Therefore, we assumed that the plantar pressure distribution was related to perceptual comfort to some extent because the human being, as an active organism, self-evaluates the perceptual information of sneakers [33]. Differences were observed in the midsole cushioning performance obtained by the mechanical/biomechanical test or the perception of comfort, which could directly affect people's choice of sports shoes. Ignoring these differences would inevitably affect the evaluation of sports shoes in terms of function. However, relevant studies on the reasons for these differences are limited. Therefore, further studies are required.

4.4. Limitations

In the present study, it is noteworthy that marker trajectories and surface electromyographic data were not collected to simplify the design by focusing on the foot loading and mimicking basketball maneuvers by limiting the experimental devices that were attached to the participants. However, future studies including electromyography results with different sports shoes in basketball players should be carried out in order to determine muscle activity [19,20,34]. Besides, it is considered that different trajectories performed by players could influence the trial times, as well as the impact on shoes [35].

5. Conclusions

No differences were observed in the impact forces and the average maximum plantar pressure between the two shoes during the three basketball-specific maneuvers. However, compared to shoe N, the plantar pressure range of shoe L was wider and showed a lower pressure at the midfoot and the lateral foot. Moreover, the comfort perception results indicated that though the general fit of the two shoes was equal, shoe L provided less overall comfort, forefoot flexibility, heel cushioning, heel stability, and heel response. Interestingly, the plantar pressure results were inconsistent with the perceptual comfort of the two shoes, which suggests that the biomechanical characteristics of the shoes themselves and the perception evaluation of the athletes should be considered in comprehensive shoe cushioning design and evaluation.

Author Contributions: X.Z., Z.L. and X.W. contributed equally. Conceptualization, W.F.; methodology, X.Z., Z.L. and X.W.; formal analysis, X.Z., Z.L., Y.Y., J.N. and X.W.; investigation, X.Z., Z.L., X.W., Y.Y., J.N. and W.F.; resources, W.F.; data curation, X.Z.; writing—original draft preparation, X.Z., Z.L., X.W. and J.N.; writing—review and editing, W.F.; project administration, W.F.; funding acquisition, W.F.

References

1. Randers, M.B.; Hagman, M.; Brix, J.; Christensen, J.F.; Pedersen, M.T.; Nielsen, J.J.; Krustrup, P. Effects of 3 months of full-court and half-court street basketball training on health profile in untrained men. *J. Sport Health Sci.* **2018**, *7*, 132–138. [CrossRef] [PubMed]
2. Nin, D.Z.; Lam, W.K.; Kong, P.W. Effect of body mass and midsole hardness on kinetic and perceptual variables during basketball landing manoeuvres. *J. Sport. Health Sci.* **2016**, *34*, 756–765. [CrossRef] [PubMed]
3. Meeuwisse, W.H.; Sellmer, R.; Hagel, B.E. Rates and risks of injury during intercollegiate basketball. *Am. J. Sports Med.* **2003**, *31*, 379–385. [CrossRef] [PubMed]
4. Irmischer, B.S.; Harris, C.; Pfeiffer, R.P.; DeBeliso, M.A.; Adams, K.J.; Shea, K.G. Effects of a knee ligament injury prevention exercise program on impact forces in women. *J. Strength Cond. Res.* **2004**, *18*, 703–707. [PubMed]
5. Chiu, H.T.; Shiang, T.Y. Effects of insoles and additional shock absorption foam on the cushioning properties of sport shoes. *J. Appl. Biomech.* **2007**, *23*, 119–127. [CrossRef] [PubMed]
6. Morlock, M.; Nigg, B.M. Theoretical considerations and practical results on the influence of the representation of the foot for the estimation of internal forces with models. *Clin. Biomech.* **1991**, *6*, 3–13. [CrossRef]
7. Blackmore, T.; Ball, N.; Scurr, J. The effect of socks on vertical and anteroposterior ground reaction forces in walking and running. *Foot* **2011**, *21*, 1–5. [CrossRef]
8. Nilsson, J.; Thorstensson, A. Ground reaction forces at different speeds of human walking and running. *Acta Physiol.* **2010**, *136*, 217–227. [CrossRef]
9. Lam, W.K.; Qu, Y.; Yang, F.; Cheung, R.T.H. Do rotational shear-cushioning shoes influence horizontal ground reaction forces and perceived comfort during basketball cutting maneuvers? *PeerJ* **2017**, *5*, 1–13. [CrossRef]
10. Wei, Q.; Wang, Z.; Woo, J.; Liebenberg, J.; Park, S.K.; Ryu, J.; Lam, W.K. Kinetics and perception of basketball landing in various heights and footwear cushioning. *PLoS ONE* **2018**, *13*, e0201758. [CrossRef]
11. Lam, W.K.; Ng, W.X.; Kong, P.W. Influence of shoe midsole hardness on plantar pressure distribution in four basketball-related movements. *Res. Sports Med.* **2017**, *25*, 37–47. [CrossRef] [PubMed]

12. Nigg, B.M.; Bahlsen, H.A.; Luethi, S.M.; Stokes, S. The influence of running velocity and midsole hardness on external impact forces in heel-toe running. *J. Biomech.* **1987**, *20*, 951–959. [CrossRef]
13. Brizuela, G.; Llana, S.; Ferrandis, R.; Garcia-Belenguer, A.C. The influence of basketball shoes with increased ankle support on shock attenuation and performance in running and jumping. *J. Sports Sci.* **1997**, *15*, 505–515. [CrossRef] [PubMed]
14. Jordan, C.; Payton, C.; Bartlett, R. Perceived comfort and pressure distribution in casual footwear. *Clin. Biomech.* **1997**, *12*, 215–220. [CrossRef]
15. Robbins, S.; Waked, E.; Krouglicof, N. Improving balance. *J. Am. Geriatr. Soc.* **1998**, *46*, 1363–1370. [CrossRef] [PubMed]
16. Hennig, E.M.; Valiant, G.A.; Qi, L. Biomechanical Variables and the Perception of Cushioning for Running in Various Types of Footwear. *J. Appl. Biomech.* **1996**, *12*, 143–150. [CrossRef]
17. Dinato, R.C.; Ribeiro, A.P.; Butugan, M.K.; Pereira, I.L.R.; Onodera, A.N.; Sacco, I.C.N. Biomechanical variables and perception of comfort in running shoes with different cushioning technologies. *J. Sci. Med. Sport* **2015**, *18*, 93–97. [CrossRef] [PubMed]
18. Lam, W.K.; Sterzing, T.; Cheung, J.T.M. Reliability of a basketball specific testing protocol for footwear fit and comfort perception. *Footwear Sci.* **2011**, *3*, 151–158. [CrossRef]
19. Roca-Dols, A.; Elena Losa-Iglesias, M.; Sanchez-Gomez, R.; Becerro-de-Bengoa-Vallejo, R.; Lopez-Lopez, D.; Palomo-Lopez, P.; Rodriguez-Sanz, D.; Calvo-Lobo, C. Electromyography activity of triceps surae and tibialis anterior muscles related to various sports shoes. *J. Mech. Behav. Biomed. Mater.* **2018**, *86*, 158–171. [CrossRef]
20. Roca-Dols, A.; Losa-Iglesias, M.E.; Sanchez-Gomez, R.; Becerro-de-Bengoa-Vallejo, R.; Lopez-Lopez, D.; Rodriguez-Sanz, D.; Martinez-Jimenez, E.M.; Calvo-Lobo, C. Effect of the cushioning running shoes in ground contact time of phases of gait. *J. Mech. Behav. Biomed. Mater.* **2018**, *88*, 196–200. [CrossRef]
21. Price, C.; Parker, D.; Nester, C. Validity and repeatability of three in-shoe pressure measurement systems. *Gait Posture* **2016**, *46*, 69–74. [CrossRef] [PubMed]
22. Nigg, B.M.; Anton, M. Energy aspects for elastic and viscous shoe soles and playing surfaces. *Med. Sci. Sports Exerc.* **1995**, *27*, 92–97. [CrossRef] [PubMed]
23. Patrek, M.F.; Kernozek, T.W.; Willson, J.D.; Wright, G.A.; Doberstein, S.T. Hip-abductor fatigue and single-leg landing mechanics in women athletes. *J. Athl. Train.* **2011**, *46*, 31–42. [CrossRef] [PubMed]
24. Thompson, M.A.; Lee, S.S.; Seegmiller, J.; Mcgowan, C.P. Kinematic and kinetic comparison of barefoot and shod running in mid/forefoot and rearfoot strike runners. *Gait Posture* **2015**, *41*, 957–959. [CrossRef] [PubMed]
25. Lieberman, D.E.; Venkadesan, M.; Werbel, W.A.; Daoud, A.I.; D'Andrea, S.; Davis, I.S.; Mang'eni, R.O.; Pitsiladis, Y. Foot strike patterns and collision forces in habitually barefoot versus shod runners. *Nature* **2010**, *463*, 531–535. [CrossRef] [PubMed]
26. Yu, L.; Fu, W.; Wei, S. Effects of basketball shoe on impact force and quadriceps vibrations during active and passive landings. *Footwear Sci.* **2011**, *3*, 96–98.
27. Zhang, S.; Clowers, K.; Kohstall, C.; Yu, Y.J. Effects of various midsole densities of basketball shoes on impact attenuation during landing activities. *J. Appl. Biomech.* **2005**, *21*, 3–17. [CrossRef]
28. Kong, P.W.; Lam, W.K.; Ng, W.X.; Aziz, L.; Leong, H.F. In-shoe plantar pressure profiles in amateur basketball players implications for footwear recommendations and orthosis use. *J. Am. Podiatr. Med. Assoc.* **2018**, *108*, 215–224. [CrossRef]
29. Nigg, B.M.; Nurse, M.A.; Stefanyshyn, D.J. Shoe inserts and orthotics for sport and physical activities. *Med. Sci. Sports Exerc.* **1999**, *31*, 421–428. [CrossRef]
30. Leong, H.F.; Lam, W.K.; Ng, W.X.; Kong, P.W. Center of Pressure and Perceived Stability in Basketball Shoes with Soft and Hard Midsoles. *J. Appl. Biomech.* **2018**, *34*, 284–290. [CrossRef]
31. Che, H.; Nigg, B.M.; de Koning, J. Relationship between plantar pressure distribution under the foot and insole comfort. *Clin. Biomech.* **1994**, *9*, 335–341. [CrossRef]
32. Park, S.K.; Lam, W.K.; Yoon, S.; Lee, K.K.; Ryu, J. Effects of forefoot bending stiffness of badminton shoes on agility, comfort perception and lower leg kinematics during typical badminton movements. *Sports Biomech.* **2017**, *16*, 374–386. [CrossRef]
33. Scanlan, A.T.; Fox, J.L.; Borges, N.R.; Tucker, P.S.; Dalbo, V.J. Temporal changes in physiological and performance responses across game-specific simulated basketball activity. *J. Sport Health Sci.* **2018**, *7*, 176–182. [CrossRef]

34. Condello, G.; Schultz, K.; Tessitore, A. Assessment of sprint and change-of-direction performance in college football players. *Int. J. Sports Physiol. Perform.* **2013**, *8*, 211–212. [CrossRef]
35. Roca-Dols, A.; Losa-Iglesias, M.E.; Sanchez-Gomez, R.; Lopez-Lopez, D.; Becerro-de-Bengoa-Vallejo, R.; Calvo-Lobo, C. Electromyography comparison of the effects of various footwear in the activity patterns of the peroneus longus and brevis muscles. *J. Mech. Behav. Biomed. Mater.* **2018**, *82*, 126–132. [CrossRef]

19

3D Device for Forces in Swimming Starts and Turns

Karla de Jesus [1,2,3,4,*], Luis Mourão [1,2,5], Hélio Roesler [6], Nuno Viriato [2,7], Kelly de Jesus [1,2,3,4], Mário Vaz [2,7], Ricardo Fernandes [1,2] and João Paulo Vilas-Boas [1,2]

1 Centre of Research, Education, Innovation and Intervention in Sport, Faculty of Sport, University of Porto, 91 Dr. Plácido Costa st., 4200-450 Porto, Portugal
2 Porto Biomechanics Laboratory, University of Porto, 91 Dr. Plácido Costa st., 4200-450 Porto, Portugal
3 Human Performance Studies Laboratory, Faculty of Physical Education and Physiotherapy, Federal University of Amazonas, 3000 Gal. Rodrigo Octávio Jordão Ramos ave., South MiniCampus, Coroado I, Manaus 69077-000, Amazonas, Brazil
4 Human Motor Behaviour Studies Laboratory, Faculty of Physical Education and Physiotherapy, Federal University of Amazonas. 3000 Gal. Rodrigo Octávio Jordão Ramos ave., South MiniCampus, Coroado I, Manaus 69077-000, Amazonas, Brazil
5 Superior Institute of Engineering of Porto, Polytechnic Institute of Porto, 431, Dr. António Bernardino de Almeida st., 4249-015 Porto, Portugal
6 Centre of Physical Education, Physiotherapy and Sports, Aquatic Biomechanics Research Laboratory, University of the State of Santa Catarina, 358 Pascoal Simone st., Coqueiros, Florianópolis 88080-350, Santa Catarina, Brazil
7 Institute of Mechanical Engineering and Industrial Management, Faculty of Engineering, University of Porto, Dr. Roberto Frias st., 4200-465 Porto, Portugal
* Correspondence: karladejesus@ufam.edu.br;

Abstract: Biomechanical tools capable of detecting external forces in swimming starts and turns have been developed since 1970. This study described the development and validation of a three-dimensional (six-degrees of freedom) instrumented block for swimming starts and turns. Seven force plates, a starting block, an underwater structure, one pair of handgrips and feet supports for starts were firstly designed, numerically simulated, manufactured and validated according to the Fédération Internationale de Natation rules. Static and dynamic force plate simulations revealed deformations between 290 to 376 $\mu\varepsilon$ and 279 to 545 $\mu\varepsilon$ in the anterior-posterior and vertical axis and 182 to 328.6 Hz resonance frequencies. Force plates were instrumented with 24 strain gauges each connected to full Wheatstone bridge circuits. Static and dynamic calibration revealed linearity (R^2 between 0.97 and 0.99) and non-meaningful cross-talk between orthogonal (1%) axes. Laboratory and ecological validation revealed the similarity between force curve profiles. The need for discriminating each upper and lower limb force responses has implied a final nine-force plates solution with seven above and two underwater platforms. The instrumented block has given an unprecedented contribution to accurate external force measurements in swimming starts and turns.

Keywords: sports engineering; biomechanics; ground reaction forces; swimming; performance

---

1. Introduction

The analysis of swimmers' performance has traditionally examined spatiotemporal variables representing the start, turn and clean swimming distance [1]. The start and turn are fundamentally different skills than free swimming, which does not necessarily indicate a similar level of start or turning performance [1]. Generally, at the elite level, it is not only swimming speed that wins the races but rather the start and turn where most expert swimmers are travelling at their fastest velocity [2,3]. For instance, the start phase of the 50 m men's freestyle at the 2019 FINA Champions Swim Series at

Budapest has showed that 15 m after the start take-off phase, the second-placed swimmer was 0.08 s slower and the final race time difference was 0.15 s. Moreover, over a 200 m event, the turn contributes 21% to total race performance and progressively more as race distance increases [4].

External forces generated during the ventral starts using instrumented starting blocks have been measured since 1971 with a uniaxial force platform placed at the edge of the pool, which had assessed horizontal forces applied by the swimmers' feet during the conventional circular arm swing technique [5]. Cavanagh et al. [6] had optimised Elliot and Sinclair's solution including eight strain gauges in a horizontal bar to measure the horizontal and vertical forces applied by the hands and feet during the grab ventral start technique. Three-dimensional forces were assessed in starts since 2003 by Naemi et al. [7] revealing that the grab start performed with hands in between feet was less stable in preventing platform twist. Horizontal forces applied by feet and hands in the backstroke start were firstly measured in 2011 (de Jesus) using a uniaxial platform and a load cell, being fixed on the starting wall and on the handgrip, respectively.

The changes in the starting block design in 2008 implied adjustments in the previously developed instrumented platforms for start (e.g., [2]) force analyses. Mason and co-authors [2] have presented an instrumented block comprised of four triaxial force sensors placed in a main force plate fixed over the starting block, inclined rear plate, handles for ventral and backstroke start and underwater platform with holes over the front surface. Recently, researchers have shown a new device to measure independently three-axial forces exerted on hands and feet in the ventral kick start technique [8], but limitations have been identified on hand placement dependence. Despite the relevant shortcomings for start analysis that the previous systems have provided, none of them are able to narrow in a unique solution for all ventral, backstroke and relay start force analysis possibilities, assuming laterality effects and independency in hands and feet force assessment. The horizontal and vertical force components determine steering start strategies, being the most assessed. However, lateral responses are essentially a controlling movement in starts [7,9,10] and it can be better understood when assessing each swimmer's limb force contribution.

The description of forces generated during swimming turns also started in the 1970s using uniaxial force plates to assess the horizontal component in tumble and open turns (e.g., [11]). Swimming turns external forces analysis using three-dimensional force plates is still scarce, with the flip technique and its variants being the most commonly investigated (e.g., [12,13]). A double underwater tri-axial force plate solution developed for independent assessment of forces applied by each foot in a backstroke start can also provide a direct measurement of the combined forces exerted during turns and the determination of foot position. Furthermore, in some turn techniques, coaches can assess laterality data if the foot location is compatible with each force platform (e.g., [13]). Mason and co-authors' underwater force platform design has a multitude of holes system to reduce wave effects [2]. However, this configuration limits the possibility to use the same force plate for water wave effect analyses [14].

Coaching and commercial ongoing-instrumented starting blocks are still lacking some final integrated solution for start and turn force analyses that could inspire new biomechanical research directions. In a competitive, rapid uptake market such as sports equipment, it is important to keep searching for new and improved designs and materials at affordable prices [15]. Commercial force plate prices are ~$20,000, which can usually be very expensive for coaches and biomechanists [16]. Beside the high prices, technical assistance issues and spare parts' availability are sources of many difficulties for labs and researchers [17]. Thus, due to the high cost of existing force plate systems, the development of simpler low cost, adjustable and accurate models for biomechanical analysis is desirable for force measurements in swimming start and turn techniques (cf. [18]).

A dynamometric unit composed by independent 3D force plates, a starting block, an underwater structure, ventral and dorsal start handgrips and feet supports is original. It presents crucial potentialities, particularly regarding forces and momenta measurement in individual ventral and backstroke starts, relays and turning techniques. As a versatile and low cost system, the force plates can be used uncoupled from the dynamometric unit to measure active (e.g., [19]) and passive swimmers' drag (e.g., [14]), and underwater gait ground reaction forces (e.g., [20]). The current study aimed to design, construct and validate an instrumented swimming start block, emphasizing geometry description, numerical simulation, sensors bonding, calibration, experimental and ecological validation procedures.

2. Materials and Methods

2.1. 3D Geometric Computer Aided Design

Force plates, the starting block, underwater structure, handgrips and feet supports were 3D designed using a solid modelling computer aided design software (SolidWorks 2012, Dassault Systèmes, SOLIDWORKS Corporation, Waltham, MA, USA). Each force plate and handgrip was framed to achieve proper sensibility with a high rigidity and reduced mass. The start block project prioritized low deformation to support seven to nine force plates, handgrips and an underwater structure. In addition, force plates, the start block, underwater structure, handgrips and feet support dimensions (Figure 1) were conditioned to comply with the Fédération Internationale de Natation rules (FINA; FR 2.7 and FR 2.10).

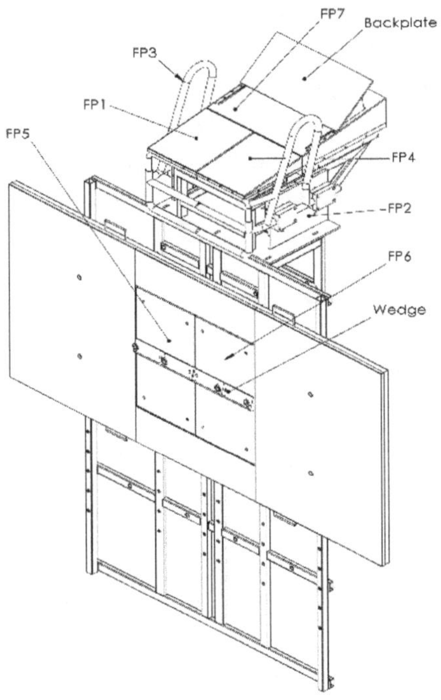

Figure 1. The seven force plates solution distributed in the start block for individual limb force-moment assessments: Each force plate (FP 1 to 7) and feet supports (back plate and wedge) are also shown.

2.2. Force Plates Spatial Layout

Contrarily to arbitrarily multiplying force platforms on the block, it is worth it to consider a minimum number of them. Such a number considers the limbs involved in the starting technique force development and the set of limb positioning on the starting block/wall. The rationale relies on the following: If a sole limb force is measured then the centre of pressure ($\overrightarrow{COP}$) lies on the limb contact area. On the other hand, if a sole platform measures simultaneously two-limb forces then the centre of pressure lies between the limbs and perhaps outside each limb contact area. Such measurement can mask postural constraints necessary for maximum performance data interpretation. The five above water force plates configuration was firstly developed for independent swimmers' upper and lower limbs kinetic analysis in individual ventral start techniques (e.g., grab and track start).

Subsets of analogous platforms have been preferable, aiming for the comparison of force plates behaviour, which implied that two pairs of platforms were similar (300 mm × 250 mm above water and 600 mm × 300 mm underwater). This resemblance provides an interchangeable ability, which might be of great importance if mass production or maintenance were considered. The fifth above water force plate is 500 mm × 440 mm, enabling support for the rear foot as used in the track start technique.

2.3. Force Plates Geometry

The main requirements of the load sensor followed Lywood et al.'s geometry [21], which consisted of instrumented rectangular section bars oriented to be most sensitive to x, y and z force and torque components (cf. [22]), obviating most cross-talk. A waterproof sensor choice enables force plates immersion into the bottom of the swimming pool (~2 m). Sensor locus, distant from the centre anchorage points, allows a better interpolation approach. As the Roesler [20] platform design complied with these previous requirements, it was selected to serve as the testing tool.

It has already been mentioned that Roesler's [20] force plate topology allows a more accurate $\overrightarrow{COP}$ determination, as well as direct and independent 3D forces and moment measurements without interference among them [18]. Each force plate core was designed to be manufactured in galvanized steel and is essentially composed by two vertical and two horizontal beams plus two lateral boxes. The beams, contrarily to the ring or pylon, can acquire the applied load with better accuracy and precision, also allowing better minute change capture in the strain throughout the top plate and not just at the corners [23]. Above and underwater top (Figure 2a,b) and bottom (Figure 2c,d) force plates were built in duralumin to minimise force plate mass. The mounting apparatus plays a crucial role in providing accurate and reliable measurements, with the force plate top and core unattached with commercial bushings.

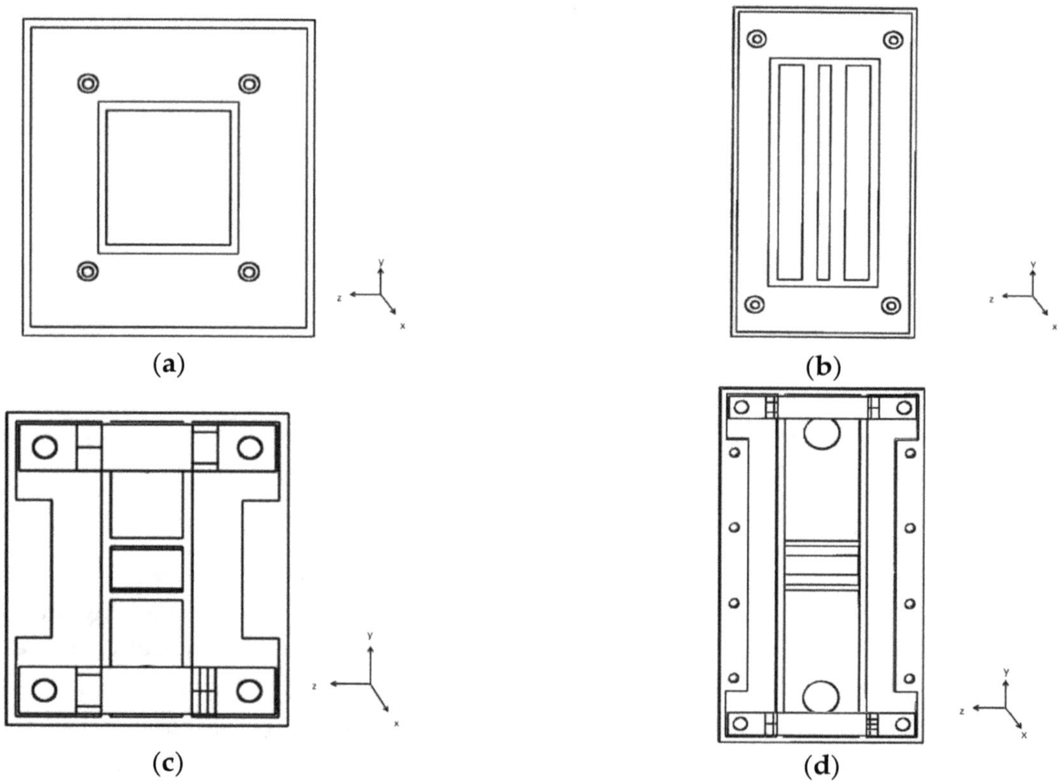

Figure 2. Above and underwater top (**a**,**b** panels) and core (**c**,**d** panels) 300 mm × 250 mm and 600 mm × 300 mm force plates top.

2.4. Start Block, Underwater Structure, Handgrips and Feet Support

Two start block projects were previously designed: (i) a bulky and solid structure and (ii) a lattice block with a declination support, which was replaced by a lattice galvanized steel structure with zero inclination due to excessive mass and reduced stability showed by the previous structures. The starting block was projected to be fixed over an underwater structure attached vertically to the swimming pool wall by front and rear edges, being similar to a previous structure used by Pereira et al. [13,14] and de Jesus et al. [24] for flip turn and backstroke start kinetics assessment. The first underwater structure included a two independent force plates support. The underwater structure evolved from a heavier to a lattice form, with its version being slighter, including holes with 100 mm distance between them placed at different heights on both force plates. It presented a flat rectangular surface for swimming turn analysis (replying the touch pad; FINA, FR 2.13), with a hollow area for underwater force plates embedding, as previously used in turn analysis [13,14].

Handgrips were projected to be independent and framed in galvanized steel, being the first design very versatile to be easily used in ventral and dorsal start technique analysis. However, the first design had shown a handgrip positioning dependency on measured strain signals that did not allow real training and competitive swimmers' movement. In fact, strain gauges would be bonded to the handgrip pipes, obliging swimmers to position their hands on a fixed place to allow comparisons (this was eliminated by the handgrips fixation on each lateral force plate top). With two force plates fixed, each one on the start block lateral, forces and moments could be measured and handgrips positioning could be located. The second handgrip project was based on a simple and outdated handgrip version (e.g., [24]), being updated for two horizontal (i.e., the highest and the lowest, 0.43 and 0.56 m above water surface, respectively) and vertical bars, following the OSB11 starting block configurations. The final handgrip prototype received fine arrangements due to the existent pipe profile. The adjustable feet support for ventral and backstroke start was framed in galvanised steel and nylon (FINA, FR 2.7 and 2.10, respectively), allowing the five rear foot authorised positions.

2.5. Finite Element Analysis

We conducted static structural simulations using modelling software for finite element analysis (Ansys v.12.1, ANSYS Inc., Canonsburg, PA, USA), thus enabling predictions on how the dynamometric unit would strain under isolated and integrated conditions. Dynamic simulations were applied to verify resonance frequency, equivalent stress, equivalent strain and deformations. Based on Roesler et al. [20] geometry and sensor location definition, a 8000 N load was vertically and antero-posteriorly applied to confirm the previously determined sensor location (Figure 3a). The 8000 N load was simulated to allow force plate use in other data collection purposes that had depicted increased ground reaction forces (e.g., long distance jump, 15.2 times body weight; [25]).

Static and dynamic force plate simulations were performed with a core, top and mounting apparatus (i.e., polyethylene bushing and screw). Simulations with the starting block and handgrips were conducted with a 2500 N (centrally located; Figure 3b) and 2000 N load (vertical and antero-posterior; Figure 3c) in the commonly used handgrip positioning for ventral and backstroke start [10]. The underwater structure with force plates vertically mounted was simulated with the gravity at sea level (i.e., 9.81 m/s^2) and values of total deformation, equivalent stress and equivalent elastic strain have also been obtained. The most refined mesh for force plates, the starting block, underwater structures and handgrip simulations was composed of pyramids and cobbled with a 1 mm length and 39,197 nodes and 12,431 elements, 76,344 nodes and 15,724 elements, 273,837 nodes and 107,653 elements, and 46,372 nodes and 17,459 elements, respectively.

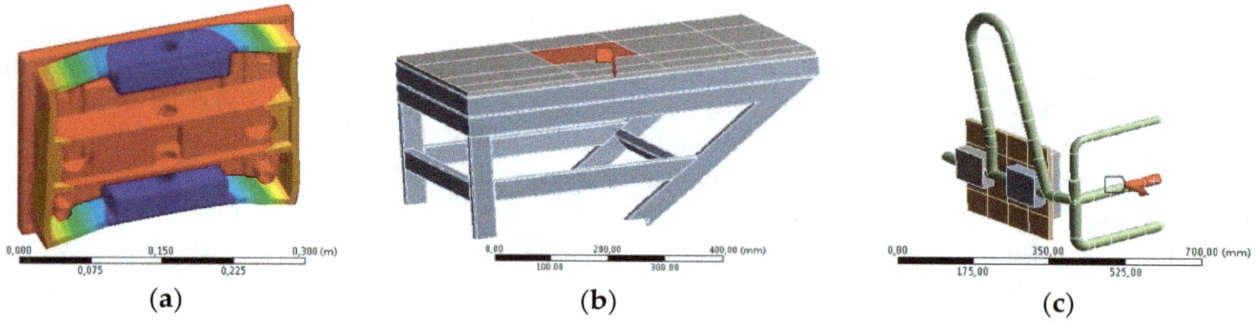

Figure 3. Strain numerical simulation in the assembled force plate (**a** panel), starting block (**b** panel), and handgrips (**c** panel).

2.6. Electrical Circuit

Following structures manufacturing, strain gauges were bonded to the platforms as sensing elements due to the previous research group background and short budget available. Each force plate was instrumented with 24 waterproof strain gauges (Kyowa, Electronic Instruments, KFW-5-120-C1-5M2B, Tokyo, Japan), arranged in six independent full Wheatstone bridges, minimising temperature effects. Those strain gauges were internally bonded to each force plate core and positioned as depicted in Figure 4a–d.

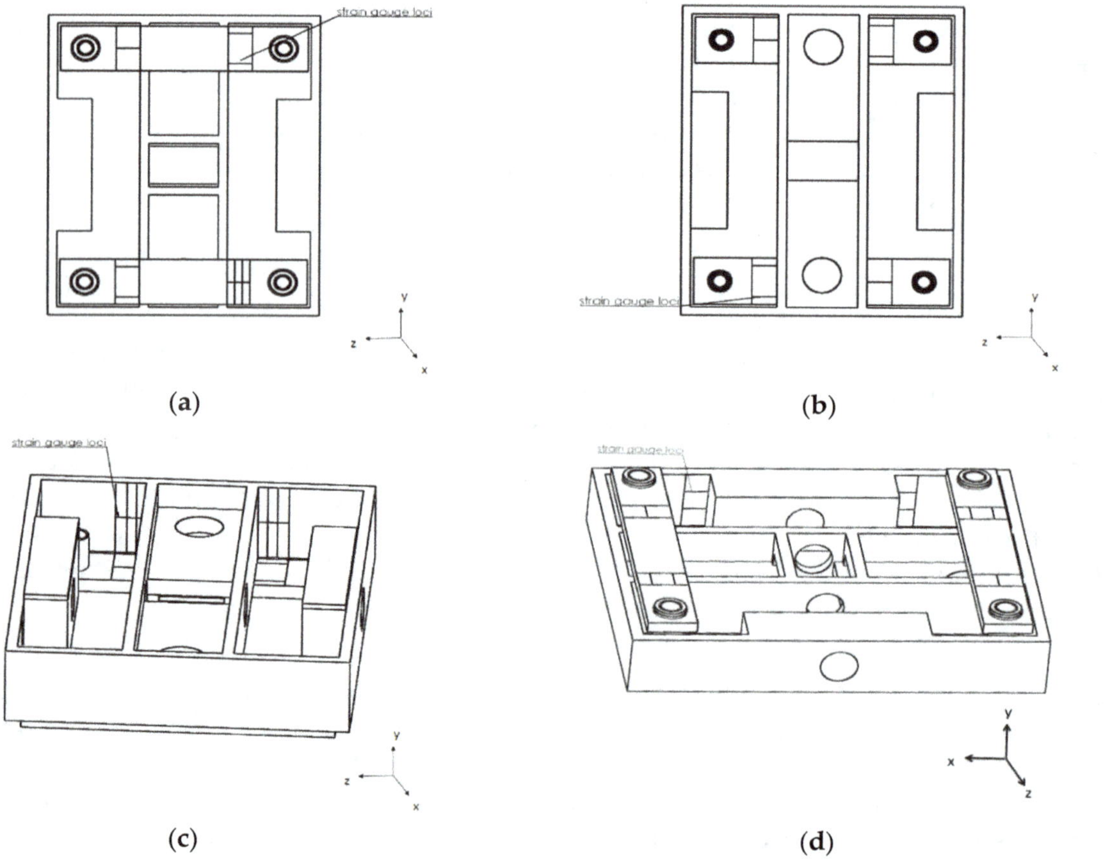

Figure 4. Strain gauge zones: Vertical force (y), antero-posterior (x) and medium-lateral (z) moment (top and bottom view, **a**,**b** panel), antero-posterior (x) force (**c** panel) and medium-lateral (z) force and vertical moment (**d** panel).

After bonding, each strain gauge received an additional protection of a two-part polybutadiene resin designed for re-enterable splice protection (Scotchcast TM re-enterable electrical insulation resin

2123, 3M TM, St. Paul, MN, USA), minimising chlorine wear. Strain gauge wires were brazed in a full Wheatstone bridge configuration (six for each force plate), silicone protected. Each full Wheatstone bridge was connected to a shielded and unfilled cable and provided data from each variable of interest (i.e., horizontal, vertical and lateral forces and momenta).

The six-shielded unfilled cables were connected to an analogue-to-digital converter module to transmit full Wheatstone bridge signals (NI9237 50 kS/s/ch 24 bit-4Channels, National Instruments Corporation, NI™, Austin, TX, USA) and to its scanner chassis (NI CompactDAQ 9172 and 9188 with 8 slots, National Instruments Corporation, NI™, Austin, TX, USA) through RJ50 connectivity, which interfaced with the computer. Strain gauges were identified by digit codes and cables wiring had also been standardised with colour code jacket terminals nearby the RJ50 plug. The dynamometric system specs included 42 strain plus two trigger channels acquiring at a 2000 Hz sampling rate.

Custom-designed data processing software was created in LabView 2013 (SP1, NI™, Austin, TX, USA) to acquire, plot and save the strain readings of each three axial force and moment of force component from each force plate. The executable file was programmed to record data in a total of 8 s (4 s before and after the trigger signal), which was a strategy implemented for the full relay start force acquisitions, anticipatory individual start (e.g., pre-activation) and turn actions (e.g., wave drag). Each force and moment of force curve profile was observed in real data time-acquisition and data acquisition files were later operated to transform strain signals into force-moment (using MatLab R2014a, The MathWorks Incorporated, Natick, MA, USA) routines for the required matricial conversion operations.

2.7. Static Calibration

Static calibration was performed on dry land before force plate proper use and applied both to a load and to an unload sequence with 10 kg individual masses (up to 50 kg in each positioning; cf. [8,18]) allowing the correspondence between strain and applied load. The vertical force component was calibrated at five positions with the use of a tension, compression machine (Instron 8804 Servohydraulic Fatigue Testing System, Instron®, Ilinois Tool Works Inc., Norwood, MA, USA) that laid the right load on each force plate top centre. On antero-posterior and lateral axis force calibration, platforms were vertically fixed on the wall and the load was applied on each centre of interest through a stainless-steel cable connection. A stainless-steel cable was fixed through holes made on the lateral of each force plate top (three per edge). Forces and moment were calibrated using the central and lateral holes (respectively).

2.8. Laboratory Experimental Validation

An experimental validation was completed comparing the results of a rigid body theoretical free rotation around a pivot point $\overrightarrow{COP}$ fall force pattern [26] and the associated strain signal pattern generated. Rigid body inertia moment of the inverted pendulum had to be assessed previously to know mass distribution to allocate its centre of mass and to calculate the centre of mass to the centre of pressure distance. This assessment implies the mass and geometrical dependency of moment of inertia and dynamic behaviour observed in force patterns generated, obviating the use of any force platform except gravity acceleration knowledge.

2.9. Ecological Experimental Validation

The instrumented start block was tested in a 25 m long and 1.90 m deep indoor swimming pool for real data acquisitions, which were then qualitatively compared with starting and turning data previously presented in the literature. All experimental procedures conformed to the requirements stipulated in accordance with The Code of Ethics of the World Medical Association (Declaration of Helsinki) and were approved accordingly by the local research ethics committee. Swimmers and parents and/or guardians (when participants were under 18 years old) provided informed written consent before data collection.

Nine well-trained, healthy and able-bodied male swimmers (mean and standard deviations: 21.09 ± 5.64 years, stature 1.74 ± 0.05 m, and body mass 71.32 ± 11.03 kg) and eight age-group male swimmers engaged on a regular basis in regional- and national-level competitions (mean ± SD: 12.4 ± 0.6 years old, 155.1 ± 13.6 cm of height, 44.6 ± 10.9 kg of body mass, 14.1 ± 5.3% of body fat, with 3.5 ± 1.4 years of experience in competitive swimming and 3.3 ± 0.7 (2–4) of Tanner maturation scale by self-evaluation) volunteered to participate in the start and turn validation study, respectively.

Swimmers performed a familiarisation period with each start and turn technique studied (cf. [27,28]). For the start protocol, each swimmer randomly performed three maximal 15 m trials of backstroke with vertical handgrips, track and one step relay starts. Swimmers performing the turn protocol were also tested in a set of three trials for the open backstroke to the breaststroke medley turning technique. Trials started and finished from the mid-pool (at 12.5 m from the turning wall) and swimmers were instructed to swim in and out at maximum speed until the 12.5 reference [13,28]. Rest periods of 2 min were observed between each repetition in both protocols.

A start signal complying with the FINA SW 4.2 rule was produced through an official device (StartTime IV acoustic start, Swiss Timing Ltd., Corgémento, Switzerland) and instrumented to simultaneously generate an auditory signal and export a pulse to the force plates with convenient signal conditioning. In the one step relay start protocol and open backstroke to breaststroke turn the starter device (without sound) was triggered 7.5 m before the incoming swimmer had touched the wall.

3. Results and Discussion

3.1. Simulations

Table 1 presents strain in antero-posterior and vertical axes (8000 N centred) and resonance frequency of the first, third and final prototypes of above water 300 mm × 250 mm, 500 mm × 440 mm and underwater 600 mm × 300 mm platforms, corroborating Roesler's [20] suggestions for strain values between 100 and 500 με. The force plates design optimisation was a compromise among maximum rigidity, minimum mass and high frequency, which allows small deformations, uncoupling, good linearity and low hysteresis (c.f. [17]). The specific force plate application determined proper resonance frequencies and the maximal vertical load was supported. The waterproof force plate used by Roesler [20], with 500 mm × 500 mm framed in galvanized steel, obtained a 35 Hz resonance frequency, which was considered sufficient for underwater applications due to over damping effects. However, in the current project, force plate versatility has been prioritized and values higher than ~140 Hz were required (cf. [20]) as they can be both used independently of the starting block and out of the water. Commercial force platforms with a natural frequency ≥150 Hz have been well accepted for triple jump ground reaction forces assessment (e.g., [25]).

Table 1. Antero-posterior and vertical strain and their resonance frequency above 300 mm × 250 mm, 600 mm × 300 mm and 500 mm × 440 mm underwater force plates of first, third and final prototypes.

Project Evolution	Static and Dynamic Simulations	300 × 250 mm	600 × 300 mm	500 × 440 mm
First	Antero-posterior (με)	323.0	470.0	297.0
	Vertical (με)	464.0	489.0	473.0
	Resonance frequency (Hz)	235.7	153.0	140.0
Third	Antero-posterior (με)	287.0	357.0	349.0
	Vertical (με)	545.0	521.0	511.0
	Resonance frequency (Hz)	323.7	197.0	177.0
Final	Antero-posterior (με)	290.0	375.0	376.0
	Vertical (με)	545.0	541.0	279.0
	Resonance frequency (Hz)	328.6	199.2	182.0

Table 2 shows results from one example of static simulation from each force plate considering all 24 strain gauge responses, which allow noticing maximal cross-talk less than 5% (cf. [20,21]). In fact, Roesler's [19] findings have shown ~3% of maximal interference among loads when 800 N had been applied. In addition, Lywood et al. [21] reported a cross-talk between orthogonal axes less than 5% for 40 N and 10 N of vertical and horizontal forces applied. The 300 mm × 250 mm force plate laterally positioned on the starting block with fixed handgrip was simulated with a 2000 N load applied vertically on the handgrips, indicating an expectable relevant lateral force (strain gauges 17, 18, 23, 24; cf. Figure 4d). When 8000 N was centrally and vertically applied on a 600 mm × 300 mm force plate, only strain gauges responsible for this measurement responded (i.e., 1 to 12, vertical force, antero-posterior and lateral moment; cf. Figure 4a,b).

Table 2. The 24 strain gauge responses when a 2000 N and 8000 N vertical load was applied on 300 mm × 250 mm and 600 mm × 300 mm force plates.

Strain Gauges	Variable	300 × 250 mm (με)	600 × 300 mm (με)
1	Lateral moment	−4.54	78.13
2	Vertical force	84.66	301.17
3	Lateral moment	−23.73	157.09
4	Lateral moment	−149.79	108.67
5	Vertical force	200.78	316.68
6	Lateral moment	83.29	93.08
7	Antero-posterior moment	−40.01	−215.51
8	Vertical force	133.75	−282.81
9	Antero-posterior moment	−74.94	−205.90
10	Antero-posterior moment	9.51	−160.94
11	Antero-posterior moment	55.70	−188.20
12	Vertical force	−72.43	−238.46
13	Antero-posterior force	−104.08	1.60
14	Antero-posterior force	93.30	0.52
15	Antero-posterior force	−177.25	0.62
16	Antero-posterior force	176.88	0.14
17	Lateral force	249.58	14.55
18	Lateral force	256.12	−10.41
19	Vertical moment	−26.40	−7.71
20	Vertical moment	−45.34	13.11
21	Vertical moment	7.09	13.10
22	Vertical moment	33.94	−8.22
23	Lateral force	−222.66	−10.20
24	Lateral force	−264.68	15.83

The starting block total deformation under a 2500 N centre vertical load was 0.00030553 m. The gravity at sea level (9.81 m/s^2) tested over the underwater structure and two force plates vertically fixed on it revealed a maximal deformation of 0.00012322 m. Moreover, using the same standard gravity at sea level, the underwater structure with force plates has showed a maximum of 0.00000813 Pa and 0.0000409 m/m, considering equivalent von-Mises stress and equivalent von-Mises elastic strain, respectively, indicating short stress gradients in the underwater structure regions. An antero-posterior 2000 N load applied both on the lowest and on the highest horizontal and vertical handgrips revealed 200, 165 and 115 maximal με. A vertical 2000 N load applied on the lowest and on the highest horizontal and vertical handgrips indicated 591, 585 and 205 maximal με.

3.2. Calibrations

The calibration regression equation for the antero-posterior and medium-lateral axis of 300 mm × 250 mm and 600 × 300 mm force plates is depicted in Figure 5a–d. Results evidenced the previously noticed linearity (R^2 ranging between 0.97 and 0.99) and non-meaningful cross-talk between orthogonal axes (small and negligible; <5%) when quantifying any couple of force plate output signals (cf. [20,21]). Calibration results of 300 mm × 250 mm force plates are depicted considering the forces applied on handgrips positioning previously simulated.

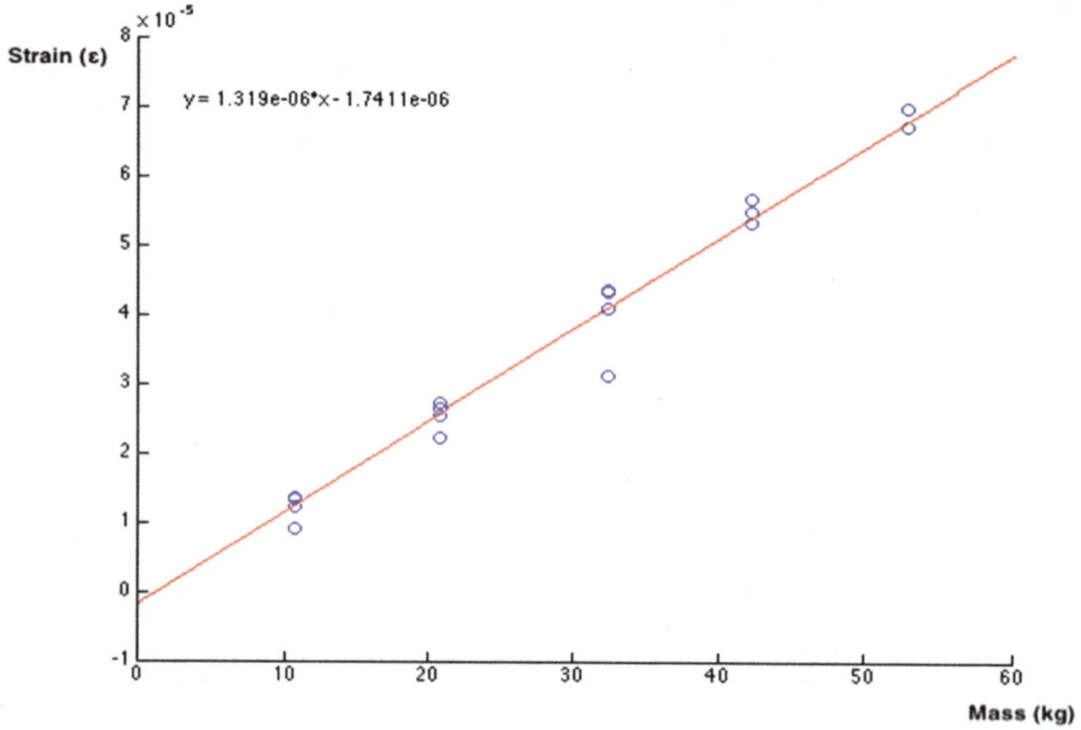

(a)

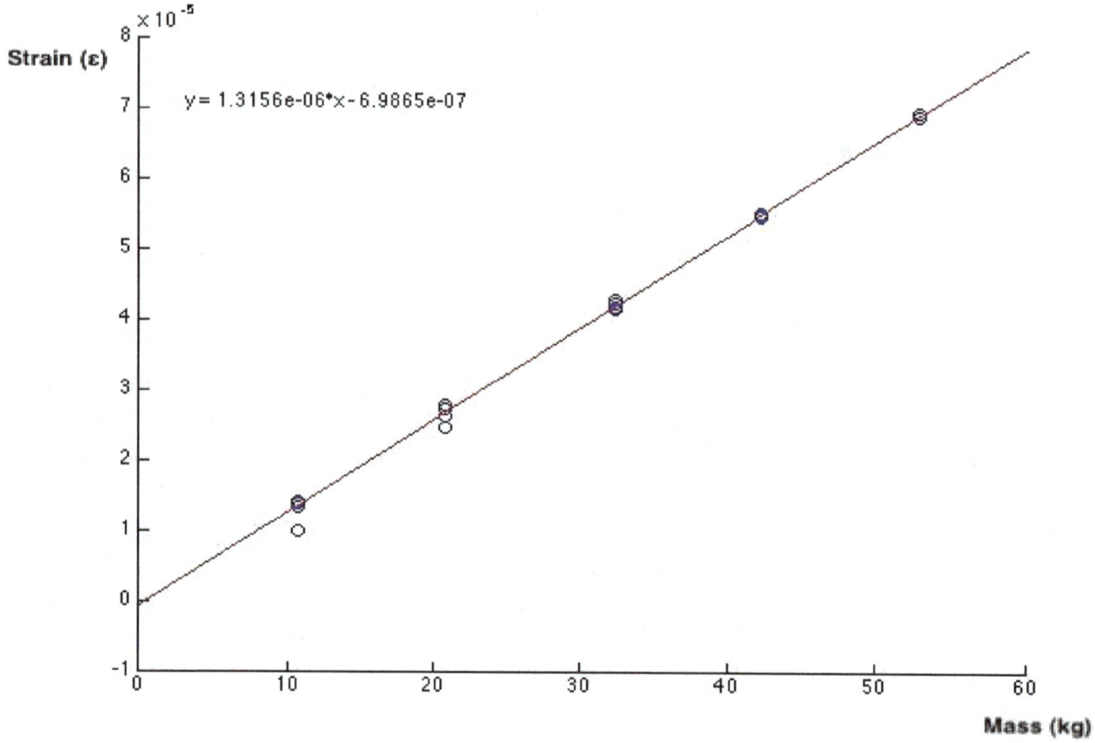

(b)

Figure 5. *Cont.*

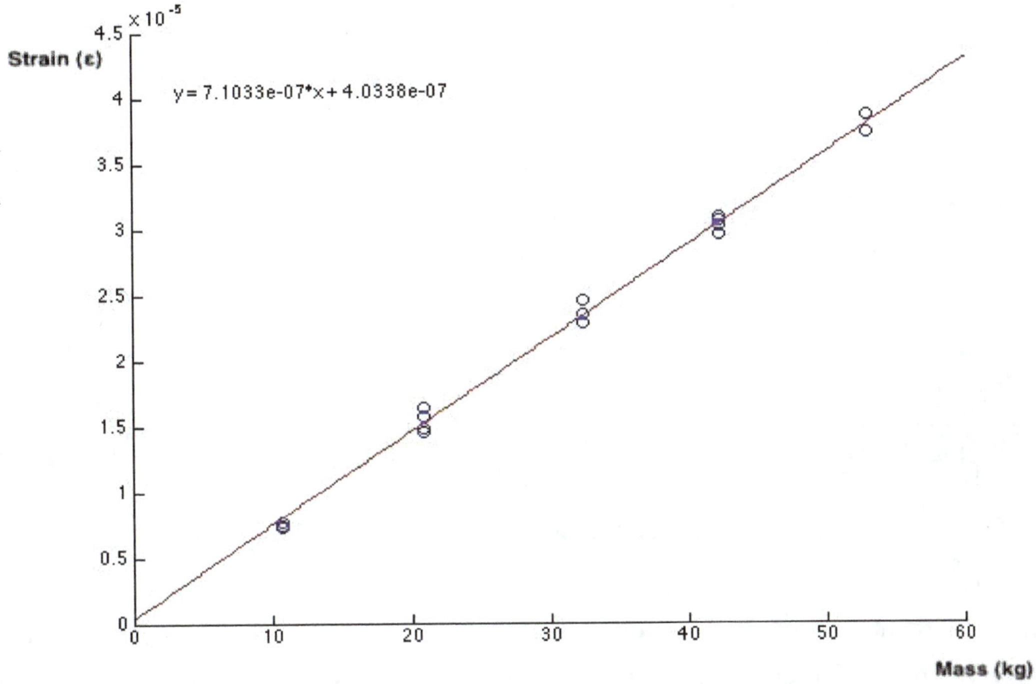

(c)

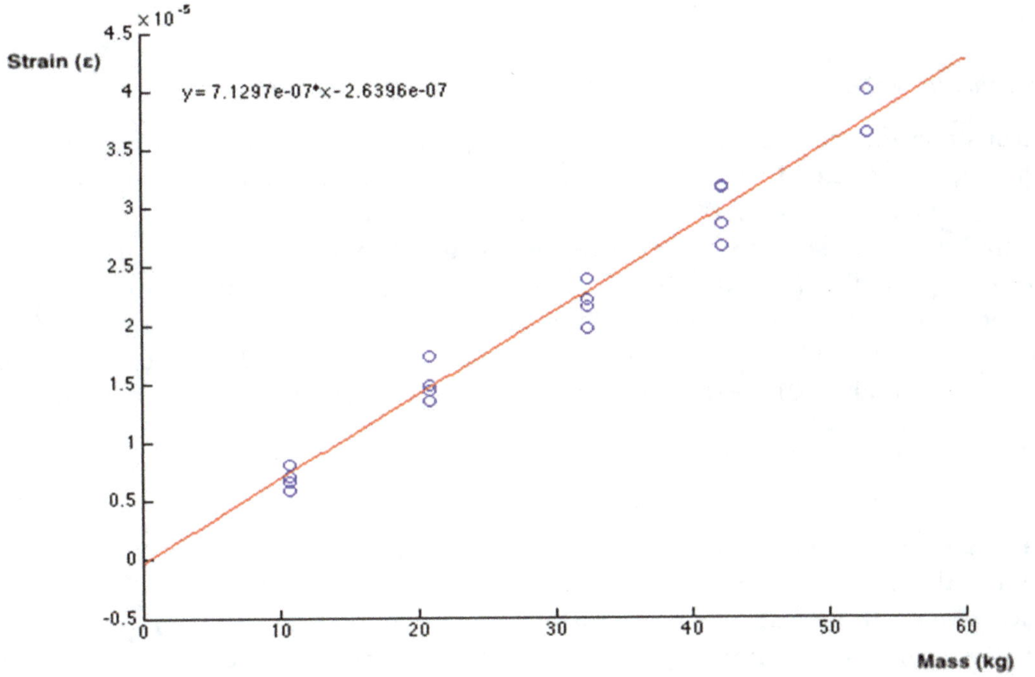

(d)

Figure 5. Force plates calibration results: 300 mm × 250 mm force plate antero-posterior force (**a** panel), medium-lateral force (**b** panel), 600 mm × 300 mm force plate antero-posterior force (**c** panel), and medium-lateral force (**d** panel).

Figure 6 presents vertical force, antero-posterior and lateral moment calibration (in normalised strain measure) for the underwater 600 mm × 300 mm force plate, evidencing linearization and cross-talk ~5% between orthogonal sensors (cf. [18,20]). The force plate design used has revealed greater sensibility in responses to the vertical loads, corroborating Lywood [21].

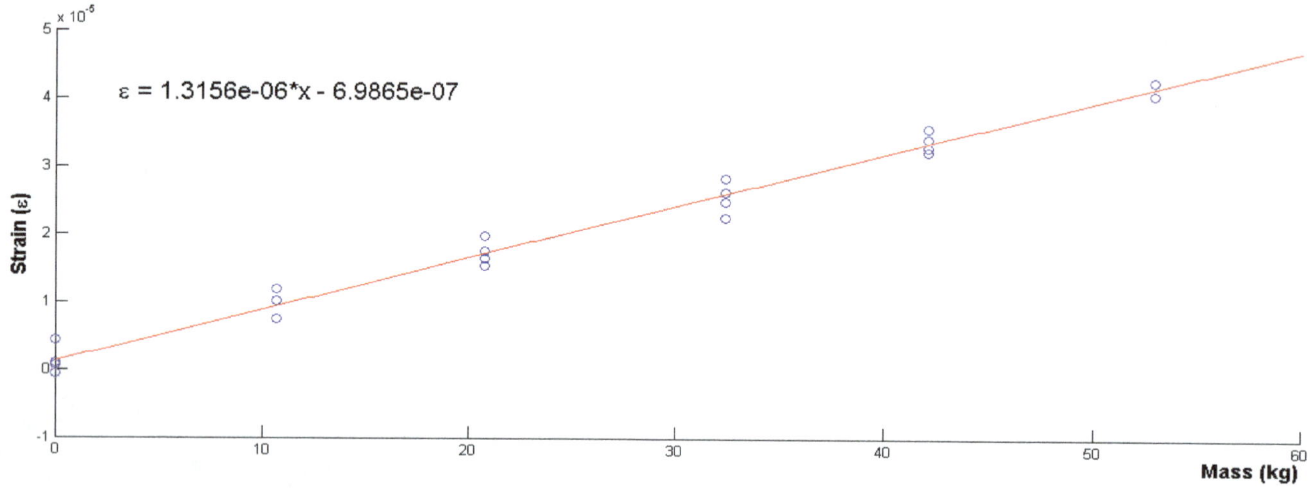

Figure 6. Force plates calibration results: 600 mm × 300 mm force plate vertical force.

Repeatability for loads above 300 N and below 40 N has revealed within 5% and 10–15% with a 95% confidence level. The $\overrightarrow{COP}$ locus was more uncertain farther from the platform centre with a reasonable radial around centre dependency.

3.3. Laboratory Experimental Validation

Due to in situ installation procedures, usage and aging, force plates accuracy may decrease, which can be propagated to the already calculated kinetic quantities. Based on these limitations, some research groups have developed systems to assess force plate accuracy using ad hoc designed in situ devices [8,26]. In the current study, static calibrations were followed by dynamical calibrations performed with a rigid body falling procedure [26], revealing homogeneity of static calibration results, particularly in the time = 0 force time curve of the falling body. The simultaneous correlation coefficient between the posterior strain filtered signal (moving average of 32 samples) and the theory generated by a previous application in MatLab R2014 (MathWorks Inc., Natick, MA,USA) has shown a value of 0.95.

3.4. Ecological Experimental Validation

The horizontal force–time curve exerted by hands and produced during a backstroke start data acquisition is similar to the one peak force profile previously presented (~0.5 BW; [24]). Most of the force–time curves displayed in backstroke start studies have analysed the horizontal component exerted on feet (e.g., [24,29]), which is similar to the dual peak force profile found in the current study (Figure 7a), with swimmers performing ~1.6 BW in the both peak forces. Vertical backstroke start forces exerted by feet have shown similar values to those found in de Jesus et al. (i.e., ~1.0 BW; [10,29]). Lateral force exerted by feet has depicted a peak force instant before the hands-off. Horizontal and vertical force–time curves exerted on feet and hands obtained in the new track start technique performed with the back plate (Figure 8) have registered similar rear (~800 N and ~1000 N) and front foot (~800 N and 600 N; cf. [1,8]) as well as hand force profiles (~150 N and ~800 N; cf. [8]). Previous studies have evidenced that the test–retest reliability of the kinetic gait parameters in the aquatic environment presented poor (medial lateral force component) to excellent reliability (vertical and antero-posterior force component; [30]).

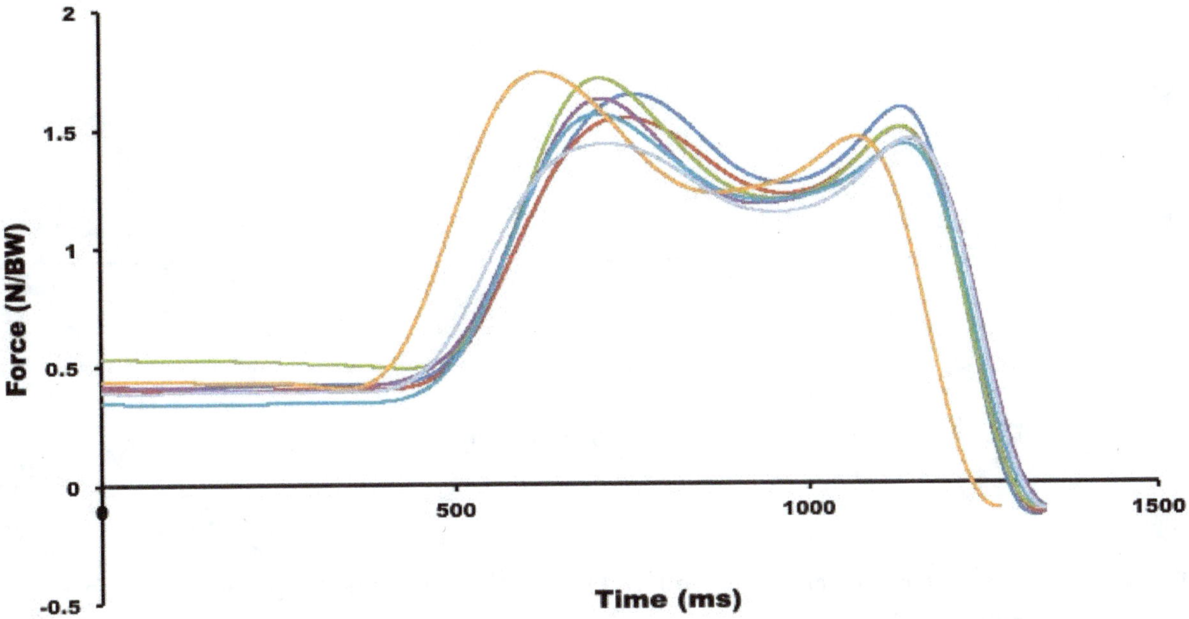

(a)

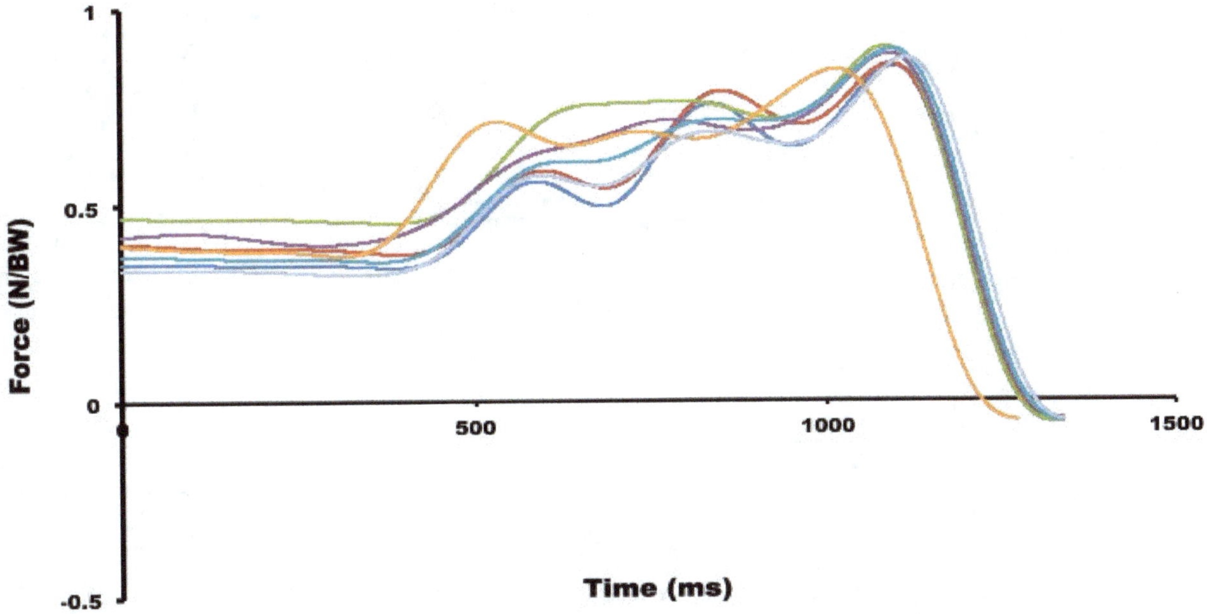

(b)

Figure 7. *Cont.*

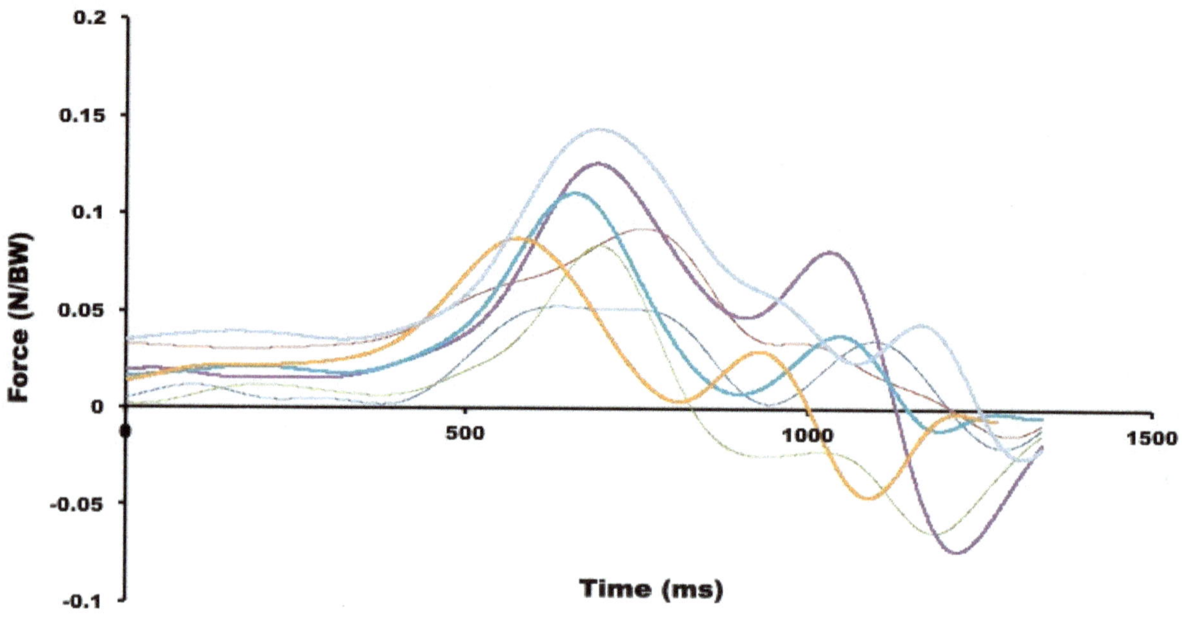

(c)

Figure 7. Backstroke start horizontal (**a** panel), vertical (**b** panel) and lateral (**c** panel) forces from seven trials of one swimmer (**c** panel).

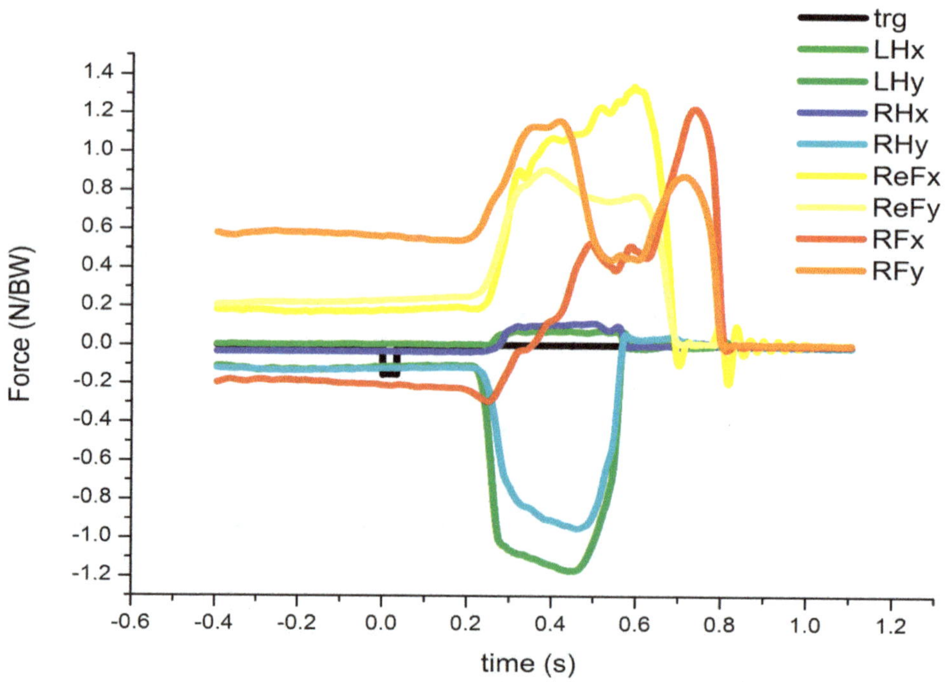

Figure 8. Individual antero-posterior (x) and vertical (y) force—time curves representing forces exerted on left and right hands (LH and RH), as well as rear and front foot (ReF and RF) in the new track start technique synchronised with the trigger (trg).

In relay start techniques, the horizontal force–time curve exerted on the feet and obtained during one step start technique (Figure 9) revealed a similar finding as obtained by Takeda et al. [31], although these authors had not measured right and left forces exerted on each foot.

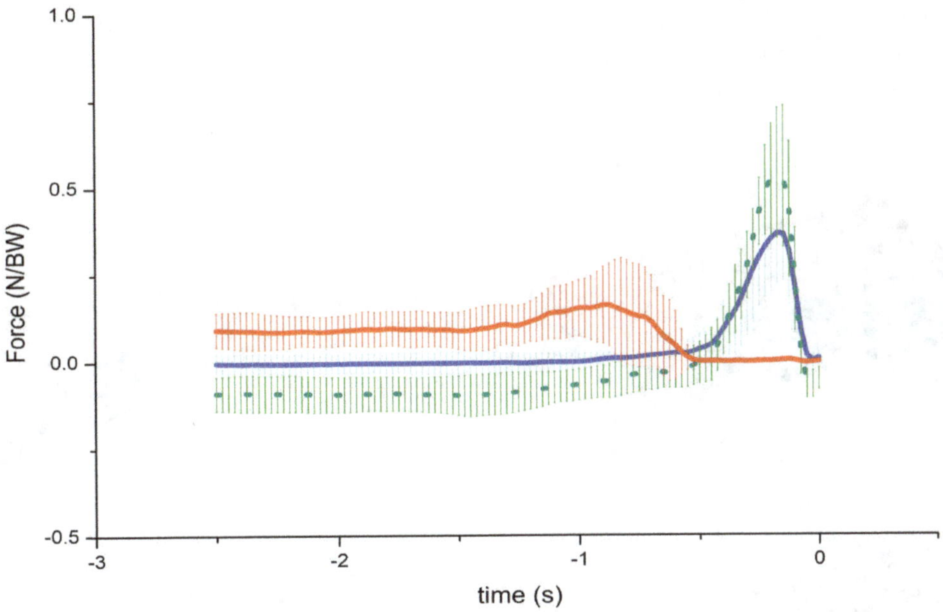

Figure 9. Horizontal force–time curve profiles from eight swimmers at the one step relay start technique: Rear foot (red line), front left and right foot (green and blue line, respectively).

Tri-axial forces measured in one underwater force plate during the open backstroke to breaststroke changeover have evidenced two distinct turn phases, the hand contact (~4.60 to 5.50 s) followed by swimmers' rotation (~4.80 s to 7.30 s) and the push-off (~7.30 to 7.80 s; Figure 10). Previous studies have already mentioned that the push-off phase depicted explosive lower limb movements since the first feet contact (~7.20 s) to the end of push-off (~7.80 s), which has been mainly observed in the horizontal force component [13,28]. Purdy and co-authors [31] have found ~193 N for the peak horizontal ground reaction force in female swimmers performing the open turn technique.

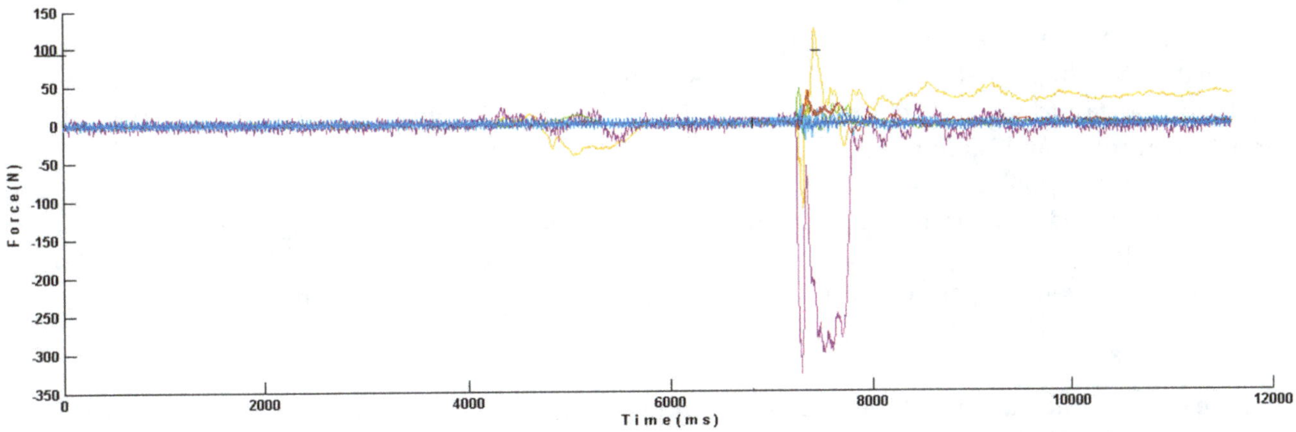

Figure 10. Individual backstroke to breaststroke open medley turning technique force–time curve with horizontal, vertical and medium-lateral components (purple, yellow and red line, respectively).

The current and the previously developed instrumented starting block configurations have shown restrictions regarding independent hand force and momentum measures with natural swimmers' hands and feet placement during all ventral start techniques. (e.g., [2,6,8]). The solution found in the current project was the replication of four more tri-axial force plates of 300 mm × 125 mm designed and numerically simulated (Figure 11a–d) to be placed in the frontal start block edge. An 800 N vertical, and 200 N medium-lateral and horizontal load were applied and registered 280.11, 109.89 and 117.34 $\mu\varepsilon$ maximal deformation and a maximal 286.45 Hz frequency. The four-force plates solution enables swimmers to grasp the top and bottom of the starting block surface, being versatile and valid to independently measure each swimmer's hand and foot forces and momenta generated regardless of the ventral starting technique used.

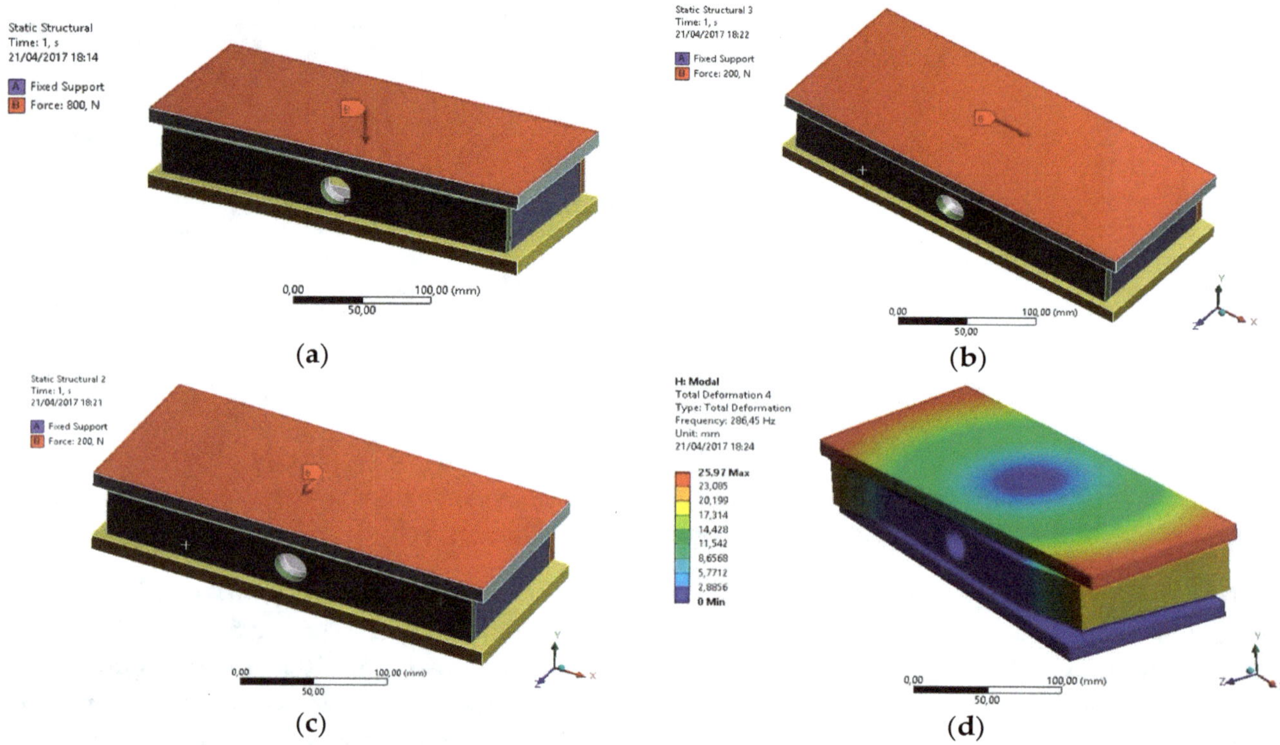

Figure 11. The four 300 mm × 125 mm force plates in static and dynamic simulation conditions for vertical, antero-posterior and medium lateral deformation (**a**–**c** panels), as well as the frequency analysis (**d** panel).

Notwithstanding the relevance of the dynamometric unit solution developed for start and turn analysis, it is recognised that future work is needed to improve main limitations: (i) finite element analysis revealed important data for project manufacturing. However, irregularities in the starting pool wall cannot be controlled and could affect measurements; (ii) despite static and dynamic calibration procedures, force plate linear responses were revealed, suggesting a less time-consuming in situ calibration procedure should be developed to avoid the detachment of each force plate from the dynamometric central; and (iii) increasing underwater force plate placement possibilities beyond side-by-side but also in an up and down location would cover independent feet force measurements from other turn techniques.

4. Conclusions

The dynamometric central for individual and relay swimming start and turn techniques framed according to FINA facility rules has evidenced reliable and accurate external force data. This device is ecologically valid and versatile, being able to be used in integrated or in future independent force plate analysis, as bow wave measurements in turns, passive drag and jumping techniques.

Author Contributions: Conceptualization, K.d.J. (Karla de Jesus), L.M., H.R., M.V. and J.P.V.-B.; data curation, K.d.J. (Karla de Jesus), L.M., M.V., R.F. and J.P.V.-B.; formal analysis, K.d.J. (Karla de Jesus), L.M., H.R., N.V., M.V. and J.P.V.-B.; funding acquisition, K.d.J. (Karla de Jesus), M.V., R.F. and J.P.V.-B.; investigation, K.d.J. (Karla de Jesus), K.d.J. (Kelly de Jesus), M.V., R.F., J.P.V.-B.; methodology, K.d.J. (Karla de Jesus), LM., H.R., N.V., K.d.J. (Kelly de Jesus), M.V., R.F., J.P.V.-B.; software, L.M., H.R., N.V., M.V., project administration; K.d.J. (Karla de Jesus), R.F., J.P.V.-B.; resources, K.d.J. (Karla de Jesus), R.F., J.P.V.-B.; supervision; K.d.J. (Karla de Jesus), L.M., M.V., R.F.,

J.P.V.-B.; validation; K.d.J. (Karla de Jesus), L.M., K.d.J. (Kelly de Jesus), J.P.V.-B.; visualization, K.d.J. (Karla de Jesus), R.F., J.P.V.-B.; writing—original draft, K.d.J., (Karla de Jesus), L.M., H.R., N.V., K.d.J. (Kelly de Jesus), R.F., J.P.V.-B.; writing—review and editing, K.d.J. (Karla de Jesus), L.M., M.V., R.F., J.P.V.-B.

Acknowledgments: Leandro dos Santos Coelho, Alexandre Igor Araripe Medeiros and Phornpot Chainok provided valuable feedback on manuscript drafts.

References

1. Slawson, S.E.; Conway, P.P.; Cossor, J.; Chakravorti, N.; West, A.A. The categorisation of swimming start performance with reference to force generation on the main block and footrest components of the Omega OSB11 start blocks. *J. Sports Sci.* **2013**, *31*, 468–478. [CrossRef] [PubMed]
2. Mason, B.; Mackintosh, C.; Pease, D. The development of an analysis system to assist in the correction of inefficiencies in stars and turns for elite competitive swimming. In Proceedings of the 30th International Symposium on Biomechanics in Sports, Melbourne, Australia, 2–6 July 2012; Bradshaw, E.J., Burnett, A., Hume, P.A., Eds.; International Society of Biomechanics in Sports: Melbourne, Australia, 2012; pp. 249–252.
3. Veiga, S.; Carla, A.; Frutos, P.; Navarro, E. Comparison of starts and turns of national and regional level swimmers by individualized-distance measurements. *Sports Biomech.* **2014**, *13*, 285–295. [CrossRef] [PubMed]
4. Slawson, S.; Conway, P.; Justham, L.; Le Sage, T.; West, A. Dynamic signature for tumble turn performance in swimming. *Procedia Eng.* **2010**, *2*, 3391–3396. [CrossRef]
5. Elliott, G.M.; Sinclair, H. The influence of block angle on swimming sprint starts. In *Swimming I, Proceedings of the I International Symposium of Biomechanics and Swimming, Waterpolo and Divig, Bruxelles, Belgium, 14–16 September 1970*; Lewillie, L., Clarys, J.P., Eds.; Brussel Universite Libre de Bruxelles, Laboratoire de I' effort: Bruxelles, Belgium, 1971; pp. 183–189.
6. Cavanagh, P.R.; Palmgren, J.V.; Kerr, B.A. A device to measure forces at hands during the grab start. In *Swimming II, Proceedings of the II International Symposium of Biomechanics in Swimming, Brussels, Belgium*; Lewillie, L., Clarys, J.P., Eds.; Tokyo Universitaire Park Press: Baltimore, MD, USA; London, UK, 1975; pp. 43–50.
7. Naemi, R.; Arshi, A.R.; Ahadian, A.; Barjasteh, B. 3D kinematic and kinetic analyses of two methods for grab start technique. In Proceedings of the 19th International Symposium on Biomechanics in Sports, Melbourne, Australia, 26–29 June 2001; Blackwell, J.R., Sanders, R.H., Eds.; International Society of Biomechanics in Sports: San Francisco, CA, USA, 2001; pp. 96–99.
8. Takeda, T.; Sakai, S.; Takagi, H.; Okuno, K.; Tsubakimoto, S. Contribution of hand and foot force to take-off velocity for the kick-start in competitive swimming. *J. Sports Sci.* **2017**, *35*, 565–571. [CrossRef] [PubMed]
9. Vantorre, J.; Seifert, L.; Fernandes, R.J.; Vilas-Boas, J.P.; Chollet, D. Comparison of grab start between elite and trained swimmers. *Int. J. Sports Med.* **2010**, *31*, 887–893. [CrossRef] [PubMed]
10. De Jesus, K.; de Jesus, K.; Gonçalves, P.; Vasconcelos, M.O.; Medeiros, A.I.A.; Carvalho, D.A.D.; Fernandes, R.J.; Vilas-Boas, J.P. Lateral kinetic proficiency and asymmetry in backstroke start performed with horizontal and vertical handgrips. *Sports Biomech.* **2018**, 13–15. [CrossRef] [PubMed]
11. Nicol, K.; Krueger, F. Impulses exerted in performing several kinds of swimming turns. In *Swimming III, Proceedings of the III International Symposium of Biomechanics in Swimming, Alberta, AB, Canada*; Terauds, J., Bedingfield, E.W., Eds.; Baltimore University Park Press: Baltimore, MD, USA; London, UK, 1979; pp. 222–232.
12. Puel, F.; Morlier, J.; Avalos, M.; Mesnard, M.; Cid, M.; Hellard, P. 3D kinematic and dynamic analysis of the front crawl tumble turn in elite male swimmers. *J. Biomech.* **2012**, *45*, 510–515. [CrossRef] [PubMed]
13. Pereira, S.M.; Ruschel, C.; Hubert, M.; Machado, L.; Roesler, H.; Fernandes, R.J.; Vilas-Boas, J.P. Kinematic, kinetic and EMG analysis of four front crawl flip turn techniques. *J. Sports Sci.* **2015**, *33*, 2006–2015. [CrossRef] [PubMed]
14. Pereira, S.M.; Gonçalves, P.; Fernandes, R.J.; Machado, L.; Roesler, H.; Vilas-Boas, J.P. Graphic removal of water wave impact in the pool wall during the flip turn. In Proceedings of the XI International Symposium for Biomechanics and Medicine in Swimming, Oslo, Norway, 16–19 June 2010; Kjendlie, P.L., Stallman, R.K., Cabri, J., Eds.; Norwergian School of Sport Science: Oslo, Norway, 2010; pp. 148–150.
15. Duncan, O.; Shepherd, T.; Moroney, C.; Foster, L.; Venkatraman, P.; Winwood, K.; Allen, T.; Alderson, A. Review of Auxetic Materials for Sports Applications: Expanding Options in Comfort and Protection. *Appl. Sci.* **2018**, *8*, 941. [CrossRef]

16. Wardoyo, S.; Hutajulu, P.T.; Togibasa, O. A Development of Force Plate for Biomechanics Analysis of Standing and Walking. *J. Phys. Conf. Ser.* **2016**, *739*. [CrossRef]
17. Silva, M.G.; Moreira, P.V.S.; Rocha, H.M. Development of a low cost force platform for biomechanical parameters analysis. *Res. Biomed. Eng.* **2017**, *33*, 259–268. [CrossRef]
18. Mourão, L.; Jesus, K.; Viriato, N.; Fernandes, R.J.; Vilas-Boas, J.P.; Vaz, M. Design and construction of a 3D force plate prototype for developing an instrumented swimming start block. *J. Biomed. Eng. Inform.* **2016**, *2*, 99. [CrossRef]
19. Formosa, D.; Mason, B.R.; Burkett, B.J. Measuring active drag within the different phases of front crawl swimming. In Proceedings of the XI International Symposium on Biomechanics and Medicine in Swimming, Oslo, Norway, 16–19 June 2010; Kjendlie, L., Stallman, R.K., Cabri, J., Eds.; Norwegian School of Sport Science: Oslo, Norway, 2010; pp. 82–84.
20. Roesler, H. Turning measurements in swimming using underwater force platforms. In Proceedings of the IX International Symposium on Biomechanics and Medicine in Swimming, de Saint-Étienne, France, 16–19 June 2010; Chatard, J.C., Ed.; l' Université de Saint-Étienne: Saint-Étienne, France, 2003; pp. 243–248.
21. Lywood, D.W.; Adams, D.J.; Van Eyken, A.; Macpherson, J.M. Small, triaxial force plate. *Med. Biol. Eng. Comput.* **1987**, *25*, 698–701. [CrossRef] [PubMed]
22. Wu, G.; Siegler, S.; Allard, P. ISB recommendation on definitions of joint coordinate system of various joints for the reporting of human joint motion-part I: Ankle, hip, and spine. International Society of Biomechanics. *J. Biomech.* **2002**, *35*, 543–548. [CrossRef]
23. Wright, D.A. *Development of a Waterproof Force Plate for Pool Applications*; Ohio State University: Columbus, OH, USA, 2011.
24. De Jesus, K.; de Jesus, K.; Figueiredo, P.; Gonçalves, P.; Pereira, S.; Vilas-Boas, J.P.; Fernandes, R. Backstroke start kinematic and kinetic changes due to different feet positioning. *J. Sports Sci.* **2013**, *31*, 1665–1675. [CrossRef] [PubMed]
25. Perttunen, J.O.; Kyrolainen, H.; Komi, P.V.; Heinonen, A. Biomechanical loading in the triple jump. *J. Sports Sci.* **2000**, *18*, 363–370. [CrossRef] [PubMed]
26. Mourão, L.; de Jesus, K.; Roesler, H.; Machado, L.; Fernandes, R.; Vilas-Boas, J.P.; Vaz, M. Effective swimmer's action during the grab start technique. *PLoS ONE* **2015**, *15*, e0123001. [CrossRef] [PubMed]
27. De Jesus, K.; de Jesus, K.; Medeiros, A.; Gonçalves, P.; Figueiredo, P.; Fernandes, R.J.; Vilas-Boas, J.P. Neuromuscular activity of upper and lower limbs during two backstroke swimming start variants. *J. Sport Sci. Med.* **2015**, *14*, 591–601.
28. Chainok, P.; Lauer, J.; Zacca, R.; Barbosa, R.; Gonçalves, P.; Fernandes, R.; Vilas-Boas, J.P. Neuromuscualar activation during rotation and push-off phases of backstroke turning techniques in age-group swimmers. In Proceedings of the XXXIV International Symposium on Biomechanics in Sports, Tsukuba, Japan, 18–22 July 2016; Ae, M., Enomoto, Y., Fujii, N., Takagi, H., Eds.; International Society of Biomechanics in Sports: Tsukuba, Japan, 2016; pp. 541–544.
29. Nguyen, C.; Bradshaw, E.; Pease, D.; Wilson, C. Is starting with the feet out of the water faster in backstroke swimming? *Sports Biomech.* **2014**, *13*, 154–165. [CrossRef] [PubMed]
30. Barreto, M.S.; Dela Bela, L.F.; Dias, J.M.; Pelegrinelli, A.R.; de Campos, R.R.; Carvalho, R.G.; Taglietti, M.; Batista, J.P., Jr.; Silva, M.F.; Olkoski, M.M.; et al. Reliability of ground reaction forces in the aquatic environment. *J. Electromyogr. Kinesiol.* **2016**, *30*, 23–30. [CrossRef] [PubMed]
31. Purdy, E.; Hurley, N.; Bengry, A.; Jensen, R. Force and tie analysis of backstroke to breaststroke turns. In Proceedings of the 30th International Symposium on Biomechanics in Sports, Melbourne, Australia, 2–6 July 2012; Bradsha, E.J., Burnett, A., Hume, P.A., Eds.; International Society of Biomechanics in Sports: Melbourne, Australia, 2012; pp. 196–199.

20

Relationship between Kinematic Variables of Jump Throwing and Ball Velocity in Elite Handball Players

Abdel-Rahman Akl [1], Ibrahim Hassan [2], Amr Hassan [3,*] and Phillip Bishop [4]

1 Faculty of Physical Education-Abo Qir, Alexandria University, Alexandria 21913, Egypt
2 Faculty of Physical Education, Zagazig University, Zagazig 44519, Egypt
3 Department of Sports Training, Faculty of Sports Education, Mansoura University, Mansoura 35516, Egypt
4 Department of Kinesiology, University of Alabama, Tuscaloosa, AL 35487, USA
* Correspondence: amrahh@mans.edu.eg;

Abstract: The purpose of this pilot study was to evaluate the relationship between the kinematic variables of the right hand and left leg with ball velocity during jump-throwing phases in handball for better-informed training. We investigated ball velocity and the key kinematic variables of jump throwing during different throwing phases in three strides. Ten right-handed male handball professional players who had competed in the Egyptian Handball Super League participated in this study. Jump throwing performance was divided into three phases (cocking, acceleration and follow-through), which included eight events during the throwing. Five trials were captured for each player, and a 3D analysis was performed on the best trial. Results indicated that the velocity of the throwing hand was the most important variable during jump throwing, which was correlated with ball velocity during the three phases of performance in four events: Initial contact (IC) (r = 0.66*), initial flight (IF) (r = 63*), maximum height of the throwing hand (Max-HH) (r = 0.78*) and ground contact (GC) (r = 0.83*). In addition, the initial flight was the most important event in which players need to be using the best angles during performance, particularly the shoulder angle.

Keywords: jump throwing ability; 3D motion analysis; acceleration

---

1. Introduction

Team handball is an Olympic sport played worldwide at a professional level in several countries. Recently, handball has received increased attention in research studies, especially in biomechanics [1–8].

Jump throwing is an essential task in handball and is used frequently from different positions when a player shoots at the goal. As has been mentioned in earlier studies, handball players perform about 48,000 throws during the season, with the mean throwing speed of 130 km·h^{-1} [9], they and commonly use (73–75% of the time) jump throwing throws during the competition [5,7]. Hence, jump throwing and players' ability to accelerate the ball with the arm throw are vital demands during a handball game.

During jump throwing in handball, ball velocity and jump height range are key factors for better throwing performance [10]. Thus, most studies have investigated ball velocity [5,11,12].

Kinematic variables contribute to the velocity of the ball in order to find the fundamental procedures for improving handball players. As such, previous studies have documented the kinematic results of jump throwing performance in handball. Wagner, Buchecker, von Duvillard and Muller [7] found a significant difference of ball velocity, body height and weight between elite and lower performance levels. As well as, Wagner, Pfusterschmied, von Duvillard and Müller [5] compared the ball velocity and throwing accuracy between jump and standing throws. In addition, van den Tillaar and Ettema [8] investigated the contribution of upper-extremity, trunk, and lower-extremity movements, and van den

Tillaar [2] compared the range of motion with throwing kinematic variables. Plummer and Oliver [1] investigated the effects of fatigue on kinematic and kinetic changes of upper-extremity jump throwing.

Many kinematic experiments have studied ball throwing for team handball players and investigated the movement phases during the ball throwing [7,8,13,14]. Few studies have examined the kinematic variables effects and established relationships with ball velocity using 3D biomechanical tools. The handball coaches tend to focus on improving the throwing velocity for players [15].

Thus, through the investigation in the biomechanics of throwing velocity in elite handball players for the purpose of providing guidance to coaches and players desiring to improve this key aspect of performance, previous studies have shown a distinctive contribution of a velocity–accuracy trade-off and have concluded that kinematic variable as displacement along the velocity accuracy is achieved as an important contributed factor of decision-making. Therefore, ball velocity is considered the main factor for high quality jump throwing towards the goal [2,16,17].

In this regard, Stirn, et al. [18] opined that there are many factors contributing to the final velocity of the ball at release. To evaluate these factors, different demanding and time-consuming acquisition and analysis methods are required, including kinematic and electromyography assessments. Wagner, Pfusterschmied, von Duvillard and Müller [5] argued that the lower extremity in this type of skill plays an important role to drive the upper-extremity during performance. Therefore, throwing performance is considered to be the final outcome of an efficient kinetic chain.

The drive leg step before the take-off during the throwing jump skill could be an essential part of throwing to provide a support for the transfer of momentum through the pelvis and trunk to the dominant throwing arm. The kinematic investigation of the current study should be helpful for identifying the optimum jumping throwing mechanics. Consequently, we evaluated the relationship between ball velocity and some kinematic variables to identify key variables which should contribute to improving jump throwing performance.

Few studies have examined kinematic variable effects and established relationships with ball velocity using 3D biomechanical tools. Our goal for this study was to evaluate the correlation between key variables and throwing velocity, with the goal of providing information useful to coaches and players for improving jump-throwing performance. Therefore, we hypothesized that there would be positive and strong relationships between the kinematic variables of the right hand and left leg with ball velocity, and we determined key kinematic variables of jump throwing.

2. Materials and Methods

2.1. Subjects

Ten right-handed male handball players participated in current study (age: 20.8 ± 1.21 years; body mass: 82.8 ± 8.57 kg; height: 189.6 ± 8.65 cm, training experience: 9 years). They were part of a professional team which competed in the Egyptian Handball Super League. The study was approved by the institutional ethics committee of studies and research, and each player's consent was obtained.

2.2. Procedures

After a 15-min warm-up including general and shoulder-specific mobility exercises, as well as stretching and familiarization with the protocol, participants performed jump-throws after three running steps while positioned in front of the goal. Players were instructed to throw the ball as fast as possible. A total of five successful attempts were recorded for each player, with a one-minute rest between attempts. The best attempt, according to velocity of the ball, was selected for 3D analysis. The jump throwing skill was broken into three phases: The cocking phase, the acceleration phase, and the follow-through phase. Eight events were identified, beginning with the touch down (this event was determined when the jump leg touched the force platform starting the take-off).

The second event was the maximum ground reaction force (this event was designated as when the peak ground reaction force was achieved). Next was take-off (this event was designated as when the jump leg left the force platform). Maximum arm cocking was designated as when the arm reached the maximum back swing. Maximum height of center of mass was defined as when the center of mass achieved maximum height.

The maximum height of throwing arm was defined as when the throwing hand was at the maximum height. Ball release was defined as when the ball was released from the throwing arm, and the last event was landing, which was designated as when the player touched down from flight during performance (Figure 1).

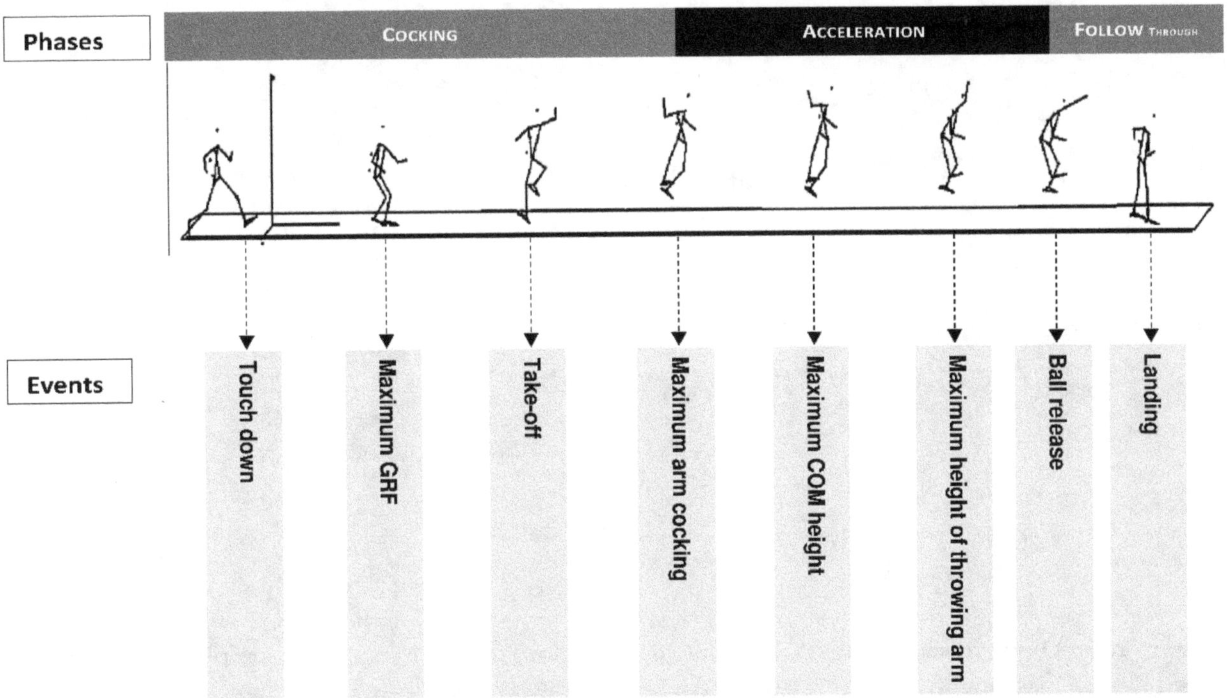

Figure 1. Jump throwing phases (cocking phase, acceleration phase, follow-through phase), and events (touch down, maximum ground reaction force (GRF), take-off, maximum arm cocking, maximum height of center of mass (COM), maximum height of throwing arm, ball release, and landing) during performance.

The kinematic variables of the right-hand (throwing arm) were measured using a 3-D motion capture system (Simi Reality motion analysis V. 9.0.6, eight synchronized Basler scA640-120gc-High-Speed Cameras were used at a 100 Hz frequency) that tracked the position of the reflective markers on anatomical landmarks according to the Hanavan model [19,20], (Figure 2). The 3D coordinates were the X (medio–lateral), Y (anterior–posterior) and Z (vertical) directions. Throwing performance was evaluated by the ball velocity [21], which was calculated by creating a rigid body of the ball using software and tracked. The angular kinematics of the joints were derived from relative angles between the two relevant segments (sagittal plane). A strain gage force platform (MP4060®, Bertec Corporation, Columbus, OH, USA) was used to determine the touch down and maximum ground reaction force events. The standard setting of software for filtering were used, and differentiation was used to calculate the kinematics variables [22].

2.3. Statistical Analysis

The Pearson coefficient of correlation was used to determine the strength of the relationships between each kinematic variable and ball velocity during each of the jump throwing phases (Table 1). Asterisk signs above the number represent significant differences between kinematic variables and ball velocity, and (*) indicates $p \leq 0.05$ for statistical procedures (SPSS 21, V. 21 Statistics for Windows. IBM Corp, Armonk, NY, USA).

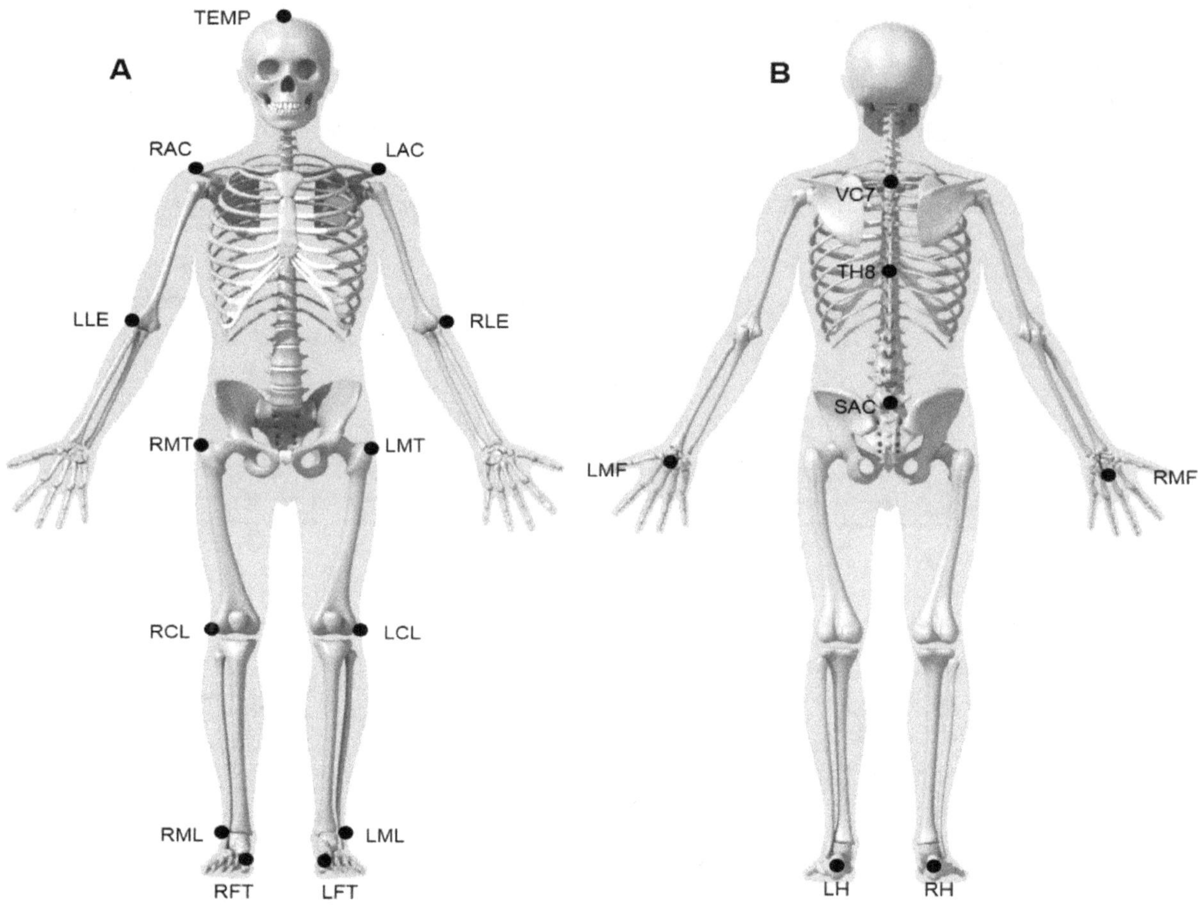

Figure 2. Full body marker set in (**A**) anterior (**B**) posterior view. The markers were placed at tempus head (TEMP), acromion left/right (LAC, RAC), epicondylus lateralis (elbow lateral) left/right (LLE, RLE), trochanter major left/right (LMT, RMT), Condylus lateralis left/right (LCL, RCL), malleolus lateralis left/right (LML, RML), foot tip left/right (LFT, RFT), vertebra C7 (VC7), vertebra Th8 (TH8), mid spina Iliaca posterior superior (SAC), middle finger base joint left/right (LMF, RMF), and heel left/right (LH, RH).

3. Results

The relationships between kinematic variables and ball velocity are shown in Tables 1 and 2 during each jump throwing phase (see Figure 1).

Table 1 provides the Pearson correlation coefficients between ball velocity and kinematic variables (displacement, velocity, and acceleration) at three investigated phases for eight events. No significant correlation was seen between ball velocity and right-hand kinematic variables during the cocking phase (displacement) and the acceleration phase (acceleration).

During the cocking phase, the ball velocity showed moderate correlations with the right arm velocity at initial contact (IC) (Y and R coordinates) (r = 0.66, r = 0.63) and initial flight (IF) (Y) (r = 0.63). Furthermore, there was a relatively strong correlation (r = 0.72) between the right arm acceleration at maximum ground reaction force (Max-GRF) (Y) and ball velocity. Through the acceleration phase, right arm displacement at maximum height of body (GC—ground contact) during flight (Max-GCH) (Y) had the highest correlation coefficients during this phase (r = 0.83) with ball velocity, and at release ball (RB) (Y) a strong correlation (r = 0.77) was observed. Likewise, ball velocity had moderate and strong correlations with the right arm displacement at maximum height of the throwing hand (Max-HH) (R) and RB (R), (r = 0.67 and r = 0.79, respectively). In addition, strong and moderate correlations were seen during the acceleration phase between velocity of the right hand and the ball velocity at Max-HH (Y) and Max-HH (R), (r = 0.78 and r = 0.70, respectively). As shown in Table 1 during the follow-through phase, the kinematic variables of the right hand such as the displacement at GC (Y, R) and velocity at GC (Y) had the highest correlation coefficients (r = 0.84, r = 0.88, and r = 0.83, respectively). A moderate correlation was observed between ball velocity and the right-hand acceleration (r = 0.68) at GC (Y) during this phase.

Table 1. Correlation between right-hand center of mass kinematic variables and ball velocity during jump throwing phases in handball. N = 10.

Variables (Unit)	Coordinates	Cocking Phase				Acceleration Phase			Follow-Through Phase
		IC	Max-GRF	IF	Max-BC	Max-GCH	Max-HH	RB	GC
Displacement (m)	X	−0.23	0.10	0.15	0.21	0.05	0.14	−0.04	−0.11
	Y	−0.27	0.32	0.34	0.57	0.83 *	0.63	0.77 *	0.84 *
	Z	0.56	−0.43	−0.27	−0.00	0.13	0.04	−0.25	−0.04
	R	0.49	−0.54	−0.21	0.04	0.22	0.67 *	0.79 *	0.88 *
Velocity (m/s)	X	−0.41	−0.05	0.15	−0.18	0.27	−0.28	−0.37	−0.39
	Y	0.66 *	0.20	0.63 *	0.22	0.51	0.78 *	−0.40	0.83 *
	Z	0.22	−0.00	−0.18	0.21	0.27	0.43	−0.51	0.50
	R	0.63 *	−0.04	0.09	0.26	0.41	0.70 *	0.04	−0.04
Acceleration (m/s^2)	X	0.56	0.62	−0.02	0.01	−0.05	−0.50	0.22	−0.34
	Y	0.40	0.79 *	0.24	−0.35	0.24	0.35	−0.57	0.68 *
	Z	−0.59	0.31	0.28	−0.40	0.26	0.08	0.43	0.30
	R	0.17	−0.54	−0.22	−0.42	0.11	−0.01	0.44	0.17

Note: Coordinates: X (medio–lateral), Y (anterior–posterior), Z (vertical), and R (resultant); IC: Initial contact (end of last step); Max-GRF: Maximum Ground Reaction force; IF: Initial flight; Max-BC: Maximum back cooking; Max-GCH: Maximum height of body GC during flight; Max-HH: Maximum height of the throwing hand GC during flight; RB: Release ball; GC: Ground contact; * Correlation were considered significant at $p < 0.05$.

Table 2. Correlation between right hand and left leg angular variables and ball velocity during jump throwing phases in handball.

Joint (Unit)	Variables (Unit)	Cocking Phase				Acceleration Phase			Follow-Through Phase
		IC	Max-GRF	IF	Max-BC	Max-GCH	Max-HH	RB	GC
Right elbow	Angle (°)	−0.21	0.22	0.08	0.03	−0.07	−0.64 *	−0.29	−0.33
	Velocity (°/s)	−0.20	−0.30	0.05	−0.41	−0.07	−0.11	−0.56	−0.03
	Acceleration ($°/s^2$)	0.44	−0.05	−0.05	0.25	0.20	0.55	−0.28	0.19
Right shoulder	Angle (°)	0.49	−0.51	−0.32	−0.38	−0.45	−0.31	−0.32	−0.63
	Velocity (°/s)	0.30	−0.32	0.69 *	−0.18	0.13	−0.37	−0.67 *	0.27
	Acceleration ($°/s^2$)	−0.59	0.31	0.67 *	0.55	0.28	−0.07	0.25	−0.21
Left hip	Angle (°)	0.07	0.33	0.41	0.32	0.28	0.36	0.22	0.73 *
	Velocity (°/s)	0.44	−0.27	−0.51	−0.05	−0.37	0.35	−0.21	−0.26
	Acceleration ($°/s^2$)	−0.30	−0.65 *	−0.67 *	0.24	−0.44	−0.23	−0.26	−0.14
Left knee	Angle (°)	0.16	−0.57	−0.01	−0.29	0.23	0.28	−0.07	−0.34
	Velocity (°/s)	0.46	−0.26	0.13	−0.02	0.28	−0.26	−0.09	−0.67 *
	Acceleration ($°/s^2$)	−0.15	−0.51	−0.18	0.22	−0.50	−0.33	0.08	−0.52
Left ankle	Angle (°)	−0.71 *	−0.80 *	0.30	0.01	−0.17	−0.10	−0.50	−0.57
	Velocity (°/s)	−0.03	0.06	0.38	−0.09	0.36	−0.61	0.08	−0.45
	Acceleration ($°/s^2$)	0.56	0.16	−0.53	−0.01	0.13	−0.19	0.37	−0.30

Note: IC: Initial contact (end of last step); Max-GRF: Maximum ground reaction force; IF: Initial flight; Max-BC: Maximum back cooking; Max-CGH: Maximum height of body GC during flight; Max-HH: Maximum height of the throwing hand GC during flight; RB: Release ball; GC: Ground contact; * Correlation were considered significant at $p < 0.05$.

The Pearson correlation coefficients between ball velocity with the right hand and left leg angular variables (angle, velocity, acceleration) during the three phases can be seen in Table 2. There were no significant correlation coefficients observed between the ball velocity and the kinematic variables of right elbow during all phases except a moderate negative performance score (r = −0.64) of angle at Max-HH during the acceleration phase. Likewise, during the follow-through phase, the velocity of the left knee had a moderate negative correlation (r = −0.67) at GC. Right shoulder velocity and acceleration had a moderate correlation with ball velocity at IF during the cocking phase (r = 0.69, r = 0.67, respectively). At RB during the acceleration phase, the right shoulder velocity had a moderate negative correlation (r = −0.67). Left hip acceleration during the cocking phase had a moderate negative correlation with ball velocity at Max-GRF and IF (r = −0.65, r = −0.67, respectively), and the angle of the left hip had a strong correlation (r = 0.73) at GC during the follow-through phase. The angle of left ankle during the cocking phase had a strong negative correlation with performance at IC and Max-GRF (r = −0.71, r = −0.80, respectively).

4. Discussion

The current study examined the relationships between ball velocity and kinematic variables during the jump throwing of elite handball players. The main aim was to determine the relationships between ball velocity and right hand (throwing hand) linear kinematics, as well as right arm and left leg (take-off leg) angular kinematics during three investigated phases over eight events.

The results in Table 1 show that the kinematic variables at maximum ground reaction force, maximum height of body center of gravity during flight, release ball and ground contact events were correlated strongly with ball velocity. These findings support a previous study which indicated important kinematic variables of the standing throw in handball [23].

The analysis of the cocking phase in our study indicated a moderate correlation between ball velocity and the velocity of the right hand at IC (Y, R) and IF (Y). This finding indicates that the primary velocity of elbow and the initial flight with the ball increased the ball velocity. During the same phase, the right-hand acceleration had a strong correlation with ball velocity at Max-GRF (Y). This strong correlation indicates that the Max-GRF during the jump throwing improved the horizontal velocity of the right hand (elbow and wrist joint) before ball release, which led to improving the arm swing during throwing.

The displacement of the right hand during the acceleration phase was strongly correlated with ball velocity at Max-CGH (Y), RB (Y) and RB (R). In addition, the Max-HH (R) during this phase correlated moderately with the ball velocity. This finding implies that maximum height of body GC and the dominant throwing hand increase the kinematic requirements of the hip and shoulder to maintain a high velocity of ball and performance; van den Tillaar and Ettema [24] showed some kinematic changes during overarm throwing related to the elbow extension and internal rotation.

Furthermore, the velocity of the right hand correlated strongly with Max-HH (Y) and moderately with Max-HH (R). The positive correlation with ball velocity and maximum heights of the throwing hand (Y, R) coordinates during the acceleration phase implies that arm motion continues until ball release time, which generates a ball rotation around the central axis, increases and generates the required release ball velocity. This supports the study of Werner, et al. [25], who suggested that the arm acceleration phase is the dynamic phase between the maximum external shoulder rotation and the instant of ball release.

During the follow-through phase, the results indicated that a higher correlation between ball velocity and the displacement of the right hand at GC (Y and R), and the velocity of the right hand had a high correlation at GC (Y). However, a moderate correlation was seen during this phase with the acceleration of the right hand at GC (Y). A strong correlation of displacement and velocity were found during this phase, so we suggest that when players perform the jump throw, they must increase their movement horizontally to enable forward movement at the landing. Hirashima, et al. [26] indicated that the ability of skilled throwers to optimize the throwing arm event of inertia during the arm cocking and arm acceleration phases highlights the importance of the arm movement to reach a high ball velocity.

Our findings in Table 2 indicate that the moderate negative correlation between ball velocity and the right elbow angle during the Max-HH event. This finding indicates that the smaller angle at the elbow joint assists in the improvement of a higher ball velocity at release for longer throwing. This finding supports previous studies [8,15,23], which indicated that the elbow extension and internal rotation velocity were factors for fast shoulder throwing, wherein about 73% of the contribution of ball velocity was based on the maximal internal rotation velocity of the shoulder and maximal elbow extension during the throw.

A moderate correlation was seen between the ball velocity and the right shoulder velocity and acceleration variables at IF during the cocking phase. In addition, a moderate correlation was observed between the right shoulder velocity at RB and ball velocity during the acceleration phase. This finding indicates that player who moves forward at take-off also maintains a higher projection angle with the wrist hyperextension at the ball release, which leads to a higher flight time style. This result is seen in the correlation between ball velocity and the releasing of ball during the acceleration phase. During the acceleration phase, the maximal angular velocities of the elbow extension, wrist flexion, and the internal rotation of the shoulder joint make a substantial contribution to overarm throwing in team handball [23].

The left hip and right hand had moderate correlations with ball velocity at Max-GRF and with IF events during the cocking phase. During the follow-through phase at GC, a strong correlation was observed between the angle of the left hip and ball velocity. These negative correlations with ball velocity during the cocking phase indicated that handball players were using a greater angle of projection to reach for optimum position before releasing the ball and generate a required power with the throwing arm. Thus, higher velocities of the arm joints could be produced [23], which could result in higher external rotation while throwing. This finding confirmed that the movement of the large body segments such as legs and trunk assist with the reduction of energy in the throwing arm in order to reduce the loads, especially on the shoulder and elbow [25,27,28].

The ball velocity had a moderate correlation with the velocity of the left knee at GC during the follow-through phase and the left ankle angle at the IC and Max-GRF events during the cocking phase (Table 2). The negative correlation between left knee velocity with ball velocity implies that players had a greater knee flexion in the follow-through phase for preparation for landing. Olsen, et al. [29] and Koga, et al. [30] reported that landing after a jump throwing with the knee near full extension was important to prevent ACL injuries in team handball players.

It should be noted that these findings were derived from a small sample of homogenous elite handball players. We selected elite players because we wanted data from high-level performance. A small sample was used in this pilot study in order to evaluate the utility of this approach. Finding strong and moderate correlations in a small, homogenous sample suggests that these findings are very conservative. We hope that future investigations will expand on these preliminary findings.

A limitation was that the sample size in the present study was small (ten right-handed male handball players), and we analyzed the best attempt of the five successful performed attempts. All our participants were elite, meaning that our sample was homogenous, making correlations more challenging to identify. We were willing to accept these limitations in this pilot study because our goal was to identify the correlations for top performers, since it was assumed that these participants represent the best performances. However, future investigations should recruit a larger number of participants and/or increase the number of attempts.

5. Conclusions

Based on the main findings from this study, the velocity of the right hand at IC and IF events (anterior–posterior direction) correlated with ball velocity during the cocking phase as a preparation phase that accelerates the arm throwing. The increases in right-hand acceleration at Max-GRF, Max-HH events (anterior-posterior direction) led to the improvement of the horizontal velocity of the right hand (elbow and wrist joint) before the RB event achieved the highest ball velocity. Furthermore, the results indicated that the change in angular variables of shoulder joint are greater than those of the elbow. Thus, we recommend that, in training programs, coaches focus on increasing their player's movement horizontally to enable forward movement at the landing when evaluating the performance level of handball players.

Also, we recommend that coaches to use special power and reaction time exercises to reduce the dominant foot contact time at the jump moment and before throwing the ball. This would allow the player to jump higher before the ball release event and keep the maximum velocity of the ball while throwing performance.

Author Contributions: Conceptualization, A.-R.A. and I.H.; methodology, A.-R.A., I.H. and A.H.; software, A.-R.A.; validation, A.-R.A., I.H., P.B. and A.H.; formal analysis, A.-R.A.; investigation, A.-R.A. and I.H.; resources, A.-R.A.; data curation, A.-R.A. writing—original draft preparation, A.-R.A., I.H. and A.H.; writing—review and editing, P.B.; visualization, A.H.; supervision, P.B.; project administration, A.-R.A.

References

1. Plummer, H.A.; Oliver, G.D. The effects of localised fatigue on upper extremity jump shot kinematics and kinetics in team handball. *J. Sports Sci.* **2017**, *35*, 182–188. [CrossRef] [PubMed]
2. Van den Tillaar, R. Comparison of range of motion tests with throwing kinematics in elite team handball players. *J. Sports Sci.* **2016**, 1–7. [CrossRef] [PubMed]
3. Serrien, B.; Clijsen, R.; Blondeel, J.; Goossens, M.; Baeyens, J.P. Differences in ball speed and three-dimensional kinematics between male and female handball players during a standing throw with run-up. *BMC Sports Sci. Med. Rehabil.* **2015**, *7*, 27. [CrossRef] [PubMed]
4. Setuain, I.; Millor, N.; Gonzalez-Izal, M.; Gorostiaga, E.M.; Gomez, M.; Alfaro-Adrian, J.; Maffiuletti, N.A.; Izquierdo, M. Biomechanical jumping differences among elite female handball players with and without previous anterior cruciate ligament reconstruction: A novel inertial sensor unit study. *Sports Biomech. Int. Soc. Biomech. Sports* **2015**, *14*, 323–339. [CrossRef] [PubMed]
5. Wagner, H.; Pfusterschmied, J.; von Duvillard, S.P.; Müller, E. Performance and kinematics of various throwing techniques in team-handball. *J. Sports Sci. Med.* **2011**, *10*, 73–80.
6. Wagner, H.; Buchecker, M.; von Duvillard, S.P.; Müller, E. Kinematic Comparison of Team Handball Throwing with Two Different Arm Positions. *Int. J. Sports Physiol. Perform.* **2010**, *5*, 469–483. [CrossRef] [PubMed]
7. Wagner, H.; Buchecker, M.; von Duvillard, S.P.; Muller, E. Kinematic description of elite vs. Low level players in team-handball jump throw. *J. Sports Sci. Med.* **2010**, *9*, 15–23.
8. Van den Tillaar, R.; Ettema, G. A three-dimensional analysis of overarm throwing in experienced handball players. *J. Appl. Biomech.* **2007**, *23*, 12–19. [CrossRef]
9. Almeida, G.P.; Silveira, P.F.; Rosseto, N.P.; Barbosa, G.; Ejnisman, B.; Cohen, M. Glenohumeral range of motion in handball players with and without throwing-related shoulder pain. *J. Shoulder Elb. Surg. Am. Shoulder Elb. Surg.* **2013**, *22*, 602–607. [CrossRef]
10. Bayios, I.A.; Anastasopoulou, E.; Sioudris, D.; Boudolos, K.D. Relationship between isokinetic strength of the internal and external shoulder rotators and ball velocity in team handball. *J. Sports Med. Phys. Fit.* **2001**, *41*, 229.
11. García, J.A.; Sabido, R.; Barbado, D.; Moreno, F.J. Analysis of the relation between throwing speed and throwing accuracy in team-handball according to instruction. *European Journal of Sport Science* **2013**, *13*, 149–154. [CrossRef]
12. Wagner, H.; Pfusterschmied, J.; Von Duvillard, S.P.; Muller, E. Skill-dependent proximal-to-distal sequence in team-handball throwing. *J. Sports Sci.* **2012**, *30*, 21–29. [CrossRef] [PubMed]
13. Meister, K. Injuries to the shoulder in the throwing athlete. Part one: Biomechanics/pathophysiology/classification of injury. *Am. J. Sports. Med.* **2000**, *28*, 265–275. [CrossRef] [PubMed]
14. Wagner, H.; Finkenzeller, T.; Wurth, S.; von Duvillard, S.P. Individual and team performance in team-handball: A review. *J. Sports Sci. Med.* **2014**, *13*, 808–816. [PubMed]

15. Debanne, T.; Laffaye, G. Coaches' Beliefs and Knowledge: Training Programs Used by French Professional Coaches to Increase Ball-throwing Velocity in Elite Handball Players. *Int. J. Sports Sci. Coach.* **2013**, *8*, 557–570. [CrossRef]
16. Van den Tillaar, R.; Ettema, G. A comparison between novices and experts of the velocity-accuracy trade-off in overarm throwing. *Percept. Mot. Ski.* **2006**, *103*, 503–514. [CrossRef] [PubMed]
17. Van den Tillaar, R.; Ettema, G. Influence of instruction on velocity and accuracy of overarm throwing. *Percept. Mot. Ski.* **2003**, *96*, 423–434. [CrossRef] [PubMed]
18. Stirn, I.; Carruthers, J.; Sibila, M.; Pori, P. Frequent Immediate Knowledge of Results Enhances the Increase of Throwing Velocity in Overarm Handball Performance. *J. Hum. Kinet.* **2017**, *56*, 197–205. [CrossRef]
19. Akl, A.-R.; Salem, M. Effects of center of mass kinematics on ball velocity during jump throwing in handball. *MOJ Appl. Bionics Biomech.* **2018**, *2*, 219–221. [CrossRef]
20. Hanavan, E.P., Jr. *A mathematical model of the human body*; USAF Institute of Technology: Greene County, OH, USA, 1964.
21. Rivilla-Garcia, J.; Grande, I.; Sampedro, J.; van den Tillaar, R. Influence of opposition on ball velocity in the handball jump throw. *J. Sports Sci. Med.* **2011**, *10*, 534–539.
22. Hanley, B.; Tucker, C.B.; Bissas, A. Differences between motion capture and video analysis systems in calculating knee angles in elite-standard race walking. *J. Sports Sci.* **2017**, 1–6. [CrossRef]
23. Van den Tillaar, R.; Ettema, G. A force-velocity relationship and coordination patterns in overarm throwing. *J. Sports Sci. Med.* **2004**, *3*, 211–219.
24. Van den Tillaar, R.; Ettema, G. A comparison of kinematics between overarm throwing with 20% underweight, regular, and 20% overweight balls. *J. Appl. Biomech.* **2011**, *27*, 252–257. [CrossRef] [PubMed]
25. Werner, S.L.; Fleisig, G.S.; Dillman, C.J.; Andrews, J.R. Biomechanics of the elbow during baseball pitching. *J. Orthop. Sports Phys. Ther.* **1993**, *17*, 274–278. [CrossRef]
26. Hirashima, M.; Yamane, K.; Nakamura, Y.; Ohtsuki, T. Kinetic chain of overarm throwing in terms of joint rotations revealed by induced acceleration analysis. *J. Biomech.* **2008**, *41*, 2874–2883. [CrossRef]
27. Fleisig, G.S.; Andrews, J.R.; Dillman, C.J.; Escamilla, R.F. Kinetics of baseball pitching with implications about injury mechanisms. *Am. J. Sports Med.* **1995**, *23*, 233–239. [CrossRef]
28. Grezios, A.K.; Gissis, I.T.; Sotiropoulos, A.A.; Nikolaidis, D.V.; Souglis, A.G. Muscle-contraction properties in overarm throwing movements. *J. Strength Cond. Res. Natl. Strength Cond. Assoc.* **2006**, *20*, 117–123.
29. Olsen, O.E.; Myklebust, G.; Engebretsen, L.; Bahr, R. Injury mechanisms for anterior cruciate ligament injuries in team handball: A systematic video analysis. *Am. J. Sports Med.* **2004**, *32*, 1002–1012. [CrossRef]
30. Koga, H.; Nakamae, A.; Shima, Y.; Iwasa, J.; Myklebust, G.; Engebretsen, L.; Bahr, R.; Krosshaug, T. Mechanisms for noncontact anterior cruciate ligament injuries: Knee joint kinematics in 10 injury situations from female team handball and basketball. *Am. J. Sports Med.* **2010**, *38*, 2218–2225. [CrossRef]

Permissions

All chapters in this book were first published by MDPI; hereby published with permission under the Creative Commons Attribution License or equivalent. Every chapter published in this book has been scrutinized by our experts. Their significance has been extensively debated. The topics covered herein carry significant findings which will fuel the growth of the discipline. They may even be implemented as practical applications or may be referred to as a beginning point for another development.

The contributors of this book come from diverse backgrounds, making this book a truly international effort. This book will bring forth new frontiers with its revolutionizing research information and detailed analysis of the nascent developments around the world.

We would like to thank all the contributing authors for lending their expertise to make the book truly unique. They have played a crucial role in the development of this book. Without their invaluable contributions this book wouldn't have been possible. They have made vital efforts to compile up to date information on the varied aspects of this subject to make this book a valuable addition to the collection of many professionals and students.

This book was conceptualized with the vision of imparting up-to-date information and advanced data in this field. To ensure the same, a matchless editorial board was set up. Every individual on the board went through rigorous rounds of assessment to prove their worth. After which they invested a large part of their time researching and compiling the most relevant data for our readers.

The editorial board has been involved in producing this book since its inception. They have spent rigorous hours researching and exploring the diverse topics which have resulted in the successful publishing of this book. They have passed on their knowledge of decades through this book. To expedite this challenging task, the publisher supported the team at every step. A small team of assistant editors was also appointed to further simplify the editing procedure and attain best results for the readers.

Apart from the editorial board, the designing team has also invested a significant amount of their time in understanding the subject and creating the most relevant covers. They scrutinized every image to scout for the most suitable representation of the subject and create an appropriate cover for the book.

The publishing team has been an ardent support to the editorial, designing and production team. Their endless efforts to recruit the best for this project, has resulted in the accomplishment of this book. They are a veteran in the field of academics and their pool of knowledge is as vast as their experience in printing. Their expertise and guidance has proved useful at every step. Their uncompromising quality standards have made this book an exceptional effort. Their encouragement from time to time has been an inspiration for everyone.

The publisher and the editorial board hope that this book will prove to be a valuable piece of knowledge for researchers, students, practitioners and scholars across the globe.

List of Contributors

Kao-Shang Shih
Department of Orthopedic Surgery, Shin Kong Wu Ho-Su Memorial Hospital, Taipei 111, Taiwan
School of Medicine, College of Medicine, Fu Jen Catholic University, New Taipei City 242, Taiwan

Shu-Yu Jhou and Ching-Chi Hsu
Graduate Institute of Applied Science and Technology, National Taiwan University of Science and Technology, Taipei 106, Taiwan

Wei-Chun Hsu and Jun-Wen Chen
Graduate Institute of Biomedical Engineering, National Taiwan University of Science and Technology, Taipei 106, Taiwan

Jui-Chia Yeh and Yi-Chun Hung
Footwear & Recreation Technology Research Institute, Taichung 407, Taiwan

Pablo González-Frutos
Faculty of Health Sciences, Universidad Francisco de Vitoria, 28223 Madrid, Spain0

Santiago Veiga, Javier Mallo and Enrique Navarro
Health and Human Performance Department, Technical University of Madrid, 28040 Madrid, Spain

Herbert Wagner
Department of Sport and Exercise Science, University of Salzburg, Schlossallee 49, Hallein-Rif, 5400 Salzburg, Austria

Cristina Cortis
Department of Human Sciences, Society and Health, University of Cassino e Lazio Meridionale, Viale dell'Università, 03043 Cassino FR, Lazio, Italy

Philip X. Fuchs and Andrea Fusco
Department of Sport and Exercise Science, University of Salzburg, Schlossallee 49, Hallein-Rif, 5400 Salzburg, Austria
Department of Human Sciences, Society and Health, University of Cassino e Lazio Meridionale, Viale dell'Università, 03043 Cassino FR, Lazio, Italy

Saioa Etxaleku and Iosu Sesma
TDN, Orthopedic Surgery and Advanced Rehabilitation Center, Clinical Research Department, Pol Mutilva C/V nave 3, 31192 Mutilva, Spain

Mikel Izquierdo
Navarrabiomed, Complejo Hospitalario de Navarra (CHN)-Universidad Pública de Navarra (UPNA), Navarra Institute for Health Research (IdiSNA), 31008 Pamplona, Spain

Igor Setuain
TDN, Orthopedic Surgery and Advanced Rehabilitation Center, Clinical Research Department, Pol Mutilva C/V nave 3, 31192 Mutilva, Spain
Navarrabiomed, Complejo Hospitalario de Navarra (CHN)-Universidad Pública de Navarra (UPNA), Navarra Institute for Health Research (IdiSNA), 31008 Pamplona, Spain

Eder Bikandi
Athletic Club, Mazarredo Zumarkalea, 23. 48009 Bilbao, Bizkaia, Spain

Jaime García Arroyo
TEN Centre, C/San Julian nº 8 Majadahonda, 28220 Madrid, Spain

Iñigo Sarriegi
Southampton FC, Staplewood Football Development & Support Centre, Marchwood, Southampton SO40 4WR, UK

Violeta Sánchez-Migallón, Alvaro López-Samanes, Pablo Terrón-Manrique and Vicente Fernández-Ruiz
Exercise Physiology Group, School of Physiotherapy, Faculty of Health Sciences, Universidad Francisco de Vitoria, Pozuelo de Alarcón, 28049 Madrid, Spain

Esther Morencos
School of Exercise and Sports Sciences, School of Health Sciences, Universidad Francisco de Vitoria, Pozuelo de Alarcón, 28049 Madrid, Spain

Archit Navandar
Faculty of Sport Sciences, Europea de Madrid University, Villaviciosa de Odón, 28670 Madrid, Spain

Victor Moreno-Pérez
Center for Translational Research in Physiotherapy, Department of Pathology and Surgery, Miguel Hernández University, 03202 Elche, Alicante, Spain

Javier Peláez Barrajón, Enrique Navarro and Alejandro F. San Juan
Department of Health and Human Performance, Sport Biomechanics Laboratory, Facultad de Ciencias Actividad Física y Deporte—INEF, Universidad Politécnica de Madrid, 28040 Madrid, Spain

Estrella Armada-Cortés
Department of Health and Human Performance, Sport Biomechanics Laboratory, Facultad de Ciencias Actividad Física y Deporte—INEF, Universidad Politécnica de Madrid, 28040 Madrid, Spain
Department of Physical Activity and Sports Science, Faculty of Sport Sciences, University of Castilla-La Mancha, 45071 Toledo, Spain

José Antonio Benítez-Muñoz
Department of Health and Human Performance, LFE Research Group, Facultad de Ciencias Actividad Física y Deporte—INEF, Universidad Politécnica de Madrid, 28040 Madrid, Spain

Mark King, Harley Towler and Romanda Dillon
School of Sport, Exercise, and Health Sciences, Loughborough University, Loughborough LE11 3TU, UK

Stuart McErlain-Naylor
School of Sport, Exercise, and Health Sciences, Loughborough University, Loughborough LE11 3TU, UK
School of Health and Sports Sciences, University of Suffolk, Ipswich IP3 8AH, UK

Grażyna Olchowik and Agata Czwalik
Department of Biophysics, Medical University of Lublin, K. Jaczewskiego 4, 20-090 Lublin, Poland

Clemente Rocha
CBIOS (Research Center for Biosciences and Health Technologies), School of Health Sciences and Technologies, Lusófona University, 1749-024 Lisboa, Portugal

Henrique Silva and Luís Monteiro Rodrigues
CBIOS (Research Center for Biosciences and Health Technologies), School of Health Sciences and Technologies, Lusófona University, 1749-024 Lisboa, Portugal
Department of Pharmacological Sciences, Faculty of Pharmacy, University of Lisboa, 1649-003 Lisboa, Portugal

Hugo A. Ferreira
IBEB Institute of Biophysics and Biomedical Engineering, Faculty of Sciences, University of Lisboa, 1749-016 Lisboa, Portugal

Jadwiga Pietraszewska, Anna Burdukiewicz and Aleksandra Stachoń
Department of Physical Anthropology, University School of Physical Education, Paderewskiego 35 Avenue, 51-612 Wrocław, Poland

Artur Struzik
Department of Team Sport Games, University School of Physical Education, Mickiewicza 58 Street, 51-684 Wrocław, Poland

Bogdan Pietraszewski
Department of Biomechanics, University School of Physical Education, Mickiewicza 58 Street, 51-684 Wrocław, Poland

Ying Gao
Department of Sports Science, College of Education, Zhejiang University, Hangzhou 310028, China
Faculty of Sport and Health Sciences, University of Jyväskylä, 40700 Jyväskylä, Finland

Lars A. Kristensen, Thomas S. Grøndberg, Mike Murray and Gisela Sjøgaard
Department of Sports Science and Clinical Biomechanics, University of Southern Denmark, DK-5230 Odense, Denmark

Karen Søgaard
Department of Sports Science and Clinical Biomechanics, University of Southern Denmark, DK-5230 Odense, Denmark
Department of Clinical Research, University of Southern Denmark, DK-5230 Odense, Denmark

Kennedy Freitas Pereira Alves, Ana Paula de Lima Ferreira, Luana Caroline de Oliveira Parente, François Talles Medeiros Rodrigues, Thais Vitorino Marques, Gabriel Barreto Antonino, Luiz Carlos de Melo, Débora Wanderley Villela, Marcelo Renato Guerino, Wagner Souza Leite, Shirley Lima Campos and Maria das Graças Rodrigues de Araújo
Department of Physical Therapy, Universidade Federal de Pernambuco (UFPE), Recife-PE 50670 901, Brazil

Larissa Coutinho de Lucena
Faculdade Nova Esperança (FACENE), João Pessoa-PB 58067-698, Brazil

Redha Taiar
GRESPI, Université de Reims Champagne-Ardenne, 51100 Reims, France

Bruno Dino Bodini, Pietro Serafin, Jacopo A. Vitale, Antonio Serafin and Francesco Negrini
IRCCS Istituto Ortopedico Galeazzi, Via Riccardo Galeazzi 4, 20161 Milan, Italy

Giacomo Lucenteforte and Lorenzo Barone
Physical Medicine and Rehabilitation Residency Program, University of Catania, Piazza Università 2, 95124 Catania, Italy

Valerio Sansone
IRCCS Istituto Ortopedico Galeazzi, Via Riccardo Galeazzi 4, 20161 Milan, Italy
Department of Biomedical Sciences for Health, Università degli Studi di Milano, Via Mangiagalli 31, 20133 Milan, Italy

Claudia Figueiredo Azeredo, Patrícia de Castro de Paiva and Aline Reis da Silva
Programa de Pós-graduação em Saúde, Medicina Laboratorial e Tecnologia Forense, Universidade do Estado do Rio de Janeiro, Rio de Janeiro, RJ 20950-003, Brazil
Laboratório de Vibrações Mecânicas e Práticas Integrativas, Departamento de Biofísica e Biometria, Instituto de Biologia Roberto Alcântara Gomes e Policlínica Piquet Carneiro, Universidade do Estado do Rio de Janeiro, Rio de Janeiro, RJ 20950-003, Brazil

Adriana Lírio Pereira da Silva, Juliana Pessanha-Freitas, Mario Bernardo-Filho, Luiz Felipe Ferreira-Souza, Rubens Guimarães Mendonça
Laboratório de Vibrações Mecânicas e Práticas Integrativas, Departamento de Biofísica e Biometria, Instituto de Biologia Roberto Alcântara Gomes e Policlínica Piquet Carneiro, Universidade do Estado do Rio de Janeiro, Rio de Janeiro, RJ 20950-003, Brazil

Leandro Azeredo
Departamento de Fisioterapia, Hospital Central da Polícia Militar, Rio de Janeiro, RJ 20211-270, Brazil

Arlete Francisca-Santos and Bruno Bessa Monteiro de Oliveira
Laboratório de Vibrações Mecânicas e Práticas Integrativas, Departamento de Biofísica e Biometria, Instituto de Biologia Roberto Alcântara Gomes e Policlínica Piquet Carneiro, Universidade do Estado do Rio de Janeiro, Rio de Janeiro, RJ 20950-003, Brazil
Faculdade Bezerra de Araújo, Rio de Janeiro, RJ 23052-180, Brazil

Mário Fritsch Neves
Programa de Pós-Graduação emCiências Médicas, Faculdade de Ciências Médicas, Universidade do Estado do Rio de Janeiro, Rio de Janeiro, RJ 20551-030, Brazil

Camila Leite Bernardes-Oliveira
Programa de Pós-graduação em Saúde, Medicina Laboratorial e Tecnologia Forense, Universidade do Estado do Rio de Janeiro, Rio de Janeiro, RJ 20950-003, Brazil
Programa de Pós-Graduação emCiências Médicas, Faculdade de Ciências Médicas, Universidade do Estado do Rio de Janeiro, Rio de Janeiro, RJ 20551-030, Brazil

Laisa Liane Paineiras-Domingos, Danúbia da Cunha de Sá-Caputo and Eliane de Oliveira Guedes-Aguiar
Laboratório de Vibrações Mecânicas e Práticas Integrativas, Departamento de Biofísica e Biometria, Instituto de Biologia Roberto Alcântara Gomes e Policlínica Piquet Carneiro, Universidade do Estado do Rio de Janeiro, Rio de Janeiro, RJ 20950-003, Brazil
Faculdade Bezerra de Araújo, Rio de Janeiro, RJ 23052-180, Brazil
Programa de Pós-Graduação emCiências Médicas, Faculdade de Ciências Médicas, Universidade do Estado do Rio de Janeiro, Rio de Janeiro, RJ 20551-030, Brazil

Ygor Teixeira-Silva
Laboratório de Vibrações Mecânicas e Práticas Integrativas, Departamento de Biofísica e Biometria, Instituto de Biologia Roberto Alcântara Gomes e Policlínica Piquet Carneiro, Universidade do Estado do Rio de Janeiro, Rio de Janeiro, RJ 20950-003, Brazil
Programa de Pós-Graduação emCiências Médicas, Faculdade de Ciências Médicas, Universidade do Estado do Rio de Janeiro, Rio de Janeiro, RJ 20551-030, Brazil

Márcia Cristina Moura-Fernandes and Eloá Moreira-Marconi
Laboratório de Vibrações Mecânicas e Práticas Integrativas, Departamento de Biofísica e Biometria, Instituto de Biologia Roberto Alcântara Gomes e Policlínica Piquet Carneiro, Universidade do Estado do Rio de Janeiro, Rio de Janeiro, RJ 20950-003, Brazil
Programa de Pós-Graduação em Fisiopatologia Clínica e Experimental, Instituto de Biologia Roberto Alcântara Gomes, Universidade do Estado do Rio de Janeiro, Rio de Janeiro, RJ 20550-900, Brazil

José Alexandre Bachur
Cursos de Medicina e Fisioterapia da Universidade de Franca, Franca, SP 14401-426, Brazil

Vinicius Layter Xavier
Departamento de Estatística, Instituto de Matemática e Estatística, Universidade do Estado do Rio de Janeiro, Rio de Janeiro, RJ 20550-900, Brazil

Daniel Lago Borges
Hospital Universitário, Universidade Federal do Maranhão, São Luís do Maranhão, MA 65080-805, Brazil

Ana Cristina Lacerda and Vanessa Amaral Mendonça
Faculdade de Ciências Biológicas e da Saúde, Universidade Federal dos Vales do Jequitinhonha e Mucuri, Diamantina, MG 39100-000, Brazil

Anelise Sonza
Programa de Pós-graduação em Fisioterapia, Universidade do Estado de Santa Catarina, Florianópolis, SC 88080-350, Brazil

Alessandro Sartorio
Istituto Auxologico Italiano, IRCCS, Experimental Laboratory for Auxo-Endocrinological Research, Division of Metabolic Diseases & Auxology, 28824 Milan and Verbania, Italy

Francisco J. Dominguez-Muñoz, Miguel A. Hernández-Mocholi and Santos Villafaina
Physical Activity and Quality of Life Research Group (AFYCAV), Faculty of Sport Science, University of Extremadura, 10003 Cáceres, Spain

Luis J. Manso
School of Engineering and Applied Sciences, Aston University, Birmingham B4 7ET, UK

Daniel Collado-Mateo
Centre for Sport Studies, Rey Juan Carlos University, 28943 Fuenlabrada, Spain

Jose C. Adsuar
Health Economy Motricity and Education (HEME), Faculty of Sport Science, University of Extremadura, 10003 Cáceres, Spain

Narcis Gusi
Physical Activity and Quality of Life Research Group (AFYCAV), Faculty of Sport Science, University of Extremadura, 10003 Cáceres, Spain
CIBER de Fragilidad y Envejecimiento Saludable, 28029 Madrid, Spain

Chenhao Yang, Songlin Xiao, Xini Zhang, Zhen Luo, Xi Wang, Yang Yang, Jiaxin Niu and Junqing Wang
School of Kinesiology, Shanghai University of Sport, Shanghai 200438, China

Weijie Fu
School of Kinesiology, Shanghai University of Sport, Shanghai 200438, China
Key Laboratory of Exercise and Health Sciences of Ministry of Education, Shanghai University of Sport, Shanghai 200438, China

Luca von Siebenthal, Ishbel Lomax, Micah Gross and Klaus Hübner
Department of Elite Sport, Swiss Federal Institute of Sport (SFISM), 2532 Magglingen, Switzerland

Wolfgang Taube
Department of Neuroscience and Movement Science, University of Fribourg, 1700 Fribourg, Switzerland

Christoph Schärer
Department of Elite Sport, Swiss Federal Institute of Sport (SFISM), 2532 Magglingen, Switzerland
Department of Neuroscience and Movement Science, University of Fribourg, 1700 Fribourg, Switzerland

Ricardo Fernandes and João Paulo Vilas-Boas
Centre of Research, Education, Innovation and Intervention in Sport, Faculty of Sport, University of Porto, 91 Dr. Plácido Costa st., 4200-450 Porto, Portugal
Porto Biomechanics Laboratory, University of Porto, 91 Dr. Plácido Costa st., 4200-450 Porto, Portugal

Karla de Jesus and Kelly de Jesus
Centre of Research, Education, Innovation and Intervention in Sport, Faculty of Sport, University of Porto, 91 Dr. Plácido Costa st., 4200-450 Porto, Portugal
Porto Biomechanics Laboratory, University of Porto, 91 Dr. Plácido Costa st., 4200-450 Porto, Portugal
Human Performance Studies Laboratory, Faculty of Physical Education and Physiotherapy, Federal University of Amazonas, 3000 Gal. Rodrigo Octávio Jordão Ramos ave., South MiniCampus, Coroado I, Manaus 69077-000, Amazonas, Brazil
Human Motor Behaviour Studies Laboratory, Faculty of Physical Education and Physiotherapy, Federal University of Amazonas. 3000 Gal. Rodrigo Octávio Jordão Ramos ave., South MiniCampus, Coroado I, Manaus 69077-000, Amazonas, Brazil

Luis Mourão
Centre of Research, Education, Innovation and Intervention in Sport, Faculty of Sport, University of Porto, 91 Dr. Plácido Costa st., 4200-450 Porto, Portugal
Porto Biomechanics Laboratory, University of Porto, 91 Dr. Plácido Costa st., 4200-450 Porto, Portugal
Superior Institute of Engineering of Porto, Polytechnic Institute of Porto, 431, Dr. António Bernardino de Almeida st., 4249-015 Porto, Portugal

Hélio Roesler
Centre of Physical Education, Physiotherapy and Sports, Aquatic Biomechanics Research Laboratory, University of the State of Santa Catarina, 358 Pascoal Simone st., Coqueiros, Florianópolis 88080-350, Santa Catarina, Brazil

Nuno Viriato and Mário Vaz
Porto Biomechanics Laboratory, University of Porto, 91 Dr. Plácido Costa st., 4200-450 Porto, Portugal
Institute of Mechanical Engineering and Industrial Management, Faculty of Engineering, University of Porto, Dr. Roberto Frias st., 4200-465 Porto, Portugal

Abdel-Rahman Akl
Faculty of Physical Education-Abo Qir, Alexandria University, Alexandria 21913, Egypt

Ibrahim Hassan
Faculty of Physical Education, Zagazig University, Zagazig 44519, Egypt

Amr Hassan
Department of Sports Training, Faculty of Sports Education, Mansoura University, Mansoura 35516, Egypt

Phillip Bishop
Department of Kinesiology, University of Alabama, Tuscaloosa, AL 35487, USA

Index

www.ingramcontent.com/pod-product-compliance
Lightning Source LLC
LaVergne TN
LVHW081022210926
848485LV00004B/924
* 9 7 8 1 6 4 6 4 6 6 2 0 7 *